Clinical Radiology

Clinical Radiology

Editor: Coby Hawkins

AMERICAN
MEDICAL PUBLISHERS
www.americanmedicalpublishers.com

AMERICAN
MEDICAL PUBLISHERS
www.americanmedicalpublishers.com

Cataloging-in-Publication Data

Clinical radiology / edited by Coby Hawkins.
p. cm.
Includes bibliographical references and index.
ISBN 979-8-88740-008-2
1. Medical radiology. 2. Diagnosis, Radioscopic. 3. Diagnostic imaging.
4. Radiotherapy. I. Hawkins, Coby.
R895 .C55 2023
616.075 7--dc23

American Medical Publishers,
41 Flatbush Avenue,
1st Floor, New York,
NY 11217, USA

ISBN 979-8-88740-008-2 (Hardback)

Contents

Preface IX

Chapter 1 **Impact of the COVID-19 Pandemic on Radiotherapy Supply** 1
Francesco Tramacere, Artor Niccoli Asabella, Maurizio Portaluri, Corinna Altini, Cristina Ferrari, Lilia Bardoscia and Angela Sardaro

Chapter 2 **Malaysian Nurses' Knowledge of Radiation Protection** 5
Aisyah Mohd Rahimi, Intan Nurdin, Shahrina Ismail and Azira Khalil

Chapter 3 **Diagnostic Accuracy Studies in Radiology: How to Recognize and Address Potential Sources of Bias** 13
Athanasios Pavlou, Robert M. Kurtz and Jae W. Song

Chapter 4 **Early Radiologic Diagnosis of Pulmonary Infection in Febrile Neutropenic Patients: A Comparison of Serial Chest Radiography and Single CT Chest** 23
Wanaporn Burivong, Thanatorn Sricharoen, Apichart Thachang, Sunsiree Soodchuen, Panitpong Maroongroge and Vichit Leelasithorn

Chapter 5 **From Radiological Manifestations to Pulmonary Pathogenesis of COVID-19: A Bench to Bedside Review** 30
Amin Saburi, U. Joseph Schoepf, Kyle A. Ulversoy, Ramezan Jafari, Fatemeh Eghbal and Mostafa Ghanei

Chapter 6 **Image Quality and Dose Comparison of Single-Energy CT (SECT) and Dual-Energy CT (DECT)** 42
Ramin Ghasemi Shayan, Maryam Oladghaffari, Fakhrosadat Sajjadian and Mona Fazel Ghaziyani

Chapter 7 **Prevalence, Spectrum and Outcomes of Single Coronary Artery Detected on Coronary Computed Tomography Angiography (CCTA)** 53
Rashid Al Umairi and Maryam Al-khouri

Chapter 8 **Proportion of Variant Anatomy of the Circle of Willis and Association with Vascular Anomalies on Cerebral CT Angiography** 60
Roy Munialo Machasio, Rose Nyabanda and Timothy Musila Mutala

Chapter 9 **Contribution of Computed Tomography Scan to the Diagnosis of Spinal Tuberculosis in 14 Cases in Assaba, Mauritania** 67
Boushab Mohamed Boushab, Noukhoum Kone and Leonardo K. Basco

Chapter 10 **Health Insurance Ownership and Quality of Computed Tomography Requests: Experience from a Peripheral Referral Hospital in Cameroon** 73
Joshua Tambe, Yannick Onana, Sylviane Dongmo, Georges Nguefack-Tsague and Pierre Ongolo-Zogo

Chapter 11 **Real-Life Diagnostic Accuracy of MRI in Prenatal Diagnosis.......... 79**
Manuel Recio Rodríguez, Cristina Andreu-Vázquez, Israel J. Thuissard-Vasallo, Raquel Cano Alonso, Carmina Bermejo López, Ines Tamarit Degenhardt and Pilar Martínez Ten

Chapter 12 **Comparative Study of Multiple High-Signal-Intensity Spots on 3D and 2D Magnetic Resonance Sialography for Patients with Sjögren's Syndrome.......... 91**
Yusuke Shimada, Ikuho Kojima and Masahiro Iikubo

Chapter 13 **What Radiologist Should Know about MRI Translational Forces and Hazard: An Ex-Vivo Simulation of Retained Metallic Shrapnel.......... 99**
Ali Kanj, Ibrahim Ghosn, Assaad Mohanna and Georges Rouhana

Chapter 14 **Hearing Thresholds Changes after MRI 1.5T of Head and Neck.......... 104**
Maryam Bahaloo, Mohammad Hossein Davari, Mohammad Sobhan, Seyyed Jalil Mirmohammadi, Mohammad Taghi Jalalian, Mohammad Javad Zare Sakhvidi, Farimah Shamsi, Sam Mirfendereski, Abolfazl Mollasadeghi and Amir Houshang Mehrparvar

Chapter 15 **Postcontrast Fluid-Attenuated Inversion Recovery (FLAIR) Sequence MR Imaging in Detecting Intracranial Pathology.......... 108**
Ajit Mahale, Shaloo Choudhary, Sonali Ullal, Merwyn Fernandes and Sonali Prabhu

Chapter 16 **Comparison of MRI and CT in the Evaluation of Unilateral Maxillary Sinus Opacification.......... 117**
Elise Chua, Annakan V. Navaratnam, Dominic St Leger, Vincent Lam, Samit Unadkat and Alexander Weller

Chapter 17 **4DCT Scanning Technique for Primary Hyperparathyroidism: A Scoping Review.......... 127**
Steven Raeymaeckers, Maurizio Tosi and Johan De Mey

Chapter 18 **Assessment of the Local Exposure Level during Adult Chest X-Rays at the Ngaoundere Regional Hospital, Cameroon.......... 139**
Guiswe Gnowe, Henri Paul Ekobena Fouda, Mbo Amvene Jéremie, Takmou Pascal and Bonaventure Babinne Graobe

Chapter 19 **Preprocedural Hypertension is Not a Risk Factor for Postoperative Bleeding following Image-Guided Core Needle Breast Biopsy.......... 144**
Ninad Salastekar, Alexis Saunders, Kushal Patel and Katherine Willer

Chapter 20 **Stromal Fibrosis of the Breast: A Spectrum of Benign to Malignant Imaging Appearances.......... 148**
Lara Nassar, Amro Baassiri, Fatima Salah, Andrew Barakat, Elie Najem, Fouad Boulos and Ghina Berjawi

Chapter 21 **Ketamine Use in Hysterosalpingography (the Jimah Procedure): A Follow-Up of Bilateral Tubal Evaluation of 27 Infertile Women at a Teaching Hospital, Ghana.......... 154**
Bashiru Babatunde Jimah, Anthony Baffour Appiah, Benjamin Dabo Sarkodie and Dorothea Anim

Chapter 22 **Hysterosalpingography Findings and Jimah Ratio of the Uterine Cavity in Women with Infertility in Central Region, Ghana.......... 160**
Bashiru Babatunde Jimah, Philip Gorleku and Anthony Baffour Appiah

Chapter 23 **Developing of a Mathematical Model to Perform Measurements of Axial Vertebral Rotation on Computer-Aided and Automated Diagnosis Systems, Using Raimondi's Method** **167**
José Hurtado-Aviles, Joaquín Roca-González, Konstantsin Sergeevich Kurochka, Jose Manuel Sanz-Mengibar and Fernando Santonja-Medina

Chapter 24 **Predicting Molecular Subtypes of Breast Cancer with Mammography and Ultrasound Findings: Introduction of Sono-Mammometry Score** **176**
Sana Shaikh and Afshan Rasheed

Chapter 25 **A Review of Doses for Dental Imaging in 2010–2020 and Development of a Web Dose Calculator** **188**
Hawon Lee and Andreu Badal

Chapter 26 **Preoperative Portal Vein Embolization in Hepatic Surgery: A Review about the Embolic Materials and their Effects on Liver Regeneration and Outcome** **206**
Jose Hugo M. Luz, Filipe V. Gomes, Elia Coimbra, Nuno V. Costa and Tiago Bilhim

Chapter 27 **An Experimental Intervention Study Assessing the Impact of a Thin Silicone Gel Surface Overlay on Interface Pressure** **215**
Seth Kwadjo Angmorterh, Andrew England, Sonia Aboagye, Eric Kwasi Ofori and Peter Hogg

Chapter 28 **The Association between the Pulmonary Arterial Obstruction Index and Atrial Size in Patients with Acute Pulmonary Embolism** **224**
Taraneh Faghihi Langroudi, Maryam Sheikh, Mohammadreza Naderian, Morteza Sanei Taheri, Amir Ashraf-ganjouei and Isa Khaheshi

Permissions

List of Contributors

Index

Preface

Radiology is a medical specialty that involves the use of radiation for diagnosing and treating diseases. Clinical radiology systems make use of both ionizing radiation such as X-rays and non-ionizing radiation such as ultrasound. Radiology helps in capturing pictures or images of the structures in the body. Diagnostic radiology and interventional radiology are the broad two areas within radiology. Diagnostic imaging is used for diagnosing, monitoring, and screening conditions such as broken bones, heart conditions, and blood clots. The objective of interventional radiology techniques such as MRI and CT Scans is to guide medical procedures in the process of inserting catheters, wires and other small instruments and tools within the body. Some important techniques of radiology are positron emission tomography (PET) scan, nuclear medicine tests such as thallium cardiac stress test, thyroid scan and bone scan, magnetic resonance angiography (MRA), and computed tomography (CT) scan. This book provides significant information with respect to radiology for developing a good understanding of the subject. It presents researches and studies performed by experts across the globe. This book will serve as a reference to a broad spectrum of readers.

All of the data presented henceforth, was collaborated in the wake of recent advancements in the field. The aim of this book is to present the diversified developments from across the globe in a comprehensible manner. The opinions expressed in each chapter belong solely to the contributing authors. Their interpretations of the topics are the integral part of this book, which I have carefully compiled for a better understanding of the readers.

At the end, I would like to thank all those who dedicated their time and efforts for the successful completion of this book. I also wish to convey my gratitude towards my friends and family who supported me at every step.

Editor

1

Impact of the COVID-19 Pandemic on Radiotherapy Supply

Francesco Tramacere,[1] Artor Niccoli Asabella,[2] Maurizio Portaluri,[1] Corinna Altini,[3] Cristina Ferrari,[3] Lilia Bardoscia,[4] and Angela Sardaro[5]

[1]*Radiation Oncology, Department of Radiotherapy, O. Policlinic "A. Perrino", Strada Statale 7 per Mesagne, Brindisi 72100, Italy*
[2]*Nuclear Medicine Unit, A. O. Policlinic "A. Perrino", Strada Statale 7 per Mesagne, Brindisi 72100, Italy*
[3]*Nuclear Medicine Unit, Interdisciplinary Department of Medicine, University of Bari Aldo Moro, Piazza Giulio Cesare 11, Bari 70124, Italy*
[4]*Radiotherapy Unit, Clinical Cancer Centre, AUSL-IRCCS, Reggio Emilia, Italy*
[5]*Section of Radiology and Radiation Oncology, Interdisciplinary Department of Medicine, University of Bari Aldo Moro, Piazza Giulio Cesare 11, Bari 70124, Italy*

Correspondence should be addressed to Corinna Altini; corinna.altini@hotmail.it

Academic Editor: Daniele La Forgia

Background. The impetuous entrance of the COVID-19 pandemic in Italy in March 2020, after the onset and diffusion in China, found the health system widely unfit to face the large amount of infected patients. The matter of this investigation was to evaluate how pandemic fear and guidelines for limiting the diffusion of SARS-CoV-2 virus could have impacted the regular supply of radiotherapy (RT) and the outcome of the treatments. *Materials and Methods.* From March 9, 2020, to May 29, 2020, a register has been established to record patients that cancelled or postponed the RT appointment. The reasons were as follows: (1) patients whose appointments were postponed by the staff according to national guidelines; (2) patients who asked themselves to postpone the appointment; (3) patients who interrupted the treatment for causes directly or indirectly related to the pandemic; (4) patients who cancelled their care path. *Results.* A total number of 277 patients started regular RT, and 384 respected their computed tomography (CT) simulation appointment, but 60 of them had alteration of their therapeutic pathway. Among these, 18 cancelled their appointment. 42 patients asked to postpone their procedure. Twenty-seven out of 42 adduced directly or indirectly SARS-CoV-2 infection related reasons. *Conclusions.* The COVID-19 pandemic affected the regular RT delivery to oncologic patients, owing to the delay or cancellation of procedures with the likely effect to observe worsening of local disease control and reduced survival rates in the future.

1. Introduction

At the onset of the COVID-19 pandemic in Italy, i.e., at the beginning of March 2020, radiotherapy (RT) treatments were included in the list of the specialties which had to be guaranteed to all patients with cancer for whom there was indication and they should not have been canceled, contrary to what happened for other medical procedures considered nonurgent [1]. This decision was due to the shortage of resources of personnel which imposed many wards to be converted into coronavirus disease-19 (COVID-19) wards, with the aim to provide beds and adequate healthcare to the extremely increasing number of patients with SARS-CoV-2 symptomatic infection. Nonetheless, recommendations from the national scientific society Italian Association of Radiotherapy and Clinical Oncology (AIRO) suggested to postpone some nonurgent and deferrable RT treatments for patients with better prognosis (e.g., breast and prostate cancer) and evaluate the ratio risk/benefit in each case; to prefer hypofractionation schemes where indicated; and to use pharmacological treatments at home for the relief of symptoms of similar efficacy of radiotherapy. Furthermore, such guidelines suggested not to start treatment in SARS-CoV-2-positive patients and to stop it if the patients became symptomatic or positive during RT delivery. In this last case, the recommendations suggest to evaluate each case in order to complete or not the treatment, and in affirmative decision, it could happen through the permission of Health Authority, a high-level protection of the staff, and careful disinfection of the treatment room [2]. This hypothesis is not supported by any scientific evidence.

During the COVID-19 pandemic, consultations were conducted by means of telematic tools, and follow-up visits were postponed for patients who declared themselves as without evidence of oncologic disease in order to minimize patients' exposure to viral diffusion without compromising oncological outcomes. In any case, the COVID-19 pandemic produced the cancellation of appointments, postponing of procedures, and treatments' interruption. We described this phenomenon in a Radiation Oncology Department in Southern Italy. The matter of the investigation was to evaluate the impact of pandemic fear or guidelines for limiting the diffusion of SARS-CoV-2 infection on the regular supply of radiotherapy and treatment outcomes.

2. Materials and Methods

From March 9, 2020, to May 29, 2020, a total number of 277 cancer patients started RT as regularly programmed, and 384 patients respected their planning CT scan appointment, but 60 patients changed their therapeutic pathway. The characteristics of the recorded patients are reported in Table 1 and Figure 1.

From the start of COVID-19 rapid spread in Italy, since the enactment of the Italian Government official recommendation statements (reference), and once AIRO tips for the management of oncological patients in the context of the COVID-19 pandemic were available [2], a register has been established to record patients who cancelled or delayed their RT appointment. Anthropometric data (sex and age), information on cancer (time of diagnosis, histology, stage of disease, and therapeutic approach—multimodal or RT alone), intent of RT (radical vs. adjuvant vs. neoadjuvant), association with pharmacological therapy, phase of the RT program involved (first access and/or CT simulation and/or RT start and/or RT delivery), the reasons for postponing or refusing the appointment, and the time of the delay request were collected.

The motivation for postponing/refusing the RT appointment was then gathered in 3 different groups: (1) delay disposed by the radiation oncologist in accordance with national and international principles and recommendations; (2) delay for patient's request; (3) delay or interruption directly or indirectly due to COVID-19 infection.

The RT workflow consisted in treatment decision during the first access of patients at the Radiation Oncology Department, followed by CT simulation, treatment planning, and plan approval with quality assurance, and finally in treatment delivery. The definition of the treatment program and informed consent, CT simulation, and RT delivery required patient presence. We did not postpone the first consultations (treatment decision phase) for patients who needed definitive, immediate treatment for symptomatic, extensive, and/or locally advanced malignancies. We considered the delay for some CT simulations and nonurgent or deferral treatments such as localized, low-risk prostate cancer or patients with intermediate-high-very high risk disease undergoing androgen deprivation therapy, adjuvant RT for early stage, hormone-sensitive breast cancer, and those for adjuvant purposes in general, especially for elderly patients, always trying to respect the timing indicated by international guidelines and recommendations. The appointment scheduling for visits and planning CT scan were scattered across the day to minimize the number of people present in the waiting rooms at the same time [3, 4].

Table 1: Description of patients' characteristics.

	M	F	M + F
Sex	28	32	60
Median age	69 years (50–87)	64 years (50–87)	68 years (29–87)
Delay	21	21	42
Refuse	7	11	18
Radical	12	4	17
Adjuvant	9	23	32
Palliative	6	5	11

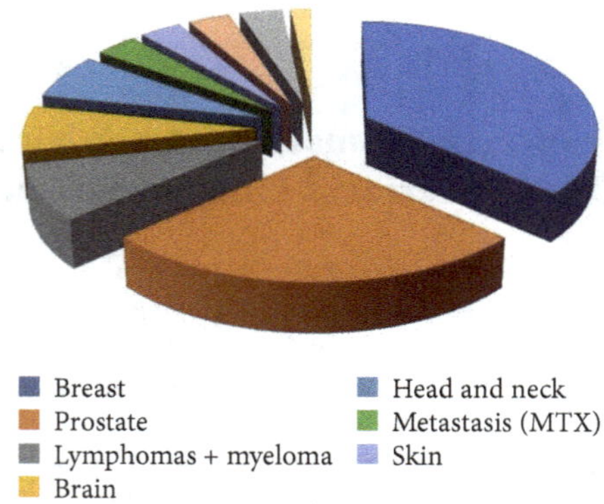

Figure 1: Diagnosis distribution.

3. Results

From March 9, 2020, to May 29, 2020, 721 cancer patients in total were listed in our dedicated register. Among these, 277 patients started RT as regularly programmed, 384 patients respected their planning CT scan appointment, but 60 patients changed their therapeutic pathway. The characteristics of the recorded patients are reported in Table 1.

Eighteen (30%) out of 60 patients cancelled their appointment (Table 2), while 42 (70%) of them postponed the programmed radiation treatment (Table 3).

Among the former group, 6 (10%) patients were recruited for palliative treatment, and the remaining 12 (20%) were candidates for radical (two, 3.3%) and adjuvant (ten, 16.7%) RT, respectively.

Tables 2 and 3 also provide the intent of RT prescription per patient, sex, age, and the reason for the delay. Median age was slightly higher in the subgroup of RT cancellation than in the RT delay group (72 vs. 68 years).

Table 2: Description of patients who refused radiotherapy.

	M	F	M + F
Median age	72 years (52–86)	72 years (46–84)	72 years (46–84)
Radical	2	-	2
Adjuvant	2	8	10
Palliative	3	3	6
Motivation 1	3	-	3
Motivation 2	2	5	7
Motivation 3	2	6	8

Table 3: Description of patients who delayed radiotherapy.

	M	F	M + F
Median age	68 years (50–87)	60 years (29–86)	63 years (20–87)
Radical	11	4	15
Adjuvant	7	15	22
Palliative	3	2	5
Motivation 1	3	0	3
Motivation 2	5	7	12
Motivation 3	13	14	27

Table 4: Oncologic diagnosis of patients.

Breast	22
Prostate	16
Lymphomas + myeloma	5
Brain	4
Head and neck	4
Metastasis (MTX)	2
Skin	2
Bladder	2
Gynecological	2
Lung	1

Table 5: Mean time of delay in patients with the postponed procedure according to the intent of treatment and motivation.

	Median (min–max) days of delay
Radical	25 (4–74)
Adjuvant	30 (5–112)
Palliative	30 (13–126)
Motivation 1	37 (30–60)
Motivation 2	30 (10–82)
Motivation 3	24 (4–126)
Overall	27.5 (4–126)

When adjusted for patients' sex, median age was 63 years for women and 68 years for men. Patients candidates to adjuvant RT were the most represented in both the aforementioned subgroups (32 53%). Diagnosis of breast and prostate cancer was the most frequent (38/60, 63%) (Table 4).

Motivation 3 (COVID-19-related delay or interruption) was found to be the most frequent reason for procedure delay or interruption (27 vs. 15) (Table 3). In detail, such motivations consisted in fever at the triage point at the entrance of the hospital, positive or ongoing SARS-CoV-2 test for suspected infections, positive SARS-CoV-2 antibody serologic test, positive tests in relatives, and subsequent quarantine. Moreover, among prostate cancer patients, delay of staging or restaging choline PET/CT performance was a further cause of appointment rescheduling. Stratification of RT procedures for oncological intent showed that median time interval of delay was substantially equivalent among the selected subgroups, with an overall median delay interval of 27.5 days (range: 4–126) and median time to delay of 25 days (range: 4–74) for radical RT and 30 days (range: 5–112 and 131–126, respectively) for adjuvant and palliative RT (Table 5).

In this setting, motivation 3 was associated with a median 24 days (range: 4–126) of delay, compared to 37 days (range: 30–60) for motivation 1 (radiation oncologist decision) and 30 days (range: 10–82) for motivation 2 (patients' request). The postponing request involved mostly the date of CT-simulation procedure (26/42, 60%), with 15 (40.6%) cases in the adjuvant RT subgroup.

4. Discussion

The impetuous entrance of the COVID-19 pandemic in Italy in March 2020, after the onset and diffusion in China, found the health system largely unfit to face the large amount of infected patients [4–6]. Although social distancing and the need for staff preservation to avoid severe shortage by SARS-CoV-2 infection and related impairment of the full functioning of radiation therapy facilities were recommended in national guidelines and international praxis adopted in Asiatic countries, at the onset of the pandemic in the radiotherapy department, some authors reminded correctly that "suboptimal delivery of radiotherapy (including delays, interruptions, or omissions) has been demonstrated to compromise both local control and survival." [78] They further recalled that "the findings of a systematic review demonstrate that delaying the initiation of adjuvant radiotherapy >8 weeks after surgery doubles the risk of local recurrence in patients with breast cancer. Furthermore, a meta-analysis conducted by the Early Breast Cancer Trialists' Collaborative Group indicates that radiotherapy reduces the risk of local recurrence, with 3.8% absolute reduction in 15-year risk of breast cancer mortality (from 25.2% to 21.4%; $P = 0.00005$)." [9]

It can be expected for sure that the median delay of 30 days we registered in the present observational study, which should be added to the waiting time generally registered in Italy between the first evaluation and the start of RT, will produce, in the medium/long term, adverse effects to the patients in terms of worse local control of the disease and lower survival rates. This effect cannot be measured at the moment, but the large amount of literature reporting the negative impact of longer treatment time and waiting time in radiotherapy is well known. Because the majority of the patients performed an adjuvant treatment for breast tumor (22/60) or a radical one for prostate tumor (16/60), which are cancer diseases with low mortality rate and need long time to develop a local recurrence, it is impossible to evaluate the impact on the outcome of the delay in this small group of patients.

In our series, there was a shorter postponing time for radical patients compared to those presenting for adjuvant or palliative irradiation because of the urgency of the need for RT start. The adjuvant patients were the majority in the postponing group, likely because their care pathway had been ensured in part by the surgical time. This is in line with the American Society for Radiation Oncology (ASTRO) and the European Society for Radiotherapy and Oncology (ESTRO) consensus statements for risk-adapted RT strategies during the COVID-19 pandemic, with the aim to protect patients and healthcare professionals from potential exposure and at the same time ensure high-quality treatments both for saving lives and for palliative purposes [11].

It is noteworthy that the median age of patients who refused or required to postpone RT was higher (72 vs. 68 years) than the overall series. Such findings support that the fear of SARS-CoV-2 infection was widely spread in the elder population.

In the analyzed group, 18/60 (30%) patients refused to start treatment, and to date, we had no further updates concerning their medical choices since they were not traceable either by the authorized contact person. Such findings were cause for concern, especially for the two (10%) patients needing for radical treatment. We supposed the "palliative" group was likely to be managed at home with the palliative medical approach, instead. Among the motivations attributed to the delay or refusal of RT, some of them regarded the waiting for staging or restaging diagnostic procedures, such as choline-F PET/CT for prostate cancer patients, propaedeutic to the start of primary or postoperative RT on the prostate/prostate bed, rather than ablative, stereotactic RT for nodal and/or bone oligometastases. It is well known that, during the lockdown, many medical activities were performed only on an emergency basis although the governmental provisions established that oncologic patients had a priority in the diagnostic and therapeutic pathway, but this could not be observed because the pandemic absorbed a large part of technological and human resources.

5. Conclusion

Our findings seemed to confirm that different reasons, directly or indirectly related to the COVID-19 pandemic, impacted on the regular supply of radiotherapy, determining delay or cancellation of procedures with the likely effect to observe, in the future, worse local control of the disease and survival rates in these oncological patients.

Authors' Contributions

FT and ANA designed the study. MP wrote the manuscript. CA and CF carried out data collection and analysis. AS supervised the work and revised the manuscript. All authors read and approved the manuscript.

References

[1] Ministero della Salute–Allegato 1-Raccomandazioni per la gestione dei pazienti oncologici e onco-ematologici in corso di emergenza da COVID-19, 2020, http://www.salute.gov.it/imgs/C_17_pagineAree_5373_3_file.pdf.

[2] Associazione Italiana di Radioterapia Oncologica. Documento di indirizzo per la valutazione e la gestione del rischio dei pazienti e degli operatori nei reparti di radioterapia oncologica in corso di diffusione del COVID-19, 2020, https://www.radioterapiaitalia.it/wp-content/uploads/2020/03/v-2-Documento-AIRO-COVID-19-24-03-2020.pdf.

[3] M. Krengli, E. Ferrara, F. Mastroleo, M. Brambilla, and U. Ricardi, "Running a radiation Oncology department at the time of coronavirus: an Italian experience," *Advances in Radiation Oncology*, vol. 5, no. 1, pp. 3–6, 2020.

[4] M. Portaluri, F. Tramacere, T. Portaluri, and E. A. L. Gianicolo, "Southern Italy: how the availability of radiation therapy, patient outcomes, and risk to health care providers have changed during the coronavirus disease 2019 pandemic," *Advances in Radiation Oncology*, vol. 5, no. 4, pp. 597–600, 2020.

[5] A. R. Filippi, E. Russi, S. M. Magrini, and R. Corvò, "Letter from Italy: first practical indications for radiation therapy departments during COVID-19 outbreak," *International Journal of Radiation Oncology * Biology * Physics*, vol. 107, no. 3, pp. 597–599, 2020.

[6] M. Portaluri, S. Bambace, F. Tramacere, A. Errico, S. Carbone, and T. Portaluri, "Staff and patient protection in radiation Oncology departments during coronavirus disease 2019 (COVID-19) pandemic," *Advances in Radiation Oncology*, vol. 5, no. 4, pp. 628–630, 2020.

[7] S. Wu, D. Zheng, Y. Liu, D. Hu, W. Wei, and G. Han, "Radiation therapy care during a major outbreak of COVID-19 in Wuhan," *Advances in Radiation Oncology*, vol. 5, no. 4, pp. 531–533, 2020.

[8] H. Nagar and S. C. Formenti, "Cancer and COVID-19-potentially deleterious effects of delaying radiotherapy," *Nature Reviews Clinical Oncology*, vol. 17, no. 6, pp. 332–334, 2020.

[9] J. Huang, L. Barbera, M. Brouwers, G. Browman, and W. J. Mackillop, "Does delay in starting treatment affect the outcomes of radiotherapy? A systematic review," *Journal of Clinical Oncology*, vol. 21, no. 3, pp. 555–563, 2003.

[10] S. Darby, S. Darby, P McGale et al., "Effect of radiotherapy after breast-conserving surgery on 10-year recurrence and 15-year breast cancer death: meta-analysis of individual patient data for 1001 women in 17 randomised trials," *Lancet*, vol. 378, no. 9804, pp. 1707–1716, 2011.

[11] D. J. Thomson, D. Palma, M. Guckenberger et al., "Practice recommendations for risk-adapted head and neck cancer radiotherapy during the COVID-19 pandemic: an ASTRO-ESTRO consensus statement," *Radiotherapy and Oncology*, vol. 151, pp. 314–321, 2020.

2

Malaysian Nurses' Knowledge of Radiation Protection

Aisyah Mohd Rahimi, Intan Nurdin, Shahrina Ismail, and Azira Khalil

Faculty of Science and Technology, Universiti Sains Islam Malaysia, 71800 Nilai, Negeri Sembilan, Malaysia

Correspondence should be addressed to Azira Khalil; azira@usim.edu.my

Academic Editor: Lorenzo Faggioni

Radiology is a vital diagnostic tool for multiple disorders that plays an essential role in the healthcare sector. Nurses are majorly involved in a healthcare setting by accompanying patients during the examination. Thus, nurses tend to be exposed during inward X-ray examination, requiring them to keep up with radiation use safety. However, nurses' competence in radiation is still a concept that has not been well studied in Malaysia. The study aimed to define the level of usage understanding and radiation protection among Malaysian nurses. In this research, a cross-sectional survey was conducted among 395 nurses working in hospitals, clinics, and other healthcare sectors in Malaysia. The survey is based on the developed Healthcare Professional Knowledge of Radiation Protection (HPKRP) scale, distributed via the online Google Forms. SPSS version 25.0 (IBM Corporation) was used to analyze the data in this study. Malaysian nurses reported the highest knowledge level in radiation protection with a mean of 6.03 ± 2.59. The second highest is safe ionizing radiation guidelines with 5.83 ± 2.77, but low knowledge levels in radiation physics and radiation usage principle (4.69 ± 2.49). Therefore, healthcare facilities should strengthen the training standards for all nurses working with or exposed to radiation.

1. Introduction

The radiological examination using X-rays remains the most widely used ionizing radiation in the medical field. It is liable for the most significant human-made radiation exposure to the worldwide population [1]. Based on the United Nations Scientific Committee on the Effects of Atomic Radiation (UNSCEAR) study, approximately 4 billion X-ray examinations are conducted every year [2]. X-ray examinations are primary imaging tools for diagnosing tests that have been used for decades. They allow us to see what is in our body without performing an incision [3]. This X-ray procedure is performed quickly and painlessly. X-ray imaging is the most important imaging used in clinical settings to help doctors diagnose and monitor certain body conditions and medical health [4] in most hospitals and clinics worldwide. The invention of X-rays was a major development in medicine. X-ray imaging tests are a valuable diagnostic instrument for various procedures and examinations [5].

Ionizing radiation has been strictly controlled in that it could pose a harmful effect on human health. To protect both humans and the environment from the adverse effects of ionizing radiation, radiation safety standards have been developed [6]. Nurses can engage in a variety of medical ionizing radiation procedures. For example, when X-ray imaging involves exposing patients, it sometimes needs to be conducted in wards for patients who cannot walk to the X-ray room, exposing them to scattered radiation [7]. Deterministic effects are also referred to as tissue reactions, depending on the amounts of radiation exposure. At higher doses, health effects such as skin injury and hair loss may be more severe [7–9]. This endangers the safety of nurses and patients when exceeding the radiation threshold [10]. Besides, tumors and leukemia are the stochastic effects of radiation, arising throughout extended periods caused by genetic material changes [8, 9]. Therefore, the possible stochastic risks of ionizing radiation exposure should be known by nurses, while patients should be wary of both deterministic and stochastic risks.

The previous statement shows that nurses play a vital role in the healthcare sector since they accompany patients most of the time. Thus, during the inward radiation, they can be exposed to radiation while working behind protective barriers. There are two probable sources of radiation exposure from the occupational viewpoint [11]. The true radiation source is the X-ray tube, but workers may be inadvertently exposed to the primary beam in rare situations. The second source of radiation exposure is the patient. The interaction between the primary X-ray beam and the area of the patient's body getting imaged creates scattered radiation originating from the patient in all directions. However, in most situations, occupational exposure's key determinant is nurses' proximity to the patient as exposures are taking place. According to the WHO, IAEA, and ICRP, radiation protection should be standardized to the highest possible safety level [12, 13]. The lack of ionizing radiation awareness among nurses can cause them to be unable to effectively protect themselves and their patients [14–16].

Nurses' knowledge of the ALARA (as low as reasonably achievable) concept of radiation safety is important. ALARA is a principle of protection intended to reduce radiation doses and radioactive material releases. ALARA focuses on legal dosage limits for regulatory compliance, serving as a standard for all radiation safety programs rather than just best practice [17]. It is possible to conform to ALARA principles by knowing and using the main parameters, shielding, time, and distance. Usually, patient dosage reduction also reduces the dose to nurses [18]. In radiological practice, the design of optimized procedures is also an important part of radiation protection [19]. Hence, nurses should know radiation use and protection to ensure their safety involving ionizing radiation. However, the competence of nurses in radiation remains a poorly studied term. The previous study shows that there has been a general lack of radiation education among nurses [7, 20].

To ensure that nurses possess adequate radiation understanding, described as the person's ability to use radiation safely, it is crucial to identify their specific deficiencies and assess the current level of understanding. From the previous study conducted in Finland, nurses' radiation understanding has been assessed using the Healthcare Professional Knowledge of Radiation Safety (HPKRP) scale to assist these efforts. This scale includes an indication of three radiation knowledge areas [6, 21]. The first is radiation physics and the radiation use principle in the medical setting. In contrast, the second area is radiation protection, which protects patients and nurses from harmful ionizing radiation. Finally, there are guidelines for using medical radiation relating to national and international guidelines for safe ionizing radiation. In Malaysia, the study that addresses this issue was conducted in 2014 but not using the HPKRP scale, which encourages the need to perform a new current study [22]. Therefore, this study was conducted to investigate a cross-sectional study of Malaysian nurses' knowledge of radiation use and radiation safety using HPKRP scale items. The HPKRP scale is chosen in this research because it was developed from the previous research [6] to be used in educational, clinical practice, and research settings.

This study aimed to characterize the understanding of radiation usage and protection by Malaysian nurses. In this study, target groups were nurses who use ionizing radiation to serve in hospitals, clinics, and other healthcare sectors around Malaysia. Malaysian nurses working in the first-aid clinics, operating theatres, medical wards, and radiology departments were invited to answer the questionnaire. This study's objectives were to investigate Malaysian nurses' current radiation understanding level and identify their understanding of radiation use and protection affected by background factors.

2. Methods

2.1. Study Design. A cross-sectional questionnaire survey was conducted in which data from nurses working in random hospitals, clinics, and other healthcare sectors across Malaysia were collected simultaneously. The questionnaire was created using a Google Form divided into two sections, with 39 questions in total.

2.2. Participant and Settings. In 2019, around 108 thousand (107,830) registered nurses in Malaysia increased compared to the previous year [23]. Based on the sample size calculator, the sufficient data to generalize this research outcome on Malaysia's whole nurse population are $N = 383$ (with 95% confidence interval and 5% margin error) [24]. Therefore, random Malaysian nurses ($N = 395$) serving in first-aid clinics, operating theatres, radiology departments, and medical wards were invited to participate in the research. In Malaysia, nurses exposed to radiation every day typically work in first-aid clinics, operating theatres, and radiology departments. Inclusion requirements for nurses must have been employed in a unit where ionizing radiation can be used or exposed. Nurses received the invitations and questionnaires from the beginning of semester 1 to the middle of semester 1 in 2020.

2.3. Instrument. The self-administered questionnaire consisted of two sections. Section one consists of the background question (participant background), while section two is regarding HPKRP scale's items, further classified into another three parts. Demographic (background) questions comprise gender, age, educational level, work experience, and details about the nurses' work unit. On the contrary, the HPKRP scale helped to determine the radiation understanding of involved nurses [6]. The following radiation understanding dimensions or aspects are addressed by the three sections of scope given by (1) radiation physics and radiation use principle that contain 12 items; (2) radiation protection, which has 13 items; and (3) guidelines for safe ionizing radiation use that include 8 items. Each item is evaluated on a Likert scale from 1 to 10, where 1 denotes "no knowledge" and 10 denotes "full knowledge." The scale reflected the knowledge and understanding of the participants. The HPKRP scale was then designed to collect highly detailed information on participants' self-reported understanding and use of different radiation aspects [21]. It has been psychometrically checked and shown to have much validity of the face, content, and construction [14]. Note that Cronbach's alpha coefficients of the scale ranged from 0.93 to 0.96 with an S-CVI value of 0.83 [21]. This showed that the scale is valid to be used in the research setting.

2.4. Data Collection. Random Malaysian nurses working in first-aid clinics, operating theatres, medical wards, and radiology departments were invited to participate in the study, where 395 of them accepted the invitation. All data were collected using the Google Form, in which participants could easily access using a link throughout the distributed message. The participating nurses' response was anonymous and processed according to the published standards of good research practice.

2.5. Ethical Consideration. All participants were required to sign an informed consent form before responding to the questionnaire, which explains the introduction of this study, what it will entail, the benefits, risks and discomforts, confidentiality, payment and rewards, and the duration. The authors also stated that responses from the participants would be documented for further study. The data will be safely stored, where only researchers would have access to the data. The data will be deleted after the data analysis is finished and the final paper is accepted for publication. All participants decided to participate in the research, and none declined to answer the questionnaire.

2.6. Data Analysis. The data received from the Google Form were evaluated using SPSS version 25.0 (IBM Corporation). Demographic data were evaluated with descriptive statistics and summarized as percentages and frequency, while the data of radiation knowledge were summarized as standard deviation and mean. Moreover, a binary logistic regression and cross-tabulation were employed to analyze whether the radiation knowledge was related to any demographic variables. The outcome variables were then classified from Likert scale responses into dichotomous variables. The first variable is "0" for scores between 1.00 and 4.99, while the second variable is "1" for scores between 5.00 and 10.00, designated "lower" and "higher" knowledge, respectively [21]. The results were investigated and presented as distribution percentage and probability, where statistical significance was set at $p < 0.05$.

3. Results

Most nurses were female (360, 91.1%) aged between 18 and 27 years (155, 39.2%). The nurses had various educational backgrounds: 332 (84.1%) had diploma level education, 60 (15.2%) had a bachelor's degree, and 3 (0.8%) had a master's degree. Most nurses received medical radiation education (269, 68.1%), while only 126 out of 395 nurses did not receive medical radiation education. Most participating nurses are from first-aid clinic units, with 186 nurses (47.1%) (see Table 1).

For the dimension of radiation physics and radiation use principles (Table 2), the lowest reported knowledge is on stochastic effects of a certain radiation dose (mean: 4.07; SD: 2.84). The nurses' highest reported knowledge in this section is about the harmful effects of medical radiation (mean: 6.79; SD: 2.63). Next, for radiation protection (Table 2), the highest reported knowledge is about other personnel safety while working in a controlled area that involves radiation exposure (mean: 7.39; SD: 2.57). In contrast, the lowest reported knowledge is on the meaning of the inverse square law in radiation protection (mean: 4.41; SD: 3.13). In the third section of the HPKRP scale, which is guidelines for safe ionizing radiation use, most nurses recorded higher knowledge about the meaning of warning signs regarding radiation safety (mean: 6.99; SD: 2.77). Knowledge about dose limitation in radiation protection was the lowest reported knowledge of participating nurses (mean: 5.07; SD: 3.15).

The correlation of demographic data and radiation knowledge is shown in Tables 3–5. In this research, statistical significance was set at $p < 0.05$, implying a significant correlation between those demographic data and radiation knowledge area. The binary logistic regression and cross-tabulation analysis show that age, nurse's work unit, nurse's working experience, and medical radiation education correlate with each radiation knowledge area. Nurses aged between 28 and 37 years recorded significantly higher levels of radiation physics and radiation use principles than nurses aged 18 to 27 years ($n = 39$, $\% = 9.9$, and $p = 0.03$) (see Table 3). Also, nurses who have work experience between 10 and 14 years reported significantly higher levels of this knowledge than nurses with working experience between 0 and 4 years ($n = 29$, $\% = 7.3$, and $p = 0.04$). Besides, nurses who work in the radiology department have significantly higher radiation physics levels and radiation use principles than nurses who work in operating theatres ($n = 19$, $\% = 4.8$, and $p = 0.01$). In addition, nurses who receive medical radiation education recorded significantly higher levels of this knowledge than nurses who had not received the education ($n = 167$, $\% = 42.3$, and $p < 0.01$).

The correlation between the background data of nurses and radiation protection knowledge area can be seen in Table 4. Nurses who have completed medical radiation education recorded significantly higher levels of this knowledge area than nurses who had not completed the education ($n = 258$, $\% = 65.3$, and $p < 0.01$). The results also show that nurses' age and medical radiation education correlate with guidelines of safe ionizing radiation use (Table 5). Nurses between 28 and 37 years old scored significantly higher in this knowledge than nurses between 18 and 27 years old ($n = 57$, $\% = 14.4$, and $p < 0.01$). Again, nurses who received medical radiation education recorded significantly higher levels of this radiation knowledge area than nurses who had not received the education ($n = 240$, $\% = 60.8$, and $p < 0.01$).

TABLE 1: Demographic details of participating nurses ($N = 395$).

Background variables	n	%
Age (years)		
18–27	155	39.2
28–37	104	26.3
38–47	88	22.3
48–57	48	12.2
Gender		
Male	35	8.9
Female	360	91.1
Work experience in years		
0–4	151	38.2
5–9	56	14.2
10–14	57	14.4
15–20	52	13.2
Over 20	79	20.0
Education		
Diploma	332	84.1
Bachelor's degree	60	15.2
Master's degree	3	0.8
Working unit		
Operating theatre	70	17.7
Radiology department	20	5.1
First-aid clinic	186	47.1
Medical ward	119	30.1
Medical radiation education in hours		
No	126	31.9
Yes	269	68.1

TABLE 2: Items of HPKRP scale competence ($N = 395$).

HPKRP scale main factors and items	Mean ± standard deviation
Radiation physics and radiation use principles	4.69 ± 2.49
I know how ionizing radiation is produced	4.41 ± 2.76
I know the differences between ionizing and nonionizing radiation	4.20 ± 2.77
I know the differences between electromagnetic and ionizing radiation	4.40 ± 2.90
I know the characteristics and physical features of X-rays	4.96 ± 2.92
I know how the harmful effects of medical radiation are caused	6.79 ± 2.63
I can describe the deterministic effects of certain radiation doses	4.29 ± 2.85
I can describe the stochastic effects of a certain radiation dose	4.07 ± 2.84
I know the justification principles for medical radiation examinations	4.57 ± 2.90
I understand the equations and measures in medical radiation examinations	4.13 ± 2.82
I understand the meaning of the as low as reasonably achievable principle in radiation examinations	4.21 ± 2.98
I know the fundamental principles of radiation protection	5.89 ± 2.92
I have obtained enough education about the use of radiation in medical examinations	4.35 ± 2.72
Radiation protection and safety	6.03 ± 2.59
I know how to properly use personal radiation protection equipment (PPE)	7.29 ± 2.62
I know how to properly use the radiation protection equipment for patients	6.65 ± 2.85
I pay attention to the other personnel while working in a controlled area and using radiation	7.39 ± 2.57
I know how to document all the essential information concerning the use of radiation	5.52 ± 3.15
I am aware that information concerning a patient's radiation dose must be written down in patient records	5.44 ± 3.22
I know the protocols concerning radiation workers who are pregnant	6.85 ± 2.90
I try to promote agreed safety protocols concerning radiation dose and radiation usage in my daily work and actions	6.12 ± 3.03
I understand the factors affecting a patient's radiation dose	5.67 ± 3.09
I understand the meaning of the inverse square law in radiation protection	4.41 ± 3.13
I know how to account for differences between adult and child/adolescent patients in radiological examinations	5.27 ± 3.14
I know how to assess my actions critically and comprehensively while working with medical radiation	5.33 ± 3.03
I am aware of the radiation safety arrangements at my work	6.32 ± 2.92
I understand the meaning of radiation safety culture	6.14 ± 2.96
Guidelines of safe ionizing radiation use	5.83 ± 2.77

TABLE 2: Continued.

HPKRP scale main factors and items	Mean ± standard deviation
I know the meaning of warning signs regarding radiation safety	6.99 ± 2.77
I observe and notice the warning signs concerning radiation while working in the control area	6.97 ± 2.73
I know how radiation workers' health monitoring has been organized	6.08 ± 3.13
I am aware of the classification of radiation workers	5.47 ± 3.12
I understand the procedures for how radiation exposure in radiation workers is monitored	5.66 ± 3.11
I know how to report abnormal events in radiation usage	5.22 ± 3.15
I understand the situations in which the "abnormal event notification" must be performed	5.22 ± 3.17
I understand the principle of dose limitation in radiation protection	5.07 ± 3.15

This HPKRP scale is credited to T. Schroderus-Salo et al., "Development and validation of a psychometric scale for assessing healthcare professionals' knowledge in radiation protection."

TABLE 3: Background factors correlated with radiation physics and radiation use principles' knowledge area ($N = 395$).

Independent variable	Outcome variable				Probability (p)
	Lower knowledge		Higher knowledge		
	n	%	n	%	
Age (years)					
18–27 (ref.)					
28–37	65	16.5	39	9.9	0.03
38–47	61	15.4	27	6.8	0.14
48–57	37	9.4	11	2.8	0.06
Gender					
Male (ref.)					
Female	209	52.9	151	38.2	0.95
Work experience in years					
0–4 (ref.)					
5–9	40	10.1	16	4.1	0.58
10–14	28	7.1	29	7.3	0.04
15–20	37	9.4	15	3.8	0.33
Over 20	60	15.2	19	4.8	0.22
Education					
Diploma (ref.)					
Bachelor's degree	30	7.6	30	7.6	0.09
Master's degree	1	0.3	2	0.5	0.29
Working unit					
Operating theatre (ref.)					
Radiology department	1	0.3	19	4.8	0.01
First-aid clinic	127	32.2	59	14.9	0.52
Medical ward	55	13.9	64	16.2	0.08
Medical radiation education					
No (ref.)					
Yes	102	25.8	167	42.3	<0.01

4. Discussion

The study found that participating nurses scored higher in their radiation safety expertise than their knowledge of the other two aspects of radiation knowledge (guidelines of radiation use and radiation physics). Here, the average value on the 10-point Likert scale is 6.03. The fact that nurses have such a relatively clear knowledge of radiation safety policies is encouraging, given the importance of radiation protection to those exposed to it [25]. They indicated that staff safety is crucial when operating in a regulated area involving exposure to radiation but lack of understanding of the concept of the inverse square law of radiation protection. The participants rated their knowledge of safety radiation guidelines second best, with a mean Likert score of 5.83 (Table 2). They mentioned being adept at the use of warning signs in radiation protection. Unfortunately, they have less understanding of the concept of dose limitation in radiation safety. Deficiencies in the knowledge of radiation safety precautions and actions have been reported [15], and they should specifically be discussed to guarantee the safe use of radiation [26].

The radiation physics dimension and radiation usage principles were the lowest recorded information levels with a mean Likert scale of just 4.69 (Table 2). The data show that most participating nurses are experts about the harmful

TABLE 4: Background factors correlated with radiation protection and safety knowledge area ($N = 395$).

Independent variable	Outcome variable: Lower knowledge n	%	Higher knowledge n	%	Probability (p)
Age (years)					
18–27 (ref.)					
28–37	40	10.1	64	16.2	0.75
38–47	44	11.1	44	11.1	0.51
48–57	22	5.6	26	6.6	0.44
Gender					
Male (ref.)					
Female	125	31.6	235	59.5	0.94
Work experience in years					
0–4 (ref.)					
5–9	25	6.3	31	7.8	0.71
10–14	17	4.3	40	10.1	0.75
15–20	25	6.3	27	6.8	0.69
Over 20	42	10.6	37	9.4	0.44
Education					
Diploma (ref.)					
Bachelor's degree	20	5.1	40	10.1	0.04
Master's degree	0	0.0	3	0.8	0.99
Working unit					
Operating theatre (ref.)					
Radiology department	1	0.3	19	4.8	0.46
First-aid clinic	79	20.0	107	27.1	0.49
Medical ward	35	8.9	84	21.3	0.21
Medical radiation education					
No (ref.)					
Yes	11	2.8	258	65.3	<0.01

TABLE 5: Background factors correlated with guidelines of safe ionizing radiation use knowledge area ($N = 395$).

Independent variable	Outcome variable: Lower knowledge n	%	Higher knowledge n	%	Probability (p)
Age (years)					
18–27 (ref.)					
28–37	47	11.9	57	14.4	<0.01
38–47	52	13.2	36	9.1	0.04
48–57	26	6.6	22	5.6	0.03
Gender					
Male (ref.)					
Female	142	35.9	218	55.2	0.78
Work experience in years					
0–4 (ref.)					
5–9	27	6.8	29	7.3	0.20
10–14	21	5.3	36	9.1	0.13
15–20	33	8.4	19	4.8	0.53
Over 20	45	11.4	34	8.6	0.11
Education					
Diploma (ref.)					
Bachelor's degree	23	5.8	37	9.4	0.26
Master's degree	1	0.3	2	0.5	0.49
Working unit					
Operating theatre (ref.)					
Radiology department	1	0.3	19	4.8	0.26
First-aid clinic	89	22.5	97	24.6	0.27
Medical ward	38	9.6	81	20.5	0.60
Medical radiation education					
No (ref.)					
Yes	29	7.3	240	60.8	<0.01

effects of medical radiation but not well educated with the ALARA concept and stochastic effects of a certain radiation dose in medical radiation. The lack of knowledge of this main theory (and issues raised earlier) has been noted globally [16, 26]. Another significant outcome is that, as previously stated, nurses felt that they had not undergone adequate radiation education [16]. From the result above, it is clear that medical radiation education is significantly linked with all three areas of radiation knowledge. The need to enhance education is reinforced by further observation of a clear gap in understanding radiation safety between nurses who had not undergone radiation education. The lack of radiation education will put both nurses' and patients' health at high risk [18]. Hence, education is important to ensure that nurses successfully follow the applicable rules and procedures for the safe use of radiation [27], develop a culture of protection among users of radiation, and adhere to national and international standards.

5. Conclusion

The study shows that Malaysian nurses are well educated about radiation protection and radiation usage but lack radiation physics knowledge. This has serious implications for both patients and nurses. Training and learning by providing skills for all nurses involved in the ionizing radiation is a key for optimizing quality and education. Therefore, healthcare organizations play an important role in ensuring that all nurses in Malaysia are well educated about radiation knowledge by enhancing education requirements for all nurses who act around or are exposed to radiation. In conclusion, the findings demonstrate the value of radiation knowledge and radiation understanding and, most significantly, the function and role of education to ensure the safe use of medical radiation.

Acknowledgments

The authors would like to thank the Faculty of Science and Technology, Universiti Sains Islam Malaysia (USIM), for supporting the current study. This work was supported by the Universiti Sains Islam Malaysia Research Grant (PPPI/FST/0119/051000/17519).

References

[1] C. T. Expo, "Evaluating organ dose and radiation risk of routine CT examinations in Johor, Malaysia," *Sains Malaysiana*, vol. 45, no. 4, pp. 567–573, 2016.

[2] United Nations Scientific Committee on the Effects of Atomic Radiation, *UNSCEAR 2008 Report: Sources and Effects of Ionizing Radiation*, United Nations Scientific Committee on the Effects of Atomic Radiation, New York, NY, USA, 2010.

[3] B. Krans, "X-ray: purpose, procedure, and risks," December 2020, https://www.healthline.com/health/x-ray.

[4] W. C. Serena Low, J. H. Chuah, C. A. T. H. Tee et al., "An overview of deep learning techniques on chest X-ray and CT scan identification of COVID-19," *Computational and Mathematical Methods in Medicine*, vol. 2021, Article ID 5528144, 17 pages, 2021.

[5] A. Khalil, A. Faisal, S. C. Ng, Y. M. Liew, and K. W. Lai, "Mitral valve rigid registration using 2D echocardiography and cardiac computed tomography," in *Proceedings of the 2017 International Conference on Applied System Innovation (ICASI)*, pp. 629–632, IEEE, Sapporo, Japan, May 2017.

[6] T. Schroderus-Salo, L. Hirvonen, A. Henner et al., "Development and validation of a psychometric scale for assessing healthcare professionals' knowledge in radiation protection," *Radiography*, vol. 25, no. 2, pp. 136–142, 2019.

[7] A. Agarwal, "Radiation risk in orthopedic surgery: ways to protect yourself and the patient," *Operative Techniques in Sports Medicine*, vol. 19, no. 4, pp. 220–223, 2011.

[8] "Radiation: effects and sources," December 2020, https://wedocs.unep.org/handle/20.500.11822/7790;jsessionid1/453F5CB27020794BD3372ECAEBFF3DCB1.

[9] United Nations Scientific Committee on the Effects of Atomic Radiation, *Sources, Effects and Risks of Ionizing Radiation: UNSCEAR 2017 Report to the General Assembly with Scientific Annexes*, UN, New York, NY, USA, 2018.

[10] T. Jindal, "The risk of radiation exposure to assisting staff in urological procedures: a literature review," *Urologic Nursing*, vol. 33, no. 3, 2013.

[11] International Atomic Energy Agency, "Radiation protection in medicine: setting the scene for the next decade," in *Proceedings of an International Conference*, pp. 2–17, Bonn, Germany, December 2012.

[12] I. A. E. Agency, *Radiation Protection and Safety of Radiation Sources: International Basic Safety Standards*, International Atomic Energy Agency, Vienna, Austria, 2014.

[13] W. H. Organization, *Bonn Call-For-Action-Joint Position Statement by the IAEA and WHO*, WHO, Geneva, Switzerland, 2014.

[14] A. Yurt, B. Çavuşoğlu, and T. Günay, "Evaluation of awareness on radiation protection and knowledge about radiological examinations in healthcare professionals who use ionized radiation at work," *Molecular Imaging Radionucl. Ther*, vol. 22, no. 2, pp. 48–53, 2014.

[15] E. Jones and K. Mathieson, "Radiation safety among workers in health services," *Health Physics*, vol. 110, no. 5, pp. S52–S58, 2016.

[16] M. Alotaibi and R. Saeed, "Radiology nurses' awareness of radiation," *Journal of Radiology Nursing*, vol. 25, no. 1, pp. 7–12, 2006.

[17] I. Laboratories, "Digital Download Information and insights into radiography using your IDEXX Digital Imaging System ALARA principle for minimizing radiation exposure," p. 70045, 2009.

[18] J. Kiah and D. Stueve, "The importance of radiation safety for healthcare workers as well as patients," *CathLab Digest*, vol. 20, no. 1, 2012.

[19] *67Guidence Document for Occupational Radiation Protection.pdf*, Ketua Pengarah Kesihatan Malaysia, Putrajaya, Malaysia, 2016.

[20] IAEA, *Applying Radiation Safety Standards in Radiotherapy*, vol. 38, IAEA, Vienna, Austria, 2006.

[21] L. Hirvonen, T. Schroderus-Salob, A. Henner et al., "Nurses' knowledge of radiation protection: a cross-sectional study," *Radiography*, vol. 25, no. 4, pp. e108–e112, 2019.

[22] N. A. Yunus, M. H. R. O. Abdullah, M. A. Said, and P. E. Ch'Ng, "Assessment of radiation safety awareness among nuclear medicine nurses: a pilot study," *Journal of Physics: Conference Series*, vol. 546, no. 1, pp. 3–9, 2014.

[23] H. Nurhayati, "Malaysia: number of registered nurses 2019 | Statista," *Statista*, February 2021, https://www.statista.com/statistics/1199568/malaysia-number-of-registered-nurses/.

[24] "Sample size calculator: understanding sample sizes | SurveyMonkey," February 2021, https://www.surveymonkey.com/mp/sample-size-calculator/.

[25] T. A. N. Ahmed and S. Taha, "Radiation exposure, the forgotten enemy: toward implementation of national safety program," *The Egyptian Heart Journal*, vol. 69, no. 1, pp. 55–62, 2017.

[26] P. Cole, R. Hallard, J. Broughton et al., "Developing the radiation protection safety culture in the UK," *Journal of Radiological Protection*, vol. 34, no. 2, pp. 469–484, 2014.

[27] T. Coldwell, P. Cole, C. Edwards et al., "The advantages of creating a positive radiation safety culture in the higher education and research sectors," *Journal of Radiological Protection*, vol. 35, no. 4, p. 917, 2015.

3

Diagnostic Accuracy Studies in Radiology: How to Recognize and Address Potential Sources of Bias

Athanasios Pavlou,[1,2] Robert M. Kurtz,[3] and Jae W. Song[3]

[1]*St. Vincent's Medical Center, Bridgeport, CT, USA*
[2]*Frank H. Netter MD School of Medicine, North Haven, CT, USA*
[3]*Hospital of the University of Pennsylvania, Philadelphia, PA, USA*

Correspondence should be addressed to Jae W. Song; jae.song@pennmedicine.upenn.edu

Academic Editor: André Luiz Ferreira Costa

Accuracy is an important parameter of a diagnostic test. Studies that attempt to determine a test's accuracy can suffer from various forms of bias. As radiology is a diagnostic specialty, many radiologists may design a diagnostic accuracy study or review one to understand how it may apply to their practice. Radiologists also frequently serve as consultants to other physicians regarding the selection of the most appropriate diagnostic exams. In these roles, understanding how to critically appraise the literature is important for all radiologists. The purpose of this review is to provide a framework for evaluating potential sources of study design biases that are found in diagnostic accuracy studies and to explain their impact on sensitivity and specificity estimates. To help the reader understand these biases, we also present examples from the radiology literature.

1. Introduction

The accuracy of a diagnostic test refers to how well a test can correctly identify a specific disease. Therefore, it is a crucial parameter to consider when making a decision to perform that test in a clinical setting. Inaccurate diagnostic tests can lead to over- or undertreatment, inflated healthcare costs, and potentially patient harm [1]. Diagnostic accuracy studies attempt to evaluate a test's performance by comparing it to a gold standard. These studies can suffer from biases (e.g., spectrum bias and verification bias) that are different from those affecting studies designed to test the efficacy of therapeutic interventions. Awareness of these biases and how they can impact diagnostic accuracy measures is important. Several studies have quantitatively shown that specific biases can lead to an overestimation or underestimation of accuracy measures [2, 3]. Given that diagnostic accuracy studies help experts and policymakers to create guidelines and establish standard-of-care measures [4], it is imperative that readers be aware of these biases and how they can be addressed.

As practitioners of a diagnostic specialty, it is important for radiologists to understand how to appraise diagnostic accuracy studies. Radiologists are frequently consulted by other physicians on which imaging test to order for specific indications and serve to educate and inform others about current standards of care for the diagnostic work-up of many patients. In the era of evidence-based medicine, radiologists are encouraged to keep up with the literature as well as know how to appraise the quality of a diagnostic accuracy study. Moreover, it is equally important to know how applicable the results of a particular diagnostic accuracy study are to the radiologist's own clinical practice [5].

Guidelines and checklists often serve as useful tools to help one be comprehensive and achieve consistency. As such, the Cochrane Collaboration and Agency for Healthcare Research and Quality has recommended the use of checklists such as the Quality Assessment of Diagnostic Accuracy Studies 2 (QUADAS-2) tool [6]. This tool helps to assess the risk of bias in diagnostic studies and is organized into 4 key domains. These domains include evaluating aspects of study design related to (1) patient selection, (2) the index test, (3) reference standard, and the (4) flow and timing of subjects in a study [7]. Within each domain are specific types of study design biases that should be considered.

In this paper, we use the QUADAS-2 framework to review the study design biases within each domain (see Table 1). We will also present examples from the radiology literature.

2. Basic Concepts

The framework for developing a research question in evidence-based medicine follows the PICO model. In diagnostic accuracy studies, PICO stands for P (population), I (index test), C (comparator or reference standard), and O (outcomes). A diagnostic accuracy study compares the index test (the test under investigation) with an established reference test on a specific population and provides outcomes for comparison [8]. The degree to which the outcomes of the study represent true findings among similar individuals outside the study is determined by the validity. There are two main types of validity: internal and external (see Figure 1) [9].

2.1. Internal Validity. The extent to which the observed results are not due to methodological errors is defined as internal validity. The internal validity of a study can be threatened by bias and imprecision (see Figure 2). Bias is considered to be any systematic deviation of an estimate from the true value. If a diagnostic accuracy study suffers from bias, its sensitivity and/or specificity will be consistently under- or overestimated compared to the true value. This means that the error introduced by bias will not balance out upon repetition. Imprecision is the random error that occurs with multiple estimates of a parameter and refers to how far these estimates are from each other, not how far they are from the true value. Because of the random deviation of the estimates towards opposite directions, repetition will eventually balance out this error [11].

2.2. External Validity. External validity examines whether the findings of a study can be generalized to the population level. If the study's sample is representative of the target population, the results of the study can be generalized to the population from which the sample was drawn and even beyond that to other similar populations. This is especially important as it determines whether the results of the study can be applied in daily clinical practice [12].

Applicability is also an important consideration when evaluating diagnostic accuray studies. Careful evaluation of the PIC (Population-Index-Reference) parameters of a study will help determine the extent of applicability of a study to a reader's clinical practice. The patient demographics, selection and use of the index test, and test interpretation should be compared between the study and the reader's practice. To allow for this comparison, it is vital that diagnostic accuracy studies report their methods with completeness and transparency, preferably using standardized checklists such as the Standards for the Reporting of Diagnostic Accuracy studies (STARD) [13].

Using the PIC framework will help the reader assess the external validity as well as gain insight into the applicability of the study. For assessment of internal validity, critically appraising the study design using a four-domain framework is suggested [11]. We now review specific sources of study design biases using the QUADAS-2 framework.

3. Domain 1: Patient Selection

The goal of sampling is to ensure that the sample group is representative of the population of interest. The results of the study are contingent on the studied sample. Thus, sampling methods are a critical part of a study design. Participants should ideally be recruited from a population in a process that ensures no over- or underrepresentation of certain subpopulations [14].

3.1. Sampling Definition and Methods. Sampling is the process of selecting a group of study subjects from the target population. There are two main categories of sampling methods: probability and nonprobability sampling.

In probability sampling methods, all eligible subjects in the target population have equal chances to be selected (e.g., random sampling). The challenge with this type of sampling method is that it requires the presence of a comprehensive list or registry of all eligible patients in the target population, from which the subjects are randomly chosen using, for instance, a random number generator [14]. As such registries are rarely available in practice, clinical studies more frequently use nonprobability sampling [15].

In nonprobability sampling methods, the sample is selected in a process that does not guarantee equal chances to be selected for each eligible subject in the target population. An example of nonprobability sampling is convenience sampling, where patients are selected only based on accessibility and availability. The selection process for convenience sampling can lead to over- or underrepresentation of certain population attributes and therefore decreases the generalizability of the study results (sampling bias). A special form of convenience sampling, commonly used in clinical research, is consecutive sampling. In this sampling method, for a specified period of time, every subject who meets the predefined inclusion and exclusion criteria is recruited for the study. This sampling method prevents the researchers from "picking and choosing" subjects [15]. Analysis of 31 published meta-analyses showed that nonconsecutive sampling tended to overestimate the diagnostic accuracy of the test by 50% compared to consecutive sampling in diagnostic accuracy studies [16].

The effect of consecutive over nonconsecutive sampling can be seen in a study evaluating deep venous thrombosis (DVT) of the lower extremities. Kline et al. recruited subjects using a consecutive method to compare the diagnostic accuracy of emergency clinician-performed compression ultrasonography for DVT of the lower extremities against whole-leg venous ultrasonography and reported a sensitivity

Table 1: Types of bias in diagnostic accuracy studies and how to address them.

Bias type	How to address
Spectrum bias	Perform random or consecutive sampling; avoid excluding subjects with ambiguous results
Information bias	Implement blinding of the researchers to the results of the reference test when interpreting the index test; predetermine the thresholds when designing a study
Misclassification bias	Predict the direction and degree of deviation for the diagnostic accuracy in sensitivity analysis and adjust accordingly; create a composite reference standard
Diagnostic review bias	Implement blinding of the researchers to the results of the index test when interpreting the reference test
Incorporation bias	Address in the limitations section the possibility of overestimation of accuracy estimates and if possible, adjust accordingly
Verification bias	Use the same reference standard for all subjects and if not possible, acknowledge and measure the potential accuracy estimate error
Attrition bias	Study the characteristics of subjects lost and how they differ from those that remain; perform sensitivity analysis to calculate the range of diagnostic accuracy estimates as if all withdrawals tested positive or negative

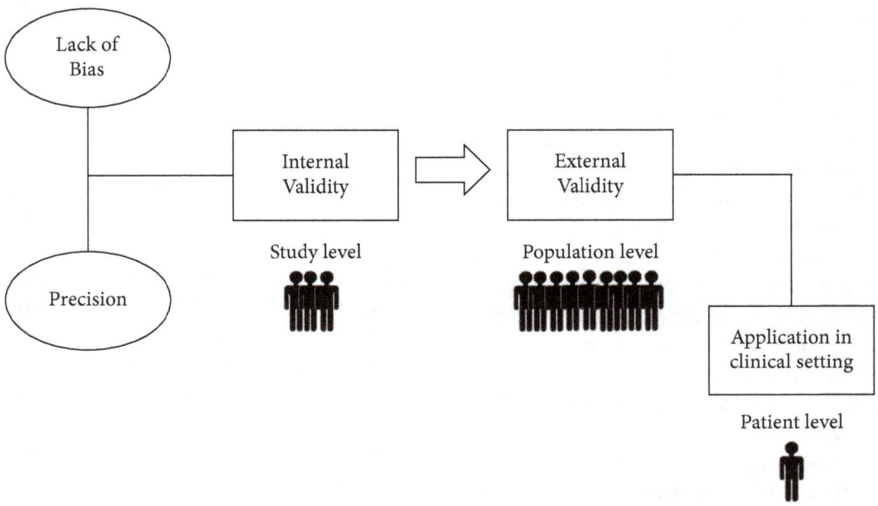

Figure 1: Internal and external validity. Precision and lack of bias dictate the internal validity of the study. External validity refers to the process of applying the study results from the study level to the population level. Radiologists can use these results in their own clinical practice for management of individual patients.

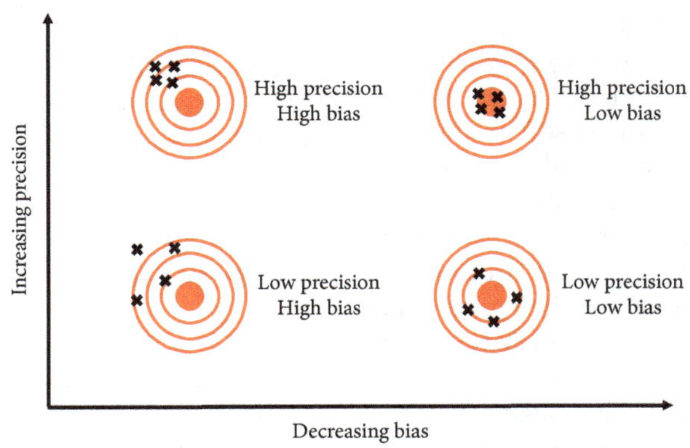

Figure 2: Precision and bias. Increasing precision reduces the random error and decreasing bias is equivalent to decreasing systematic error. The higher the precision and the lower the bias, the higher the internal validity of the study. Adapted from ELife, 7, e35718, Brandmaier, A. M. et al., Assessing reliability in neuroimaging research through intraclass effect decomposition (ICED) (2018) (modified) [10].

of 70% and specificity of 89% [17]. By contrast, other studies on the same topic reported almost perfect diagnostic accuracy (sensitivity: 100% and specificity: 91.8–100%) using a nonconsecutive sample. These higher accuracy measures could be due to excluding complex cases, excluding patients who may be difficult to perform ultrasound, or excluding ambiguous results [18, 19].

3.2. Spectrum Bias. Spectrum bias is commonly used to describe the variation in test performance across patient subgroups. Studies that utilize a limited portion of the patient spectrum can be affected by this type of bias. For example, a study that includes only high-risk patients may provide different diagnostic accuracy estimates compared to a study that includes only low-risk patients, as the test performance varies in different populations [20, 21].

An obvious source of spectrum bias is a patient selection method that leads to a sample that is not representative of the target population. Local referral practices can also remove cases from the initial distribution, narrow the spectrum of patients, and lead to bias [11]. Understanding spectrum bias is important as it can prohibit the generalization of the results from the studied sample to a wider population, especially when studying heterogeneous populations. It has been suggested that "spectrum effect" is a more appropriate term, as the estimate from a narrow spectrum of patients is valid for this specific subgroup [21].

An example of how diagnostic accuracy measurements can be influenced by the patient spectrum is seen in a meta-analysis that studied the accuracy of magnetic resonance imaging (MRI) to detect silicone breast implant rupture. The authors found that the diagnostic accuracy of MRI in studies that included patients with symptoms of implant rupture was 14 times higher compared to studies that included only asymptomatic patients and two times higher compared to studies that used both symptomatic and asymptomatic patients (screening sample) [2].

3.3. Case-Control and Cross-Sectional Study Design. In diagnostic accuracy studies, based on the way subjects are recruited, the study design is usually a case-control, cross-sectional, or cohort study design. In case-control designs, patients are sampled separately from controls, which introduces spectrum bias. This is because patients tend to be "the sickest of the sick," which leads to sensitivity overestimation, and controls tend to be the "healthiest of the healthy," which leads to specificity overestimation (see Figure 3). In cross-sectional and cohort designs, patients and controls are sampled together from a population based on the presence of a characteristic regardless of the presence of disease [3, 22]. In a study by Lijmer et al., which reviewed 184 diagnostic accuracy studies for design-related bias, case-control designs tended to overestimate the diagnostic performance of the test by threefold compared to studies with cohort design [3].

An area in radiology where the difference between case-control and cohort has been studied is Artificial Intelligence (AI). As noted by Park [23], utilizing a case-control design for the clinical validation of AI algorithms forces a binary distinction of outcomes that does not accurately represent real-world situations, where disease-simulating conditions and comorbidities may be present. As a result, the diagnostic performance of an AI algorithm may be inflated, and consequently, the generalization of study results to real-world practice may be problematic. Nevertheless, case-control studies are still typically used as initial validation methods for deep learning algorithms, as they are more convenient to perform and allow for establishment of a reference standard [23, 24].

Another limitation of the case-control design is that the positive predictive value (PPV) (probability that subjects with a positive test truly have the disease) and negative predictive value (NPV) (probability that subjects with a negative test truly do not have the disease) cannot be directly measured, as the ratio of cases to control is set by the investigator and disease prevalence is not reflected in the data (see Figure 4) [22].

4. Domain 2: Index Test

4.1. Information Bias. An important source of bias when evaluating the index test is the lack of blinding of the investigators to the results of the reference standard for each subject. Knowledge of the reference standard results may influence the interpretation of the index test results. This is also known as information bias. This type of bias can lead to larger deviations when the index test is not an objective measurement and depends on a rater's subjective assessment [25].

Aside from blinding to avoid information bias, it is important for diagnostic accuracy studies to prespecify the threshold used for the index test interpretation. A posteriori determination of a threshold in a data-driven way can lead to overestimation of test performance, especially in studies with a small number of subjects. This is because an optimal cutoff may be chosen based on the available results to favor overly optimistic measures of diagnostic accuracy [26].

For example, Kivrak et al. performed a study comparing computed tomography (CT) virtual cystoscopy with conventional cystoscopy for the diagnosis of bladder tumors, which they designed in a rigorous way to avoid introducing information bias. The authors report that the two experienced radiologists, who independently interpreted the virtual cystoscopy (the index test), were blinded to the findings of conventional cystoscopy (the reference standard). Additionally, the virtual cystoscopy was performed and interpreted prior to the conventional cystoscopy, thereby ensuring that the investigators were blinded to the results of the reference test [27].

4.2. Indeterminate Index Test Results. Patients with indeterminate or ambiguous results should not be excluded from the study, as this could limit the results to an unrepresentative spectrum of extremes and potentially introduce spectrum bias. In this case, it is preferable to transform the 2×2 table to a 3×2 table and report positive, indeterminate, and negative results separately. To ensure

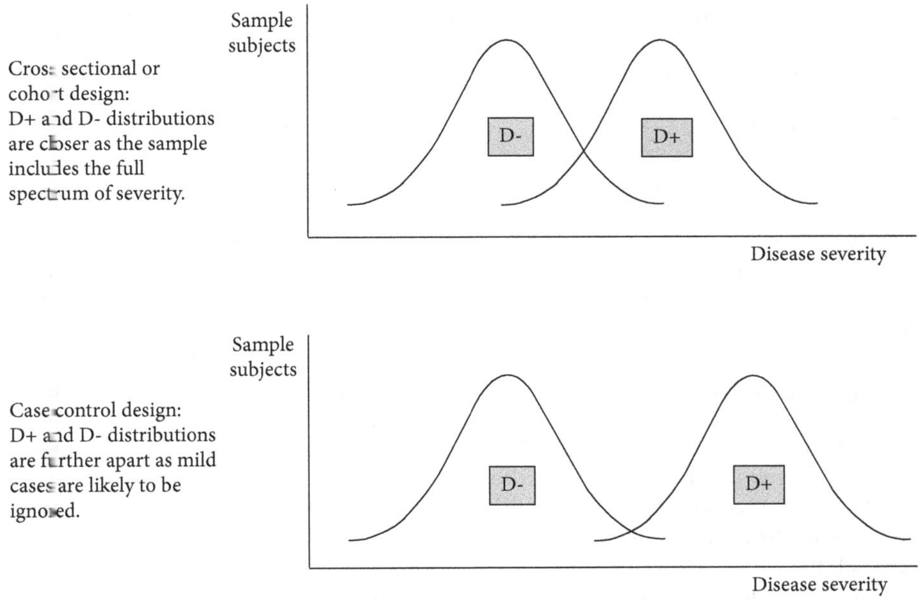

FIGURE 3: Cross-sectional study design minimizes spectrum bias as cases and controls are not sampled separately from the target population. D refers to disease status with D+ meaning disease is present and D-patients meaning disease is absent.

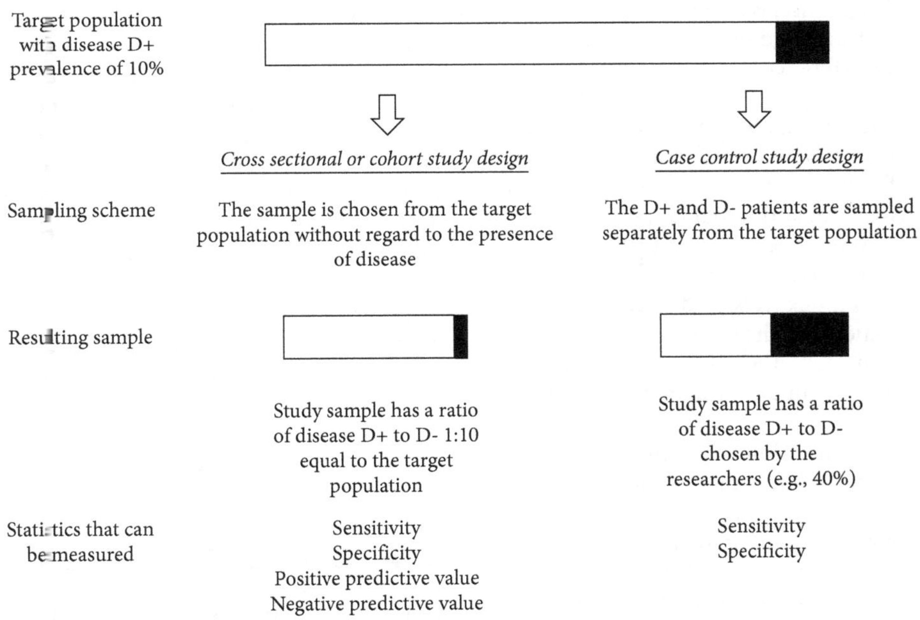

FIGURE 4: Cross-sectional and cohort designs allow for the calculation of a negative predictive value (NPV) and a positive predictive value (PPV), as they incorporate meaningful prevalence data. D refers to disease status with D+ meaning disease is present and D-patients meaning disease is absent.

that diagnostic accuracy estimates are not overestimated, a conservative "intention to diagnose" approach should be followed; indeterminate cases that test positive with the reference test are classified as false negative for the index. Indeterminate cases that test negative with the reference test are classified as false positive for the index (see Table 2). In the scenario when the reference test also yields indeterminate results, the table may be extended to a 3×3 table to ensure transparent reporting [28].

A meta-analysis by Schuetz et al. [28] pooled coronary CT angiography studies to compare how the handling of nonevaluable results affects diagnostic accuracy estimates. As CT angiography interpretation can involve nonevaluable test results especially in areas with vessel calcifications [29], the authors can consider nonevaluable vessel segments as positive or negative, exclude them from analysis, or even exclude patients with nonevaluable segments altogether. The authors in this study found that handling the test results with

Table 2: Various approaches for indeterminate index test results and their effect on sensitivity and specificity.

Indeterminate results	Sensitivity	Specificity
Excluded from analysis	Increased	Increased
Indeterminate results considered positive	Increased	Decreased
Indeterminate results considered negative	Decreased	Increased
"Intention to diagnose" approach	Decreased	Decreased

an "intention to diagnose" approach using a 3×2 table yielded lower diagnostic accuracy measures (Area Under Curve 0.93) compared to the other approaches (Area Under Curve 0.96–0.99) [28].

5. Domain 3: Reference Standard

The reference test represents the gold standard to which the index test is being compared. The assumption is that the reference standard is 100% accurate, so any disagreement with the results of the index test is attributed to the limited sensitivity or specificity of the latter. However, reference standards that perfectly differentiate between patients with and without the target condition are rare and, thus, some patients will inevitably be misclassified [30].

5.1. Misclassification Bias. Misclassification bias, which is also called imperfect gold standard bias, occurs due to errors in the reference test. The reference test may be susceptible to errors either due to its interpretation or due to technical limitations. For example, an imaging exam can give erroneous results because of inexperienced readers or due to limited resolution. If pathology is used as a reference standard, sampling error is an additional factor which could lead to false-negative results. The effect of this bias on the diagnostic accuracy estimates can vary depending on whether the reference and index tests tend to err in the same direction on the same patients or the reference and index test errors are independent of each other. As a result, sensitivity and specificity can be over- or underestimated by this type of bias [22].

An example of misclassification bias can be found in a study by Ai et al. which determined the diagnostic accuracy of chest CT for the diagnosis of Coronavirus Disease 2019 (COVID-19). The reference standard was a Reverse Transcription Polymerase Chain Reaction (RT-PCR) test, which can give false-negative results in the early stages of the disease. The authors calculated the sensitivity of chest CT for the diagnosis of COVID-19 to be 97% and the specificity 25% but acknowledged in the limitations section that, due to misclassification bias, the sensitivity may have been overestimated and the specificity may have been underestimated by solely relying on the results of a single RT-PCR test [31].

Various methods have been proposed to correct for misclassification bias. One suggestion is adjusting the accuracy estimates based on external evidence about the degree and direction of the reference standard misclassification. Other ways to minimize this bias are to combine multiple tests to a composite reference standard or validate the index test usefulness by correlating directly with future clinical events or other clinical characteristics [32].

5.2. Diagnostic Review Bias. Another important consideration when evaluating the reference standard is whether it is interpreted without the knowledge of the index test results. A positive index test may drive raters to search the reference study more carefully for evidence of disease. This is known as diagnostic review bias [25]. As pointed out by Ransohoff et al. [20], an example of this bias can be found in a study by Meadway et al. [33] which evaluated the diagnostic performance of Doppler ultrasound compared to venography. No indication was provided that the venograms were examined independently of the Doppler studies and thus it is possible that knowledge of the Doppler results affected the venogram diagnoses.

5.3. Incorporation Bias. On some occasions, the index test may be part of the reference standard. The resulting bias is called incorporation bias and leads to overestimation of the sensitivity and specificity. Incorporation bias often occurs when the reference standard relies on clinical judgment as the clinician often uses the index test to arrive at a diagnosis. This bias will result in an overestimation of diagnostic accuracy [34]. An example of this bias in the radiology literature can be found in a study by Mater et al. which evaluated the diagnostic accuracy of shunt series radiographs and CT to assess for cerebrospinal fluid shunt malfunction. The clinical decision to proceed to shunt revision, which was used as the reference standard, was made by the neurosurgeons after reviewing the radiograph and CT imaging. Despite the introduction of incorporation bias, this decision was reasonable in this study due to the lack of an independent gold standard. The authors also acknowledged this concern in the limitations section by stating possible overestimation of the sensitivity [35].

6. Domain 4: Patient Flow and Timing

Diagnostic accuracy studies should be designed taking into account time-dependent changes of the disease on the studied population and follow—as much as possible—a homogeneous approach for all subjects. Intervals between the index and reference test and disturbances in the flow of the study, such as changes in the reference test or withdrawals, are important sources of bias [7].

6.1. Timing of the Index and Reference Test. The time interval between the conduction of the index and the reference tests should ideally be as short as possible. A long period between the two could lead to misclassification bias, as the disease might improve or deteriorate during the interval time. An interval of a few days could be reasonable for chronic

Table 3: Direction of diagnostic accuracy estimates by type of bias.

Type of bias	Sensitivity [3, 16, 22, 26]	Specificity [3, 16, 22, 26]	RDOR from Rutjes et al. [16]	RDOR from Lijmer et al. [3]
Sampling bias (consecutive over nonconsecutive sampling)	Increases if complex cases are excluded Decreases if clear-cut cases are excluded	Increases if complex cases are excluded Decreases if clear-cut cases are excluded	1.5, 95% CI (1.0–2.1)	0.9, 95% CI (0.7–1.1)
Spectrum bias	Increases when severe cases are overrepresented in the patient sample ("the sickest of the sick")	Increases when healthy controls are overrepresented in the patient sample ("the healthiest of the healthy")	4.9, 95% CI (0.6–37.3)	3.0, 95% CI (2.0–4.5)
Information bias: lack of blinding	Variable	Variable	1.1, 95% CI (0.8–1.6)	1.3, 95% CI (1.0–1.9)
Information bias: post hoc definition of cutoff	Increases	Increases	1.3 95% CI (0.8–1.9)	Not studied
Misclassification bias (imperfect gold standard)	Increases if errors in index and reference test are correlated Decreases if errors in index and reference test are independent	Increases if errors in index and reference test are correlated Decreases if errors in index and reference test are independent	Not studied	Not studied
Incorporation bias	Increases	Increases	1.4, 95% CI (0.7–2.8)	Not studied
Verification bias: differential (i.e., different reference standards)	Increases if the gold standard is used for positive index results and a different reference test (e.g., noninvasive and less expensive) is used for negative index results	Increases if the gold standard is used for positive index results and a different reference test (e.g., noninvasive and less expensive) is used for negative index results	1.6, 95% CI (0.9–2.9)	2.2, 95% CI (1.5–3.3)
Verification bias: partial	Increases	Decreases	1.1, 95% CI (0.7–1.7)	1.0, 95% CI (0.8–1.3)

RDOR: Relative Diagnostic Odds Ratio. CI: confidence interval.

diseases but would be problematic for acute diseases. For reference tests that require follow-up to determine whether the disease is present, an appropriate minimum follow-up time should be set for all patients [6]. For example, a systematic review investigated the diagnostic accuracy of MRI in the diagnosis of early multiple sclerosis using clinical follow-up as reference standard. The average follow-up period in the included studies ranged from 7 months to 14 years and the authors found that studies with shorter follow-up tended to overestimate the sensitivity and underestimate specificity [36].

6.2. Verification Bias. Verification bias is a form of bias introduced when not all patients receive the gold standard (partial) or when some patients receive a different reference test than the rest (differential) [3]. In partial verification bias, if the decision is made to perform the gold standard only for positive index test cases, the sensitivity will be overestimated (fewer false negatives) and specificity will be underestimated (more false positives) [37]. The effect of differential verification depends on the quality of the different reference tests that are being used. Using a superior reference test for the positive test results and a different reference test for the negative results will overestimate both sensitivity and specificity [3]. Notably, using the same gold standard for all patients may not be clinically or ethically appropriate. If verification bias cannot be eliminated by choosing a proper study design, it should be at least acknowledged or statistically corrected by the authors [38].

An example can be found in the Prospective Investigation of Pulmonary Embolism Diagnosis (PIOPED) study, which evaluated the diagnostic accuracy of Ventilation-Perfusion (V-Q) scan using conventional angiography as a reference standard. From the 131 patients with near normal/normal results on the V-Q scan, only 57 received angiography (gold standard). For the remaining 74, an alternative reference standard was used: no evidence of pulmonary embolism during one-year follow-up. The authors calculated that if those 74 patients were included in the analysis, the NPV for near normal/normal scan would have been 96% and if not, the NPV would have been 91%. So, they concluded that the true NPV value is somewhere between those two numbers but possibly closer to the first [39].

Another area in radiology where partial verification bias has been described is Single Photon Emission Computed Tomography (SPECT) for the diagnosis of coronary artery disease [40–43]. The decision to perform coronary angiography, which is the gold standard for the diagnosis of coronary artery disease, may be affected by the result of a preceding SPECT which introduces verification bias (also called posttest referral bias). Authors have utilized mathematical formulas (e.g., Begg and Greenes [44] and Diamond [45]) to adjust for this bias leading to significant changes in calculated diagnostic accuracy parameters. Miller et al. [42] reported an unadjusted sensitivity of 98% and specificity of 13% for SPECT in coronary artery disease. After correction with the Begg and Greenes formula, the sensitivity dropped to 65% and the specificity increased to 67% which indicates that verification bias can have an effect on accuracy estimation.

6.3. Attrition Bias. An important consideration is whether all patients were included in the analysis. Withdrawals lead to over- or underestimation of accuracy estimates (attrition bias) if the patients lost to follow-up differ in some way from those who remain. It is important for studies to report withdrawals and evaluate their effect on accuracy estimates [46]. An example of the effect of withdrawals on diagnostic accuracy estimates can be found in a study by Kearl et al. which investigated the accuracy of MRI and ultrasound in the diagnosis of appendicitis. Of the 589 patients included, the reference standards, which were pathology reports, surgical diagnosis, or clinical decision for medical treatment for appendicitis, were not available for 63 patients (10.7%) due to loss to follow-up. The authors acknowledged this limitation and analyzed the effect on diagnostic accuracy. A sensitivity analysis was performed, and the diagnostic accuracy was calculated separately as if all withdrawals were positive for appendicitis as well as if all withdrawals were negative for appendicitis with the reference standard [47].

7. Direction of Accuracy Measures due to Bias

Knowing the direction of diagnostic accuracy measures is a first step in countering the effect of bias in our interpretation of study results. The general direction towards which the diagnostic accuracy estimates may deviate can be predicted and depends on the specific type of bias. Rutjes et al. [16] and Lijmer et al. [3] quantified the effect of several study design biases on diagnostic accuracy measures (see Table 3). They used the Relative Diagnostic Odds Ratio (RDOR) as a parameter to compare studies with a specific methodological shortcoming to those without. An RDOR greater than one indicates that diagnostic accuracy parameters are overestimated in the study, while an RDOR less than one indicates that diagnostic accuracy parameters are underestimated in the study. The limitation with using RDOR is that important biases that have opposing effects on sensitivity and specificity may not cause significant directional changes in RDOR, which will remain close to one. This may be the explanation why both of these studies failed to detect statistically significant changes in the RDOR for some forms of bias [3] (see Table 3).

8. Conclusion

Diagnostic accuracy studies can suffer from many forms of bias. QUADAS-2 provides a useful framework for thinking about study design biases. Patient selection, index test, reference test, and patient flow/timing are the four main domains to be evaluated in each study, as they cover the primary sources of systematic error in diagnostic accuracy studies. Potential sources of bias should be acknowledged by the authors and their effect on test performance should be estimated and reported. We are encouraged to become familiar with the biases that can be found in diagnostic accuracy studies and critically assess the studies before applying the conclusions to their own clinical practice.

References

[1] A. S. Saber Tehrani, H. Lee, S. C. Mathews et al., "25-year summary of US malpractice claims for diagnostic errors 1986–2010: an analysis from the National Practitioner Data Bank," *BMJ Quality and Safety*, vol. 22, pp. 672–680, 2013.

[2] J. W. Song, H. M. Kim, L. T. Bellfi, and K. C. Chung, "The effect of study design biases on the diagnostic accuracy of magnetic resonance imaging for detecting silicone breast implant ruptures: a meta-analysis," *Plastic and Reconstructive Surgery*, vol. 127, pp. 1029–1044, 2011.

[3] J. G. Lijmer, B. W. Mol, S. Heisterkamp et al., "Empirical evidence of design-related bias in studies of diagnostic tests," *Journal of the American Medical Association*, vol. 282, pp. 1061–1066, 1999.

[4] R. K. Owen, N. J. Cooper, T. J. Quinn, R. Lees, and A. J. Sutton, "Network meta-analysis of diagnostic test accuracy studies identifies and ranks the optimal diagnostic tests and thresholds for health care policy and decision-making," *Journal of Clinical Epidemiology*, vol. 99, pp. 64–74, 2018.

[5] Evidence-Based Radiology Working Group, "Evidence-based radiology: a new approach to the practice of radiology," *Radiology*, vol. 220, pp. 566–575, 2001.

[6] J. B. Reitsma, A. W. S. Rutjes, P. Whiting, V. V. Vlassov, M. M. G. Leeflang, and J. J. Deeks, "Chapter 9: assessing methodological quality," in *Cochrane Handbook for Systematic Reviews of Diagnostic Test Accuracy Version 1.0.0*, J. J. Deeks, P. M. Bossuyt, and C. Gatsonis, Eds., The Cochrane Collaboration, London, UK, 2009.

[7] P. F. Whiting, A. W. S. Rutjes, M. E. Westwood et al., "QUADAS-2: a revised tool for the quality assessment of diagnostic accuracy studies," *Annals of Internal Medicine*, vol. 155, pp. 529–536, 2011.

[8] S. Aslam and P. Emmanuel, "Formulating a researchable question: a critical step for facilitating good clinical research," *Indian Journal of Sexually Transmitted Diseases and AIDS*, vol. 31, pp. 47–50, 2010.

[9] C. M. Patino and J. C. Ferreira, "Internal and external validity: can you apply research study results to your patients?" *Jornal Brasileiro de Pneumologia*, vol. 44, p. 183, 2018.

[10] A. M. Brandmaier, E. Wenger, N. C. Bodammer, S. Kühn, N. Raz, and U. Lindenberger, "Assessing reliability in neuroimaging research through intra-class effect decomposition (ICED)," *eLife*, vol. 7, Article ID e35718, 2018.

[11] R. L. Schmidt and R. E. Factor, "Understanding sources of bias in diagnostic accuracy studies," *Archives of Pathology & Laboratory Medicine*, vol. 137, pp. 558–565, 2013.

[12] C. Andrade, "Internal, external, and ecological validity in research design, conduct, and evaluation," *Indian Journal of Psychological Medicine*, vol. 40, pp. 498-499, 2018.

[13] J. F. Cohen, D. A. Korevaar, D. G. Altman et al., "STARD 2015 guidelines for reporting diagnostic accuracy studies: explanation and elaboration," *BMJ Open*, vol. 6, Article ID e012799, 2016.

[14] M. Elfil and A. Negida, "Sampling methods in clinical research; an educational review," *Emergency*, vol. 5, no. 1, p. e52, 2017.

[15] K. Mathieson, "Making sense of biostatistics: probability versus nonprobability sampling," *Journal of Clinical Research Best Practices*, vol. 10, no. 8, pp. 1-2, 2014.
[16] A. W. S. Rutjes, J. B. Reitsma, M. Di Nisio, N. Smidt, J. C. van Rijn, and P. M. M. Bossuyt, "Evidence of bias and variation in diagnostic accuracy studies," *Canadian Medical Association Journal*, vol. 174, pp. 469–476, 2006.
[17] J. A. Kline, P. M. O'Malley, V. S. Tayal, G. R. Snead, and A. M. Mitchell, "Emergency clinician-performed compression ultrasonography for deep venous thrombosis of the lower extremity," *Annals of Emergency Medicine*, vol. 52, pp. 437–445, 2008.
[18] S. Farahmand, M. Farnia, S. Shahriaran, and P. Khashayar, "The accuracy of limited B-mode compression technique in diagnosing deep venous thrombosis in lower extremities," *The American journal of emergency medicine*, vol. 29, pp. 687–690, 2011.
[19] T. Jang, M. Docherty, C. Aubin, and G. Polites, "Resident-performed compression ultrasonography for the detection of proximal deep vein thrombosis: fast and accurate," *Academic Emergency Medicine*, vol. 11, pp. 319–322, 2004.
[20] D. F. Ransohoff and A. R. Feinstein, "Problems of spectrum and bias in evaluating the efficacy of diagnostic tests," *New England Journal of Medicine*, vol. 299, pp. 926–930, 1978.
[21] S. A. Mulherin and W. C. Miller, "Spectrum bias or spectrum effect? subgroup variation in diagnostic test evaluation," *Annals of Internal Medicine*, vol. 137, pp. 598–602, 2002.
[22] M. A. Kohn, C. R. Carpenter, and T. B. Newman, "Understanding the direction of bias in studies of diagnostic test accuracy," *Academic Emergency Medicine*, vol. 20, pp. 1194–1206, 2013.
[23] S. H. Park, "Diagnostic case-control versus diagnostic cohort studies for clinical validation of artificial intelligence algorithm performance," *Radiology*, vol. 290, no. 1, pp. 272-273, 2019.
[24] J. G. Nam, S. Park, E. J. Hwang et al., "Development and validation of deep learning–based automatic detection algorithm for malignant pulmonary nodules on chest radiographs," *Radiology*, vol. 290, no. 1, pp. 218–228, 2019.
[25] P. Whiting, A. W. S. Rutjes, J. B. Reitsma, A. S. Glas, P. M. M. Bossuyt, and J. Kleijnen, "Sources of variation and bias in studies of diagnostic accuracy," *Annals of Internal Medicine*, vol. 140, pp. 189–202, 2004.
[26] M. M. G. Leeflang, K. G. M. Moons, J. B. Reitsma, and A. H. Zwinderman, "Bias in sensitivity and specificity caused by data-driven selection of optimal cutoff values: mechanisms, magnitude, and solutions," *Clinical Chemistry*, vol. 54, pp. 729–737, 2008.
[27] A. S. Kivrak, D. Kiresi, D. Emlik, K. Odev, and M. Kilinc, "Comparison of CT virtual cystoscopy of the contrast material-filled bladder with conventional cystoscopy in the diagnosis of bladder tumours," *Clinical Radiology*, vol. 64, pp. 30–37, 2009.
[28] G. M. Schuetz, P. Schlattmann, and M. Dewey, "Use of 3 × 2 tables with an intention to diagnose approach to assess clinical performance of diagnostic tests: meta-analytical evaluation of coronary CT angiography studies," *BMJ*, vol. 345, Article ID e6717, 2012.
[29] C. Strong, A. Ferreira, and R. C. Teles, "Diagnostic accuracy of computed tomography angiography for the exclusion of coronary artery disease in candidates for transcatheter aortic valve implantation," *Scientific Reports*, vol. 9, Article ID 19942, 2019.
[30] C. Biesheuvel, L. Irwig, and P. Bossuyt, "Observed differences in diagnostic test accuracy between patient subgroups: is it real or due to reference standard misclassification?" *Clinical Chemistry*, vol. 53, pp. 1725–1729, 2007.
[31] T. Ai, Z. Yang, H. Hou, C. Zhan, C. Chen, and W. Lv, "Correlation of chest CT and RT-PCR testing for Coronavirus disease 2019 (COVID-19) in China: a report of 1014 cases," *Radiology*, vol. 296, pp. E32–E40, 2020.
[32] J. B. Reitsma, A. W. S. Rutjes, K. S. Khan, A. Coomarasamy, and P. M. Bossuyt, "A review of solutions for diagnostic accuracy studies with an imperfect or missing reference standard," *Journal of Clinical Epidemiology*, vol. 62, pp. 797–806, 2009.
[33] J. Meadway, A. N. Nicolaides, C. J. Walker, and J. D. O'Connell, "Value of Doppler ultrasound in diagnosis of clinically suspected deep vein thrombosis," *British Medical Journal*, vol. 4, pp. 552–554, 1975.
[34] A. Worster and C. Carpenter, "Incorporation bias in studies of diagnostic tests: how to avoid being biased about bias," *CJEM*, vol. 10, pp. 174-175, 2008.
[35] A. Mater, M. Shroff, S. Al-Farsi, J. Drake, and R. D. Goldman, "Test characteristics of neuroimaging in the emergency department evaluation of children for cerebrospinal fluid shunt malfunction," *Canadian Journal of Emergency Medicine*, vol. 10, pp. 131–135, 2008.
[36] P. Whiting, R. Harbord, C. Main, J. J. Deeks, G. Filippini, and M. Egger, "Accuracy of magnetic resonance imaging for the diagnosis of multiple sclerosis: systematic review," *BMJ*, vol. 332, pp. 875–884, 2006.
[37] A. S. Kosinski and H. X. Barnhart, "Accounting for nonignorable verification bias in assessment of diagnostic tests," *Biometrics*, vol. 59, pp. 163–171, 2003.
[38] J. M. Petscavage, M. L. Richardson, and R. B. Carr, "Verification bias an underrecognized source of error in assessing the efficacy of medical imaging," *Academic Radiology*, vol. 18, pp. 343–346, 2011.
[39] PIOPED Investigators, "Value of the ventilation/perfusion scan in acute pulmonary embolism. Results of the prospective investigation of pulmonary embolism diagnosis (PIOPED)," *Journal of the American Medical Association*, vol. 263, pp. 2753–2759, 1990.
[40] M. P. Cecil, A. S. Kosinski, M. T. Jones et al., "The importance of work-up (verification) bias correction in assessing the accuracy of SPECT thallium-201 testing for the diagnosis of coronary artery disease," *Journal of Clinical Epidemiology*, vol. 49, no. 7, pp. 735–742, 1996.
[41] C. Santana-Boado, J. Candell-Riera, J. Castell-Conesa et al., "Diagnostic accuracy of technetium-99m-MIBI myocardial SPECT in women and men," *Journal of Nuclear Medicine: Official Publication, Society of Nuclear Medicine*, vol. 39, no. 5, pp. 751–755, 1998.
[42] T. D. Miller, D. O. Hodge, T. F. Christian, J. J. Milavetz, K. R. Bailey, and R. J. Gibbons, "Effects of adjustment for referral bias on the sensitivity and specificity of single photon emission computed tomography for the diagnosis of coronary artery disease," *The American Journal of Medicine*, vol. 112, no. 4, pp. 290–297, 2002.
[43] J. A. Ladapo, S. Blecker, M. R. Elashoff et al., "Clinical implications of referral bias in the diagnostic performance of exercise testing for coronary artery disease," *Journal of the American Heart Association*, vol. 2, no. 6, Article ID e000505, 2013.

[44] C. B. Begg and R. A. Greenes, "Assessment of diagnostic tests when disease verification is subject to selection bias," *Biometrics*, vol. 39, no. 1, pp. 207–215, 1983.
[45] G. A. Diamond, "Reverend Bayes' silent majority. An alternative factor affecting sensitivity and specificity of exercise electrocardiography," *The American Journal of Cardiology*, vol. 57, no. 13, pp. 1175–1180, 1986.
[46] O. Aliu and K. C. Chung, "Assessing strength of evidence in diagnostic tests," *Plastic and Reconstructive Surgery*, vol. 129, pp. 989e–998e, 2012.
[47] Y. L. Kearl, I. Claudius, S. Behar et al., "Accuracy of magnetic resonance imaging and ultrasound for appendicitis in diagnostic and nondiagnostic studies," *Academic Emergency Medicine*, vol. 23, pp. 179–185, 2016.

4

Early Radiologic Diagnosis of Pulmonary Infection in Febrile Neutropenic Patients: A Comparison of Serial Chest Radiography and Single CT Chest

Wanaporn Burivong, Thanatorn Sricharoen, Apichart Thachang, Sunsiree Soodchuen, Panitpong Maroongroge, and Vichit Leelasithorn

Department of Radiology, Faculty of Medicine, Srinakharinwirot University, Bangkok, Thailand

Correspondence should be addressed to Wanaporn Burivong; wanaporn@g.swu.ac.th

Academic Editor: Lorenzo Faggioni

Objective. The purpose of this study is to compare the early radiologic diagnosis of pulmonary infection between serial chest radiography (chest film) and single chest computed tomography (CT chest) in the first seven days of febrile neutropenia. *Methods.* This study included 78 patients with hematologic malignancies who developed 107 episodes of febrile neutropenia from January 2012 to October 2017 and had a chest film performed within the first seven days. Demographic and radiographic data were retrospectively reviewed. Three radiologists independently and blindly evaluated chest films and CT chests. The sensitivity, specificity, and correlation of chest film with absolute neutrophil count were carried out. *Results.* A total of 222 chest films were performed during this period and found thirty-nine episodes (36.4%) of radiographic active pulmonary infection. The diagnosis of clinical positive for pulmonary infection is 44.8% (48/107). Sensitivity, specificity, positive predictive value, and negative predictive value of serial chest film in the early radiologic diagnosis of pulmonary infection are 50%, 74%, 61%, and 64%, respectively. The false-positive rate was 14%, and the false-negative rate was 22%. For single CT chest examinations, twenty-six studies were assessed, and 42.3% was indicative of radiographic active pulmonary infection. Sensitivity, specificity, positive predictive value, and negative predictive value of CT chest in the early radiologic diagnosis of pulmonary infection are 91%, 40%, 53%, and 86%, respectively. The false-positive rate was 60%. The absolute neutrophil count was not useful for predicting radiographic active pulmonary infection. *Conclusion.* Serial chest film for early radiologic diagnosis of pulmonary infection within the first seven days of febrile neutropenia has lower sensitivity with higher specificity as compared to a single CT chest. Conversely, CT chest may not only have a higher sensitivity in determining early pulmonary infection but also has a higher rate of false-positives.

1. Introduction

Patients with febrile neutropenia are particularly at high risk of infection including bacteria, fungi, and viruses [1, 2]. About 85% of patients are found in underlying hematological malignancies who received chemotherapy or underwent a hematopoietic stem cell transplant. [1]. The type and strength of chemotherapy, as well as the duration and severity of neutropenia, are the main risk factors that promote infection in these patients [3]. Infection often occurs in the gastrointestinal and respiratory tract [1, 2]. Pulmonary infection develops in about 15%. Respiratory signs and symptoms in these patients are lower than usual. Therefore, chest film is included as a part of diagnostic workup. One of the common chest infections found in these patients is invasive pulmonary aspergillosis. The chest film in this infection can show subtle or maybe undetectable findings, making its early radiographic sensitivity and specificity rather low [4]. A prior study reveals 29% of negative chest films and 71% of nonspecific abnormal radiographs in neutropenic patients with early invasive pulmonary aspergillosis [3]. More obvious radiographic findings can be seen when the neutrophil count increases. Computed tomography (CT) in febrile neutropenic patients with suspected pulmonary infection shows higher sensitivity and specificity [5]. Specific CT appearance such as mass or nodule with halo sign, cavitary lesion, and air-crescent sign can be identified and gives more suggestion of invasive pulmonary aspergillosis [5, 6]. However, due to the higher cost and radiation dose level of CT over chest film, the proper timing for CT examination is essential. Investigation too early may have negative radiographic findings, while investigation too late may cause delay diagnosis and treatment.

The purpose of this study is to compare the early radiologic diagnosis of pulmonary infection in the first seven days of febrile neutropenia between serial chest films and single CT chest by determining their relative sensitivity and specificity.

2. Materials and Methods

2.1. Study Population. This retrospective study was carried out at the Department of Radiology, Faculty of Medicine, Srinakharinwirot University, after approval from the Institutional Ethics Committee. We included patients with the underlying hematologic disease who developed febrile neutropenia (neutrophil count <500 μL and temperature >38.3°C) at HRH Princess Maha Chakri Sirindhorn Medical Center from January 1, 2012 to October 31, 2017. The inclusion criteria were patients who have chest film within the first seven days of febrile neutropenia. We excluded patients under age 15 and patients with unavailable clinical data or radiographic imaging.

2.2. Demographic Data Collection. The demographic data, age, sex, type of hematologic disease, chest symptom, and laboratory findings related to infection were recorded. Chest symptom was classified into cough, dyspnea, increased respiratory rate >20 min, decreased oxygen saturation <90%, and abnormal chest sounds such as rales, rhonchi, and decreased breath sound. Laboratory data related to infection in chest and outside chest were collected.

2.3. Radiographic Data. Three board-certified diagnostic radiologists independently and blindly reviewed chest film and CT chests within the first seven days of febrile neutropenia. Baseline chest film within three months before the episode of febrile neutropenia was also collected. Chest film opacity was classified into no opacity, new opacity, worsened opacity, stable opacity, and improvement. The chest films with no opacity, stable disease, and improvement were grouped as no radiological active pulmonary infection, while chest films with new lesions and progression were grouped as radiological active pulmonary infection. CT chest pattern was specified as pulmonary consolidation, centrilobular nodules/septal thickening, ground-glass opacity, nodule/mass, and atelectasis. Patients with CT chest findings of nodule/mass and atelectasis without other patterns were grouped as no radiological active pulmonary infection. Other CT chest findings are considered as radiological active pulmonary infection. In the cases where the radiologic interpretation was not unanimous, the agreement of two of the three radiologists was required for an interpretation to be considered final.

2.4. Statistical Analysis. The sensitivity, specificity, positive predictive value, and negative predictive value were determined by numbers of radiological active pulmonary infection from chest film and CT chest using the presence of either positive chest symptoms or positive mycobacterial study as a gold standard. Evaluation of the ability of absolute neutrophil count to differentiate positive chest films in febrile neutropenic patients was performed using area under the curve (AUC) of the receiver operating characteristic curve (ROC). Interobserver agreement of the radiographic findings on chest film and CT chest was calculated using Cohen's kappa (K) test.

3. Results

From January 2012 to October 2017, 78 patients with underlying hematologic malignancies had developed 107 episodes of febrile neutropenia. The mean age of patients was 47.9 years, with a range of 18–90 years. There were 47 male (60.3%) and 34 female (39.7%) patients. Of the 107 episodes, 41 (38.3%) had positive chest symptoms and 33 (30.8%) had laboratory data related to infection in the chest. The diagnosis of early pulmonary infection from the presence of chest symptoms or laboratory data or the combination thereof is 44.8% (48/107). Baseline characteristics of the patients, as well as chest symptoms and laboratory data, are described in Table 1.

A total of 222 chest films were performed during the first seven days of febrile neutropenia, 50% shows no opacity, while 15.8% had new lesions, 7.7% had progression, 19.8% was stable, and 7.2% found improvement on follow-up chest films. Thirty-nine episodes (36.4%) show radiographic active pulmonary infection, 14.0% was falsely positive, and 22.4% was falsely negative. Sensitivity, specificity, positive predictive value, and negative predictive value of serial chest films in the early radiologic diagnosis of pulmonary infection are 50%, 74%, 61%, and 64%, respectively.

Not all patients underwent CT chest examinations. Twenty-six single CT chest studies were performed during this period, 19 of which (73%) were positive with the following rates: pulmonary consolidation 56.0%, ground-glass attenuation 40.0%, nodular or mass lesions 32.0%, atelectasis 20%, and centrilobular nodules 4%. Ten CT chests (38.4%) were indicative of radiographic active pulmonary infection, and 60% was falsely positive. Sensitivity, specificity, positive predictive value, and negative predictive value of single CT chest in the early radiologic diagnosis of pulmonary infection are 91%, 40%, 53%, and 86%, respectively. There are 36.8% (7/19) of positive CT chest, which found no radiographic active pulmonary infection from serial chest film. Examples of serial chest film and CT chest abnormalities are presented in Figures 1–3.

Table 1: Baseline characteristics of the patients, including details of chest symptoms and laboratory data related to chest infection.

Baseline characteristic	Features	Number (%)
Gender	Male/female	47/31 (60.3/39.7)
Age (years)	Median	47.9 (range 18–90)
Hematologic malignancies	Leukemia	43 (55.1)
	Lymphoma	31 (39.7)
	Multiple myeloma	4 (5.1)
Chest symptoms	Positive/negative	41/66 (38.2/61.7)
	Shortness of breath	21 (51.2)
	Cough	19 (46.3)
	Tachypnea	15 (36.6)
	Lung signs	7 (17.1)
	Decreased breath sound	4 (9.8)
	Hypoxia	2 (4.9)
	Hemoptysis	1 (2.4)
Laboratory data related to chest infection	Positive/negative	33/74 (30.8/69.2)
	Microbial culture	18 (54.5)
	Serum galactomannan	18 (54.5)
	Influenza test	2 (6.0)

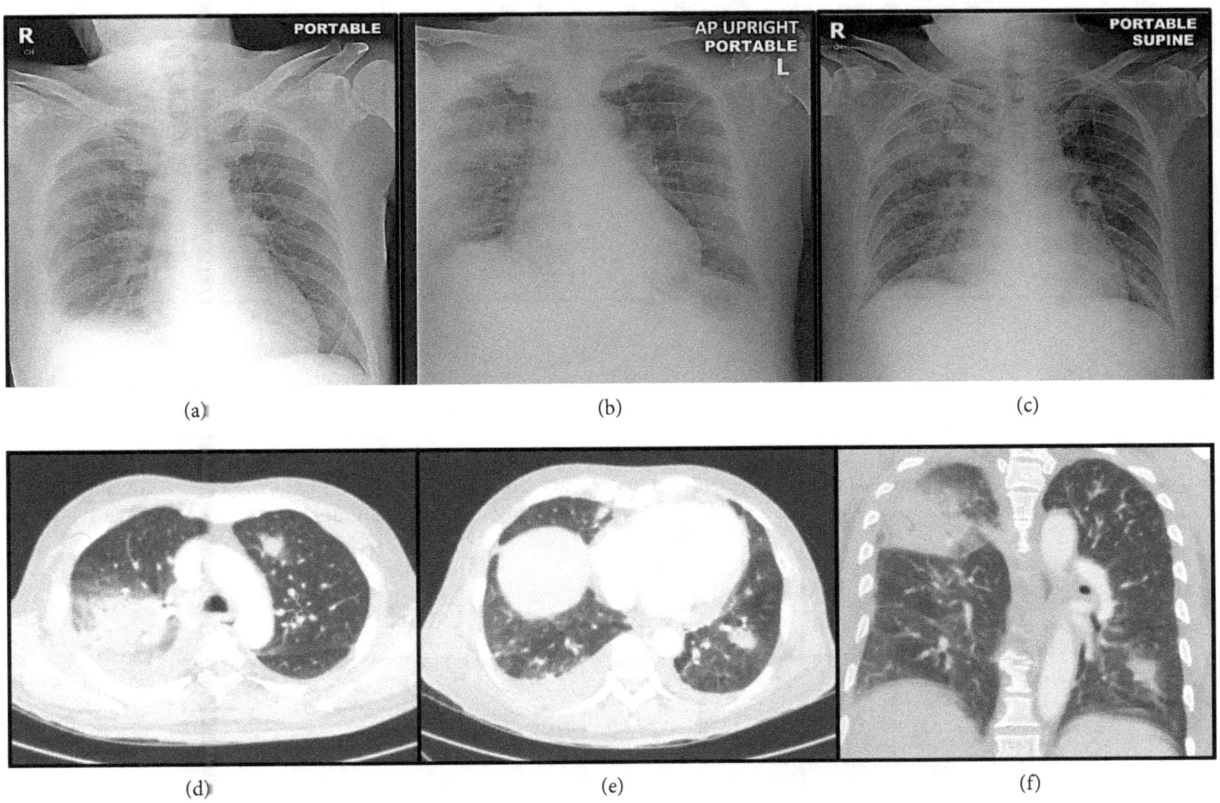

Figure 1: Images in a 58-year-old male patient with acute myeloid leukemia who had positive chest symptoms. (A) Baseline chest film shows right lower lung opacity. (B) Chest film on first day of febrile neutropenia (ANC = 0 μL) shows new opacity at right upper lung and left retrocardiac region. (C) Chest film on the fifth day of febrile neutropenia (ANC = 624 μL) shows stable opacities at right upper and left lower lungs. (D–F) Axial and coronal CT chest on third day of febrile neutropenia (ANC = 432 μL) reveals pulmonary consolidation at right upper lobe and a nodular lesion at left lower lobe. Both lesions are surrounded by a halo of ground-glass attenuation, suggesting angioinvasive pulmonary aspergillosis. This case was evaluated as true-positive chest radiograph and CT chest.

Details of consensus serial chest films and single CT chest compared to the clinical diagnosis of early pulmonary infection are summarized in Table 2.

ROC analysis shows that the absolute neutrophil count was not useful for predicting radiographic active pulmonary infection (AOC 0.483) (Figure 4).

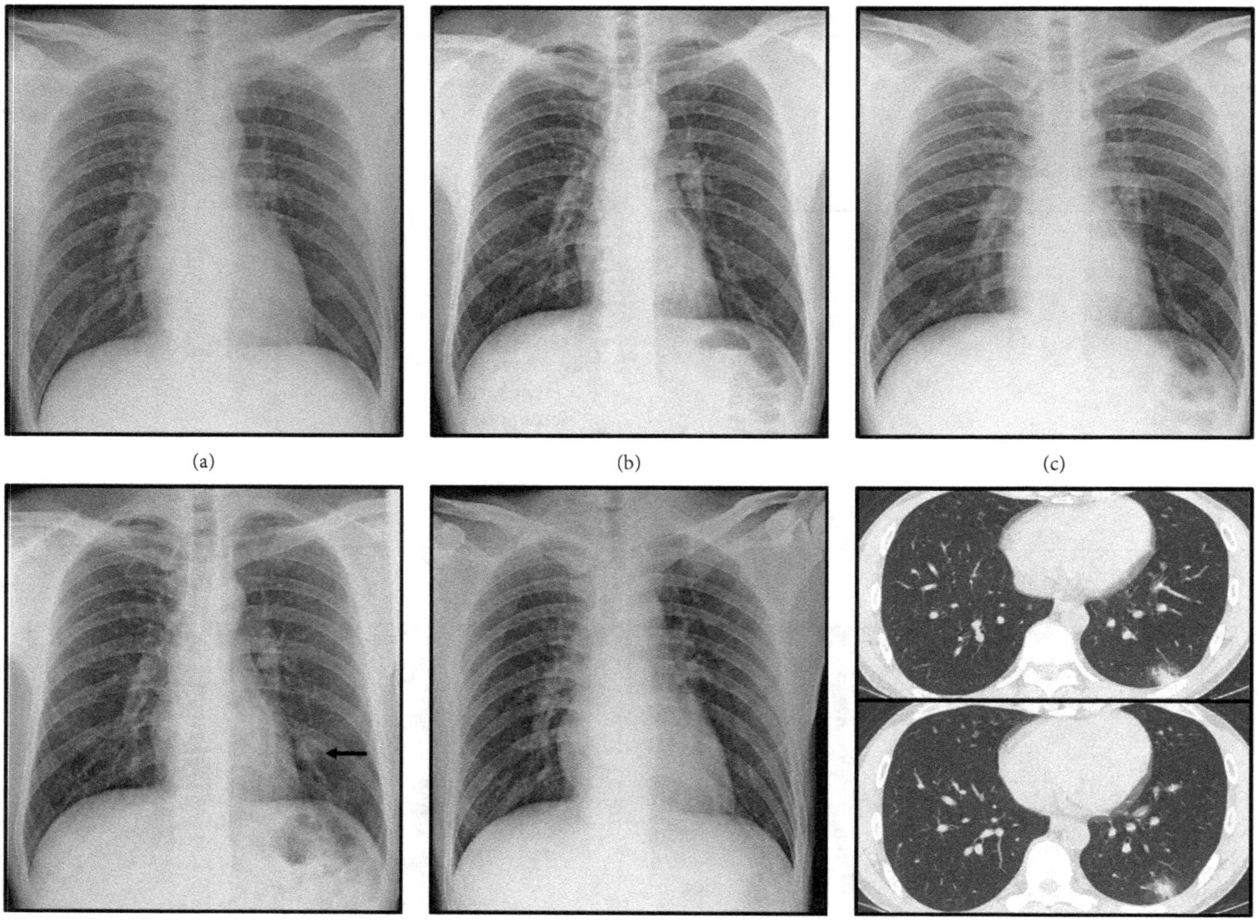

(a) (b) (c)

(d) (e) (f)

Figure 2: Images in a 37-year-old male patient with acute myeloid leukemia whose serum galactomannan test was positive. (a) Baseline chest film shows no opacity. (b) Chest film on first day of febrile neutropenia (ANC = 11 μL) shows no opacity. (c) Chest film on third day of febrile neutropenia (ANC = 17 μL) still shows no opacity. (d) Chest film on fourth day of febrile neutropenia (ANC = 0 μL) shows new opacity at left lower lung (arrow). (e) Chest film on seventh day of febrile neutropenia (ANC = 2511 μL) shows improvement of lower lung opacity. (f) Axial CT chest on the fourth day of febrile neutropenia reveals a nodular-like consolidation with surrounding ground-glass attenuation, representing a CT halo sign. This case was evaluated as true-positive chest radiograph and CT chest.

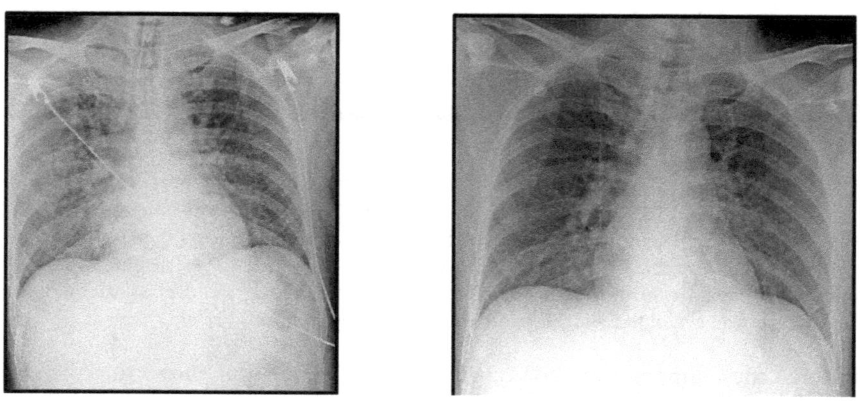

(a) (b)

Figure 3: Continued.

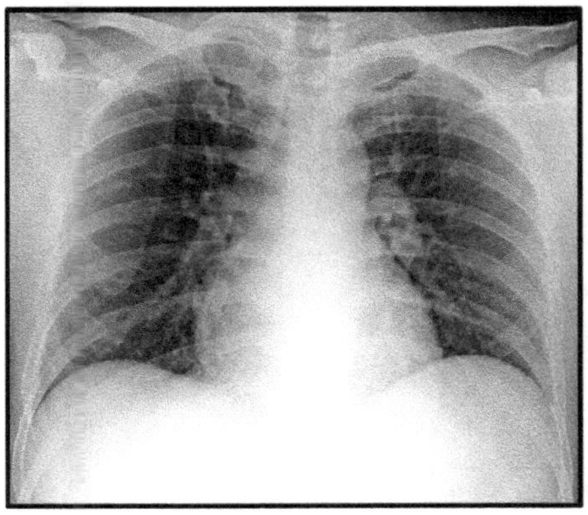

(c)

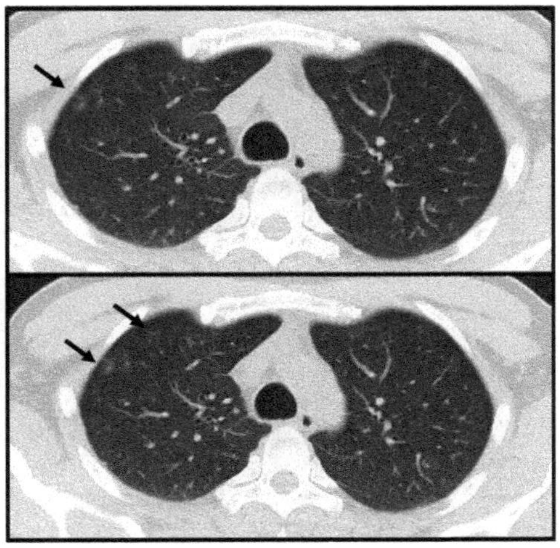

(d)

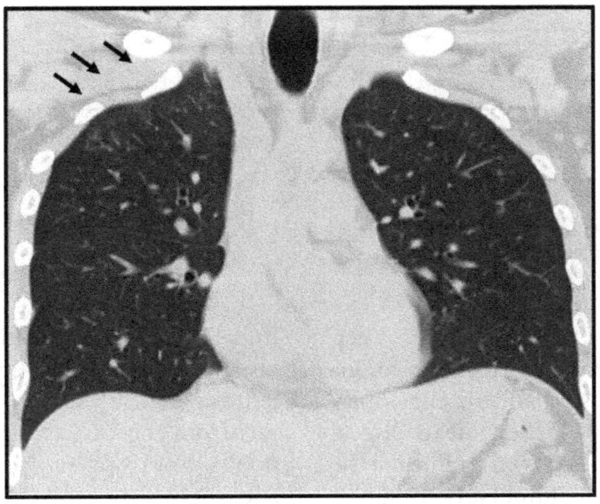

(e)

FIGURE 3: Images in a 35-year-old male with acute myeloid leukemia who had positive chest symptoms and serum galactomannan test. (A) Baseline chest film shows opacities at right upper and right lower lungs. (B) Chest film on second day of febrile neutropenia (ANC = 0 μL) shows improvement of previous opacities with no new opacity. (C) Chest film on fifth day of febrile neutropenia (ANC = 0 μL) shows no abnormal opacity. (D–E) Axial and coronal CT chest on seventh day of febrile neutropenia (ANC = 0 μL) reveals subtle ground-glass attenuation at right upper lobe (arrows). This case was evaluated as false-negative chest radiograph and true-positive CT chest.

TABLE 2: Summary of consensus chest films and CT chest compared to the clinical diagnosis of early pulmonary infection.

	Early pulmonary infection	Clinical positive ($n = 48$)	Clinical negative ($n = 59$)	
Chest film	Radiological active ($n = 39$)	24	15	PPV 61%
	No radiological active ($n = 68$)	24	44	NPV 64%
	Early pulmonary infection	Clinical positive ($n = 11$)	Clinical negative ($n = 15$)	
CT chest	Radiological active ($n = 19$)	10	9	PPV 45.8%
	No radiological active ($n = 2$)	1	6	NPV 100%

PPV, positive predictive value; NPV, negative predictive value.

The overall agreement was substantial for the detection of baseline chest film lesions (K value 0.65). For identifying the presence of a lesion, interobserver agreement was higher when using a single CT chest as compared to serial chest films (K value 0.64 and 0.55). Details of the interobserver agreement are summarized in Table 3.

4. Discussion

Patients with underlying hematologic malignancies who received chemotherapy can develop febrile neutropenia. We found leukemia, lymphoma, and multiple myeloma as underlying hematologic diseases in febrile neutropenic

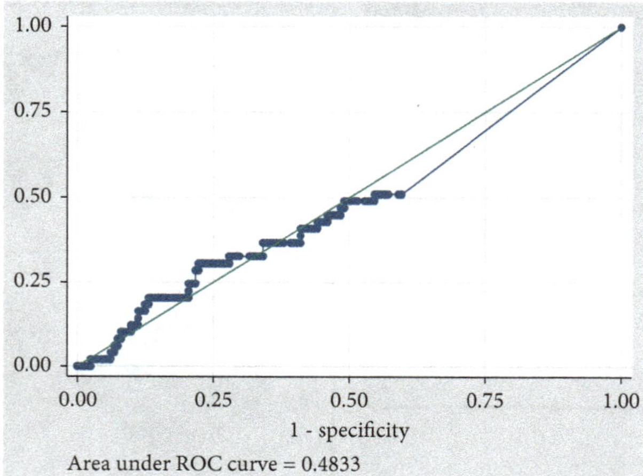

FIGURE 4: Receiver operating characteristic curve comparing the absolute neutrophil count with radiologic active pulmonary infection as predictors of pulmonary infection.

TABLE 3: Interobserver agreement in chest film and CT chest interpretation.

Radiographic interpretation	Observer 1 and 2	Observer 2 and 3	Observer 3 and 1	All
Baseline chest film	0.60	0.66	0.71	0.65
Presence of chest film active pulmonary infection	0.56	0.56	0.55	0.55
Presence of CT chest active pulmonary infection	0.61	0.69	0.62	0.64

patients, which are similar in order as Dimirel et al. [2]. When these patients develop febrile neutropenia, it leads to increased patient risk of infections, especially in the lungs. Compared to priors, our results show a higher rate of clinical pulmonary infection, likely due to patients who confirmed the diagnosis of infection outside the chest without any chest film and were therefore not included in our study population [7, 8]. The radiological active pulmonary infection compared to the clinical diagnosis of early infection in our study shows low sensitivity and moderate specificity. As compared to the study by Gerritsen et al. [9], our study reveals higher sensitivity but lower specificity. These different results may be due to different patient populations and timing of febrile episodes used for chest film interpretation. The false-negative findings are lower than in prior studies but still suggest that negative chest film does not exclude active radiologic pulmonary infection [8, 10]. The type of pulmonary infection can also affect false-negative rates in chest film. Invasive pulmonary mycoses are often not visible on chest film in the early neutropenic setting. CT chest can detect very early stage of invasive pulmonary mycoses and improve the detection rate of pulmonary infiltration [9]. Zaleska-Dorobisz et al. reported a higher sensitivity using low-dose CT chest than single chest film for detection and characterization of pulmonary abnormalities in pediatric patients with neutropenic fever. However, the higher radiation dose for CT is a concern [10]. Our single CT chest in the first seven days of febrile neutropenia shows higher sensitivity and negative predictive value than serial chest films for the detection of early pulmonary infection. Similar results were found in malignant hematological patients who received chemotherapy or underwent hematopoietic stem cell transplant (HSCT) with chest CT and chest film performed on the first day of febrile neutropenia [9]. Other studies show an increased detection rate from chest CT compared to chest film but differ in some points from our study [11–13]. However, there is a lower specificity for early pulmonary infection detection from a single CT chest than serial chest films and a high false-positive rate from the single CT chest in our study. Serial chest films can show changes or stability of the pulmonary opacities, which may improve radiologists' confidence in determining active or not active radiological infection. Conversely, a single CT chest with the presence of specific CT patterns or specific radiologic stigmata may also increase the differentiation between infectious and noninfectious pulmonary disease, as well [12]. A study by Cornetto et al. shows treatment benefit for both normal and abnormal early CT chest after HSCT [14]. However, our study did not examine this point in detail. Another detail that could cause lower than expected specificity is our categorization of nodule/mass as no radiologic active pulmonary infection for the purposes of our study, while in fact, some nodules/mass lesions are infectious processes. Therefore, a single CT chest should be helpful for neutropenic patients with fever of unknown origin.

About the relationship between absolute neutrophil count and chest film suggesting active pulmonary infection by using the ROC curve, we found the absolute neutrophil count is not a significant predictive value for radiologic active pulmonary infection. This result is defined by the low neutrophil count, which limits the inflammatory response in the chest and leads to undetectable pulmonary infiltration evidenced by radiography [7]. Deborah et al. revealed that the utility of chest film in diagnosing infection was low in the absence of respiratory symptoms. The use of serial chest film to evaluate febrile neutropenic patients with respiratory signs or symptoms can be applied [11, 13].

The variability of radiology interpretation assessed by analysis of interobserver agreement shows a similar value as informed by Gerritens et al. for chest film interpretation. The agreement for CT interpretation from our study was slightly higher [9].

There were a few limitations to this study. First, not all first seven days of febrile neutropenia have chest films and not all episodes have a CT chest. Most of the CT chests were requested if there was the presence of clinical or chest film suspicious of pulmonary abnormality. Second, our patient population does not include those with clinical diagnoses confirmed of infection outside the chest who have no chest film. Third, laboratory data related to respiratory tract infection were not reported in all patients with suspected pulmonary infection due to the retrospective nature of the study.

In conclusion, serial chest film for early radiologic diagnosis of pulmonary infection within the first seven days of febrile neutropenia has lower sensitivity with higher specificity as compared to a single CT chest. However, there is a higher false-positive rate for CT chest in determining early pulmonary infection. The number of absolute neutrophil count cannot predict the presence of radiologic active pulmonary infection from chest film. As a result, we could apply the use of serial chest films for early febrile neutropenia workup in patients with respiratory signs and symptoms, while CT chest will be more suitable when neutropenic patients have fever of unknown origin. Another advantage of serial chest film over CT chest is for the pediatric population, for which radiation dose is concern, and in low immune patients who need isolation. [15].

Acknowledgments

The authors gratefully thank Assistant Professor Dr. Kittipong Kongsomboon for his statistic suggestions. This study was supported by a research grant from the Faculty of Medicine, Srinakharinwirot University, to W. Burivong (Grant No. SWUEC/E-367/2560).

References

[1] M. Aoun, "Febrile Neutropenia," 2017, http://www.antimicrobe.org/e49.asp.

[2] A. Demirel, F. Tabak, M. C. Ar et al., "Secondary infections in febrile neutropenia in hematological malignancies: more than another febrile neutropenic episode," *Turkish Journal of Hematology*, vol. 32, no. 3, pp. 243–250, 2015.

[3] P. Niparuck, "Febrile neutropenia," 2017, https://med.mahidol.ac.th/med/sites/default/files/public/pdf/medicinebook1/Febrile%20neutropenia.pdf.

[4] R. C. Lea, E. Marchiori, R. Rodrigues, A. S. Souza, E. L. Gasparetto, and D. L. Escuissato, "Computed tomography in the assessment of angioinvasive pulmonary aspergillosis in patients with acute leukemia," *Radiologia Brasileira*, vol. 39, no. 5, pp. 327–331, 2006.

[5] B. Sanchez, M. Marti, S. M. Perez et al., Febrile Neutropenia: An Emergency for the Radiologist. Electronic Presentation Online System (EPOS), 2019, https://posterng.netkey.at/esr/viewing/index.php?module=viewing_poster&task=&pi=116931.

[6] M. Kang, D. Deoghuria, S. Varma, D. Gupta, A. Bhatia, and N. Khandelwal, "Role of HRCT in detection and characterization of pulmonary abnormalities in patients with febrile neutropenia," *Lung India*, vol. 30, no. 2, pp. 124–130, 2013.

[7] S. E. Evans and D. E. Ost, "Pneumonia in the neutropenic cancer patient," *Current Opinion in Pulmonary Medicine*, vol. 21, no. 3, pp. 260–271, 2015.

[8] G. R. Donowitz, C. Harman, T. Pope, and F. M. Stewart, "The role of the chest roentgenogram in febrile neutropenic patients," *Archives of Internal Medicine*, vol. 151, no. 4, pp. 701–704, 1991.

[9] M. G. Gerritsen, M. J. Willemink, E. Pompe et al., "Improving early diagnosis of pulmonary infections in patients with febrile neutropenia using low-dose chest computed tomography," *PLoS One*, vol. 12, no. 2, pp. 1–13, Article ID e0172256, 2017.

[10] U. Zaleska-Dorobisz, C. Olchowy, M. Łasecki et al., "Low-dose computed tomography in assessment of pulmonary abnormalities in children with febrile neutropenia suffering from malignant diseases," *Advances in Clinical and Experimental Medicine*, vol. 26, no. 4, pp. 695–701, 2017.

[11] D. S. Yolin-Raley, I. Dagogo-Jack, H. B. Niell et al., "The utility of routine chest radiography in the initial evaluation of adult patients with febrile neutropenia patients undergoing HSCT," *Journal of the National Comprehensive Cancer Network*, vol. 13, no. 2, pp. 184–189, 2015.

[12] D. Patsios, N. Maimon, T. Chung et al., "Chest low-dose computed tomography in neutropenic acute myeloid leukaemia patients," *Respiratory Medicine*, vol. 104, no. 4, pp. 600–605, 2010.

[13] C. P. Heussel, H.-U. Kauczor, G. E. Heussel et al., "Pneumonia in febrile neutropenic patients and in bone marrow and blood stem-cell transplant recipients: use of high-resolution computed tomography," *Journal of Clinical Oncology*, vol. 17, no. 3, p. 796, 1999.

[14] M. A. Cornetto, S. Chevret, S. Abbes et al., "Early lung computed tomography scan after allogeneic hematopoietic stem cell transplantation," *Biology of Blood and Marrow Transplantation*, vol. 22, no. 8, pp. 1511–1516, 2016.

[15] C. Olchowy, K. Kałwak, and U. Zaleska-Dorobisz, "Early lung computed tomography scan after allogeneic hematopoietic stem cell transplantation," *Biology of Blood and Marrow Transplantation*, vol. 22, no. 10, pp. 1908-1909, 2016.

5

From Radiological Manifestations to Pulmonary Pathogenesis of COVID-19: A Bench to Bedside Review

Amin Saburi,[1] U. Joseph Schoepf,[2] Kyle A. Ulversoy,[3] Ramezan Jafari,[1] Fatemeh Eghbal,[4] and Mostafa Ghanei[1]

[1]*Chemical Injuries Research Center, Systems Biology & Poisonings Institute, Baqiyatallah University of Medical Sciences, Tehran, Iran*
[2]*Department of Radiology and Radiological Science, Medical University of South Carolina, Charleston, SC, USA*
[3]*Augusta University/University of Georgia Medical Partnership, Athens, GA, USA*
[4]*Birjand University of Medical Sciences, Birjand, Iran*

Correspondence should be addressed to Amin Saburi; aminsaburi@yahoo.com

Academic Editor: Lorenzo Faggioni

In this review, we aim to assess previous radiologic studies in COVID-19 and suggest a pulmonary pathogenesis based on radiologic findings. Although radiologic features are not specific and there is heterogeneity in symptoms and radiologic and clinical manifestation, we suggest that the dominant pattern of computed tomography is consistent with limited pneumonia, followed by interstitial pneumonitis and organizing pneumonia.

1. Introduction

There are many studies on the radiologic manifestations of pulmonary involvement of novel coronavirus disease (named COVID-19 by the WHO) first reported from Wuhan, China. High-resolution computed tomography (HRCT) of the lung and chest X-ray are the most frequent and valuable studies to be used, but nuclear medicine scans and catheter angiography have also been used [1].

There are many HRCT findings frequently reported, including ground-glass opacity (GGO), interseptal thickening with or without the nodular pattern, subpleural sparing, and prominent vasculature. However, extensive tiny lung nodules, lymphadenopathy, pleural effusion, and pleural involvement are less frequently reported. If the previously stated findings are seen, bacterial or non-COVID-19 infections should also be kept in mind [2–4].

Almost all previous studies are focused on clinical and radiological manifestations of COVID-19, but main pulmonary pathology that explains these manifestations is less extensively discussed. It is possible to find or at least infer main pathologies based on radiologic manifestations as previously reported for similar diseases such as severe acute respiratory syndrome (SARS-CoV) or Middle East respiratory syndrome (MERS) [5].

In this review, we aim to assess previous radiologic studies on COVID-19 and to suggest pulmonary pathogenetic pathways based on radiologic findings.

2. Review of Clinical Findings

There are many reports about clinical features and epidemiologic characteristics of patients affected with COVID-19. These findings are sometimes contradictory, which may be due to population heterogeneity, differences in sample size, and selection bias. Likewise, racial and environmental characteristics in the published studies can show different results.

In one of the largest studies published in the New England Journal of Medicine, the following findings were obtained: of 1099 enrolled subjects, more than 41% were female and the mean incubation time was 4 days, less than 1% were under 15 years old (pediatric cases), and the two most frequent symptoms on admission were fever and cough. About 15% of admitted cases had severe symptoms. They reported that "the presence of any coexisting illness was more common among patients with severe disease than among those with nonsevere disease (38.7% vs. 21%)." The median age of admitted cases was 47 (35–58) y/o [6].

These findings are similar to other studies such as PingZhengMo et al.'s study who reported 155 cases with COVID-19 pneumonia. They described that the median age was 54 y/o and "Fever (81.3%), fatigue (73.2%), cough (62.6%), and myalgia/arthralgia (61.0%) were the most common symptoms" [7]. Acute respiratory distress syndrome (ARDS) was the most common indication for ICU admission in COVID-19 cases and is also the major etiology of death [8]. Age > 50 years, dyspnea, comorbidities, chest pain, cough, expectoration, increased serum inflammatory factors, and decreased lymphocytes count, specially obesity (visceral fat) were reported as risk factors for the critical phase [9, 10]. Moreover, milder and less prominent clinical symptoms were reported in pediatric patients, with a recovery period of 1-2 weeks, which is shorter than in adult cases [11].

3. Review of Radiologic Findings

In a systematic review on imaging findings of 919 patients (after excluding duplicated cases), Salehi et al. described that "Known features of COVID-19 on initial CT include bilateral multilobar ground-glass opacification (GGO) with a peripheral or posterior distribution, mainly in the lower lobes and less frequently within the right middle lobe" [8]. Likewise, bilateral GGO or patchy opacity as high as 90% was reported in these cases [12] (Figures 1(a) and 1(b)).

Although atypical imaging features such as consolidative opacities superimposed on GGO, septal thickening, bronchiectasis, pleural thickening, and subpleural involvement are less common than subpleural GGO, they are not uncommon [13]. As reported in Zhao et al.' study, more than 50% of patients show the following findings: mixed GGO and consolidation (64.4%), vascular enlargement within lesions (71.3%), and traction bronchiectasis (52.5%) [3].

One hundred and forty-nine RT-PCR confirmed positive patients in a retrospective study were included; 17 patients had normal CT on admission, and 12 cases (8%) had negative CT findings even 10 days later [14].

On the other hand, pleural effusion, pericardial effusion, lymphadenopathy, cavitation, CT halo sign, and pneumothorax were very rarely reported. The increasing size and number of GGO transforming to multifocal consolidative opacities, septal thickening (with or without the nodular pattern), and the development of a crazy-paving pattern are important markers of progression. Also, in contrast, gradual resolution of consolidative opacities and decrease in the number of lesions and involved lobes are useful as improvement markers for response to the treatment [8].

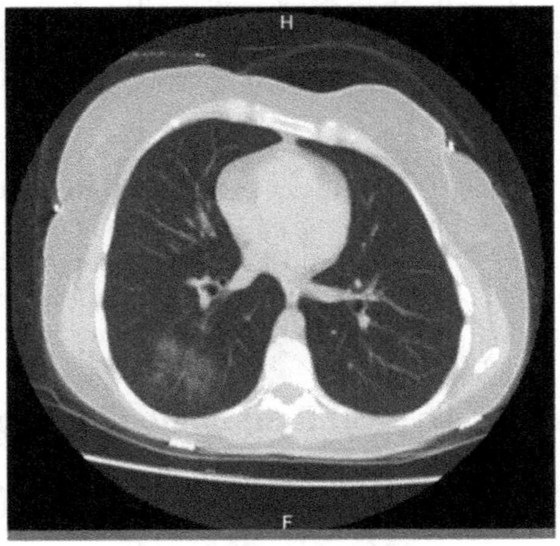

(a)

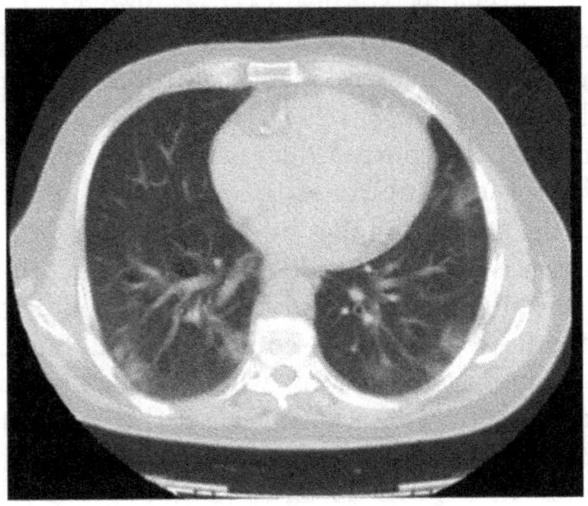

(b)

FIGURE 1: (a) Ground-glass opacities in two different cases of COVID-19 in an early stage. (b) Ground-glass opacities in two different cases of COVID-19 in an early stage.

Several radiologic signs frequently reported in bacterial pneumonia are reported in some studies [15]. For example, Zhou et al. reported vacuolar sign (45.2%), microvascular dilation sign (56.5%), fibrotic streaks (33.9%), a subpleural line (53.2%), air bronchogram (72.6%), pleural thickening (48.4%), and a pleural retraction sign (56.5%) [16].

Although patchy, peripheral, and multifocal GGO opacities are frequently reported as the main COVID-19 imaging findings, some studies have reported other findings and even normal CT scans in these patients. For example, Chung et al. distinguished that 14% of cases have no GGO or consolidation and had entirely normal chest CT examinations at presentation [17]. No CT or radiographic abnormality was found in about 18% of cases with nonsevere disease and 2.9% of cases with severe disease in Guan's study. Wu's study found that 31.25% of cases had a normal CT of both lungs, and finally, 23% of cases had a normal bilateral chest CT in the study by Xu et al. [6, 18, 19].

It is not always the case that all patients first develop GGO and later develop consolidation or other imaging features, since recently published studies report that some atypical manifestations can be seen in certain cases (e.g., elderly or pediatric cases). These unusual presentations will be discussed in the following section. The distribution of affected lobes is different in previous studies, but the posterior aspect of the lower lobes is often initially involved [15, 20].

Finally, recent insights provided by Ye et al. describe that ground-glass opacities, consolidation, a reticular pattern, and a crazy-paving pattern are typical CT manifestations of COVID-19, and in contrast, airway changes, pleural changes, fibrosis, and nodules are atypical CT manifestations [21] (Figure 2).

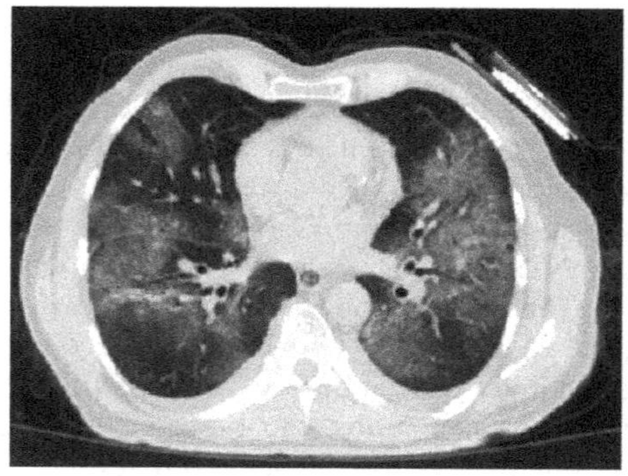

Figure 2: GGO with interlobular septal thickening in a case of COVID-19 at the subacute phase (note to pleural effusion).

4. Review of Atypical Radiologic Findings

In spite of GGOs and patchy opacities as usual findings of COVID-19 pneumonia in unenhanced chest CT, Lei et al. reported the absence of sparing of the subpleural regions in contrast to previous studies [22]. Moreover, Lin et al. published a case report of an asymptomatic case of COVID-19 pneumonia with bilateral pleural effusions, which was not previously reported [23].

Albarello et al. reported 2 cases with moderate to severe progression of lung infiltrates that included, in addition to pleural effusions, a tubular and enlarged appearance of pulmonary vessels with a sudden caliber reduction, mainly found in the dichotomic tracts, where the center of a new insurgent pulmonary lesion could be seen. Furthermore, mediastinal lymphadenopathy with short-axis oval nodes was also reported in a deteriorated case. They suggested these findings as early alert radiological signs to predict initial lung deterioration in COVID-19 cases [24].

Another study stated that, in addition to peripheral lower lobe GGOs as a routine CT manifestation, vascular thickening with a pleural parallel sign (the most valuable characteristic), intralobular septal thickening, pleural effusion, pneumatocele, pneumothorax, and less commonly halo/reversed halo sign were also seen in these cases [25, 26].

4.1. Radiologist Performance in Diagnosis of COVID-19. In addition to recognizing and diagnosing imaging findings in these patients, the radiologist should assist the clinicians in the following areas: diagnosis of underlying pulmonary abnormalities, evaluation of the severity and extent of the disease regarding architectural distortion, traction bronchiectasis, CT involvement score [3], interpretation of positive chest CT findings in some cases with negative results of PCR, especially during the first five days [27], avoiding unnecessary CT scans in patients with low probability for COVID-19 as a screening modality, distinguish unusual CT presentations from other causes according to clinical and laboratory findings, severity score determination of pulmonary involvement to distinguish critical cases from others [15], diagnosis of the complications of COVID-19, and protect radiology departments and its personnel from infections.

Severity score and classification of the disease should be performed, although its effectiveness and usefulness are not sufficiently studied. Chung et al. used a lung severity score in COVID-19 cases according to the following: "Each of the five lung lobes was assessed for degree of involvement and classified as none (0%), minimal (1%–25%), mild (26%–50%), moderate (51%–75%), or severe (76%–100%). No involvement corresponded to a lobe score of 0, minimal involvement to a lobe score of 1, mild involvement to a lobe score of 2, moderate involvement to a lobe score of 3, and severe involvement to a lobe score of 4. An overall lung total severity score was reached by summing the five lobe scores (range of possible scores, 0–20)" [17].

Based on previous evaluations, it can be concluded that patients with the following findings are more likely to progress to severe stages: architectural distortion, traction bronchiectasis, and a higher CT involvement score [3]. Also, round cystic changes might be associated with the resolving process of consolidation or could be explained by the infection causing alveolar wall damage, leading to pneumatoceles [28].

Using serial CT studies to determinate outcome and prognosis, radiologists can contribute to prognostication. Shi et al. described an evolution of three pattern types of CT findings, in which type 2 has a poor prognosis. If CT findings showed initial progression to a peak level, followed by radiographic improvement, the pattern type is type 1. A pattern of radiographic improvement across several CT scans is categorized as type 3, and progressive radiographic deterioration despite medical treatment was categorized as type 2 with poor prognosis [28].

4.2. Radiologic Findings in Time Course and Follow-Up. CT findings typically peak within 10 days of the onset of symptoms and subsequently decrease from two to five weeks, depending on the patient's clinical condition and underlying disorders. Almost always in usual cases, there are GGOs at early evaluation and then an increase in the size and number of GGOs. This progression of GGOs to multifocal consolidation, crazy-paving pattern formation, and septal thickening continues until the 10–14th day of diseases (peak of radiologic findings). Then, there is gradual resolution of consolidative opacities and a decrease in the number of involved lobes and lesions seen by 4-5 weeks.

Salehi et al. described that septal thickening, pleural thickening, bronchiectasis (usually at the later phase), pleural effusion, lymphadenopathy, pericardial effusion, CT halo sign, cavitation, and pneumothorax are seen during the progressive and complicating phase [8].

CT studies of 63 cases, with a mean age of about 50 years, show that the mean number of affected lobes on admission was more than 3 lobes. Progression from single GGO to enlarged and consolidated opacities, enlarged fibrous stripe, and increased and enlarged solid nodules were also described [29].

Bernheim et al. reviewed chest CT findings of 121 symptomatic COVID-19 cases based on the time between symptom onset and the initial CT scan. They categorized cases into 3 groups, including early (0–2 days), intermediate (3–5 days), and late (6–12 days). A normal CT was found in more than half of the cases in the early stage. With a longer time after the onset of symptoms, CT findings were more frequent, including consolidation, bilateral and peripheral diseases, greater total lung involvement, linear opacities, a crazy-paving pattern, and the reverse halo sign. Bilateral lung involvement was observed in 28% of patients in the early phase, 76% of patients in the intermediate phase, and 88% of patients in the late phase [30].

Although the development of bilateral GGOs and consolidation is frequently reported, solitary and rounded peripheral ground-glass lesions appearing 3 days after the follow-up was also reported [17].

Pan et al. postulated that based on the day of symptom onset, 4 stages of lung CT could be defined as follows: stage 1 (0–4 days), ground-glass opacities (GGO) in 75% of patients; stage 2 (5-8 days), increased the crazy-paving pattern in 53%; stage 3 (9–13 days), consolidation in 91%; and stage 4 (≥ 14 days), gradual resolution of consolidation in 75% of patients without the crazy-paving pattern [31]. Peak lung involvement was approximately on the 10th day with a mean hospitalized period of 17 days (Figure 3). The cohort excluded ARDS and hypoxemic cases, and their results are generalizable for cases with mild and moderate severity. More than the extension and distribution of GGO, it appears that the densities of GGO indicate disease progression [32]. Clinically, in addition to the densities of GGO seen on CT, monitoring of hypoxemia is a valuable indicator of severity [33].

The following findings were obtained in a study of 81 cases who were categorized based on symptom onset and the first CT scan. In group 1 (subclinical patients; scans done before symptom onset), the predominant pattern was unilateral and multifocal GGO. Lesions quickly evolved to bilateral, diffuse GGO in group 2 (scans done ≤ 1 week after symptom onset). Thereafter, the prevalence of ground-glass opacities continued to decrease in group 3 (1 to 2 weeks) and group 4 (2 to 3 weeks), and consolidation and mixed patterns became more frequent in these aforementioned groups [28].

GGOs opacities change to several subtypes during follow-up. Wang et al. demonstrated that at first, on illness days 6–11, pure GGO was the most common subtype of GGO, with rates of up to 71%, followed by GGO with irregular linear opacity (28%). The most common pattern was mixed GGO in 38% of cases until days 12–17. About 94% of cases discharged had residual manifestations on final CT scans, with GGO in 60% of cases and pure GGO in up to 74% of cases being the most common pattern and subtype [34].

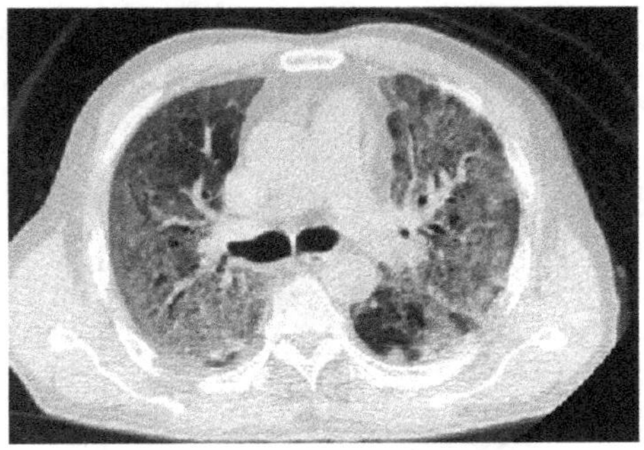

FIGURE 3: Diffuse consolidation in a case at the peak phase resembling ARDS.

In spite of all the above featured reports, it should be noted that normal CT scan findings have been frequently reported in these patients so that, in a study on 149 RT-PCR confirmed positive patients, 17 (11%) patients had normal CT on admission and 12 (8%) had negative findings even 10 days later [14].

Early CT Manifestations of 108 patients with COVID-19 pneumonia are "patchy GGO with or without consolidation involving multiple lobes, mainly in the peripheral zone, accompanied by halo sign, vascular thickening, the crazy-paving pattern, or air bronchogram sign," which is partially different from other reports that demonstrated that the above findings, except for patchy GGOs, can be seen in the early stages and the remainder in the more advanced stages [35]. The difference can be due to inclusion criteria of cases (only mild COVID-19 pneumonia is included), and there is no definite time of symptom onset and the first CT scan obtained.

CT studies of 63 confirmed patients show that 85% of patients had progressed in their disease with the following findings: increasing single GGO, enlarged and consolidated opacities, enlarging fibrous stripe, and increasing and enlarging solid nodules [29].

Zhu et al. reported CT scan findings of 50 cases. On first imaging and in the early phase, GGOs were found in 92.3% of cases, patchy consolidation and subconsolidation in 36.5%, and air bronchogram in 32.7% of cases. During hospitalization, the fibrous stripe shadow became the most usual imaging findings (75.0% within 6–9 days after admission), and the lesions distinctly resolved in 76% of cases on days 10–14 of admission [36].

The schematic review of the time course of COVID-19 CT findings is illustrated in Figure 4.

4.3. Radiologic Findings in Unusual Cases. The radiologic findings reported in the preceding sections are mainly those most commonly observed, while different radiological findings have been reported in patients with specific conditions. For example, multiple lobe involvement is more commonly reported in the elderly [37]. On the other hand, Zhu et al. reported that the ratio of central and gradient distribution of GGOs, thickening of interlobular septum,

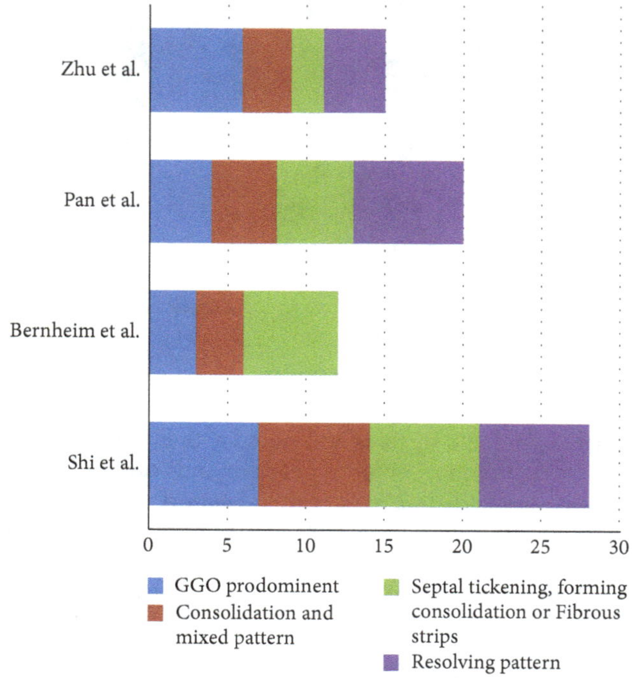

Figure 4: Comparison of CT findings in four studies with time course follow-up.

and rounded morphology were higher in cases with heart failure rather than usual cases. The ratio of central and gradient distribution of the enlargement of small pulmonary veins was also higher in heart failure cases. As expected, this enlargement disappeared after the administration of anti-heart failure medication [38].

COVID-19 has also been reported in pregnant patients with a radiologic profile similar to that of other patients [27]. However, differences have also been reported. Lie et al. demonstrated that GGO and reticulation were less common in the pregnant groups (6% and 5%) versus that of non-pregnant adults (18%). Therewith, mixed consolidation and complete consolidation were more common in pregnant groups (more than 40%) compared with 28%of the non-pregnant adults [39].

4.4. Radiologic Findings in Children vs. Adults. The disease is less symptomatic in children and is less severe, but the radiological findings reported in the pediatric age group are relatively similar to those of adults [40]. However, there are slight differences [39].

After assessment of chest CTs of 20 pediatrics cases of COVID-19, Xie et al. reported consolidation with surrounding halo sign (50%), GGOs (60%), fine mesh shadow (20%), and tiny nodules (15%), and 20% cases showed no abnormality (Figure 5). Consolidation with surrounding halo signs (suggesting underlying coinfection) was common in children with COVID-19 and unlikely to be present in adults [27]. In contrast to adults cases, pleural effusion and a "white lung-like" change is also reported in as much as 10% cases [41].

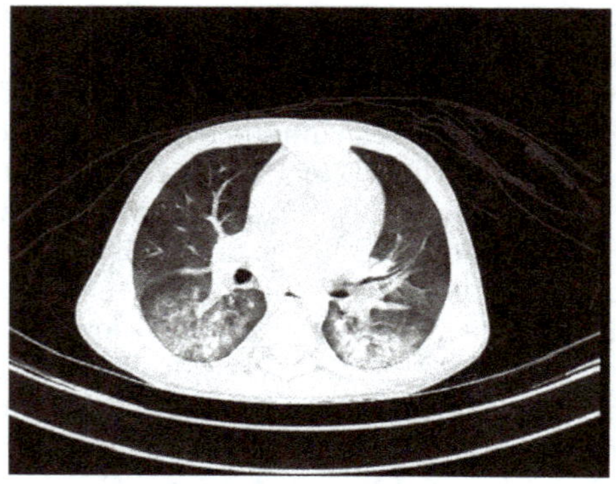

Figure 5: A 9-year-old case with the proven COVID-19 PCR test and bilateral lower lobes GGO.

Therefore, in children with suspected symptoms and clinical history, mild and sometimes unusual CT findings should be considered.

4.5. Radiologic Findings and Correlated Clinical/Paraclinical Findings. We et al. showed that a "pulmonary inflammation index (PII)" was positively correlated with the lymphocyte count, monocyte count, procalcitonin level, CRP (C-reactive protein), days of illness onset, and body temperature. These laboratory markers have been previously reported as a prognostic factor of COVID-19 in some studies. The PII, which Wu et al. used, is according to the guideline of Chongqing Radiologist Association of China and is based on distribution and severity of involved lung segments. In this scoring system, each involved lung segment is scored (with a max score of 20, which means all lobes are involved). If a lesion occupies more than 50% of a lung segment, it receives a score of 1, and if the lesion occupies less than 50%, it receives a score of 0 [42]. This scoring system can be used by the radiologist as a predictive factor of symptomatic cases, although further studies are needed to determine its value as an indicator of prognosis.

Some laboratory factors were reported to correlate with radiologic findings in these cases. The CRP, erythrocyte sedimentation rate (ESR), and lactate dehydrogenase (LDH) had a significant positive correlation with the severity of pneumonia in the first CT, and higher temperature and the severity of opacification in the first CT were considerably correlated with the progression of opacification on the follow-up CT [43]. The sensitivity of CRP, ESR, and decreased WBC was reported as high as 100%, 67%, and 80% of COVID-19 cases [16].

Reactivated cases with different laboratory findings and similar radiologic findings are reported more often than usual laboratory findings of COVID-19 cases; Ye et al. reported 5 cases of COVID-19 reactivation with typical signs of a viral infection on CT scan, but one case had progressive lymphopenia and progressive neutrophilia, and all of them had normal aminotransferase levels [44]. Just as there is a significant difference between imaging findings of young/middle age patients and the elderly, there are also different findings in the laboratory values. Liu et al. described that "The proportion of lymphocytes in the elderly group was significantly lower than that in the young and middle-aged groups, and the CRP was significantly higher in the young group" [37].

The RT-PCR false negative rate is considerable in COVID-19 and has been reported to be up to 50%. In cases with highly suspicious history of exposure and clinical and laboratory findings, chest CT was recommended. Likewise, Ai et al. stated that "the sensitivity of chest CT in suggesting COVID-19 was 97% based on positive RT-PCR results. By analysis of serial RT-PCR assays and CT scans, the mean interval time between the initial negative to positive RT-PCR results was more than 5 days." In the follow-up chest CT scans, 42% of patients showed improvement before the RT-PCR results returned as negative [45].

Besides RT-PCR, other laboratory data versus CT findings have shown acceptable sensitivity. Xu et al. reported 100% negative chest CTs in mild cases of COVID-19 with more than 50% of cases having increased CRP and 28% of cases showing changes in the WBC count [46].

In addition to the CT severity index as a predicting factor of deterioration, some laboratory findings, which include higher WBC and PMN counts, higher levels of D-dimer, creatine kinase, and creatine, are different between patients admitted to the ICU compared to those who were not admitted. All cases in both groups, however, showed bilateral lung involvement in chest CT scans. The median time from symptom onset to admission to the ICU was 10 days [47].

In addition to using chest CT to distinguish COVID-19 cases from non-COVID-19 cases, abnormal laboratory tests in AST, ALT, γ-GT, LDH, and α-HBDH can also be useful [27].

Laboratory findings will be helpful in pediatric cases, which have less obvious clinical symptoms and radiological findings when compared to adult cases. In pediatric cases, consolidation with surrounding halo signs and increased procalciton were more common when compared to adults, although pediatric patients are more susceptible to coinfection compared to adults [27].

4.6. Radiologic Findings Based on Symptoms and Severity of the Disease. Most studies review the radiologic manifestation of COVID-19 in symptomatic cases, but asymptomatic cases also have a specific radiologic pattern. Knowing this pattern can help diagnose suspicious individuals. Fifty percentage (50%) of asymptomatic carriers with a positive PCR test showed typical CT findings of ground-glass opacity, 20% presented with stripe shadowing in the lungs, and only 29% of cases showed a normal CT study [48]. Of note, many studies report that CT scanning provides positive results sooner than PCR [49, 50].

Similar to the most previous studies, Pan et al. reported that "mild COVID-19 pneumonia mainly starts as small subpleural, unilateral or bilateral GGO in the lower lobes" [31] (Figure 6). These lesions develop into subsequent consolidation and a crazy-paving pattern. The residual GGO and subpleural parenchymal bands appear gradually after two weeks, indicating a decrease in the severity of the disease (Figure 7). This engenders the question whether radiological findings can distinguish mild cases from severe disease in need of intensive care. In other words, what are the findings in computed tomography of severe predictive of intensive care transfer? We will discuss this further.

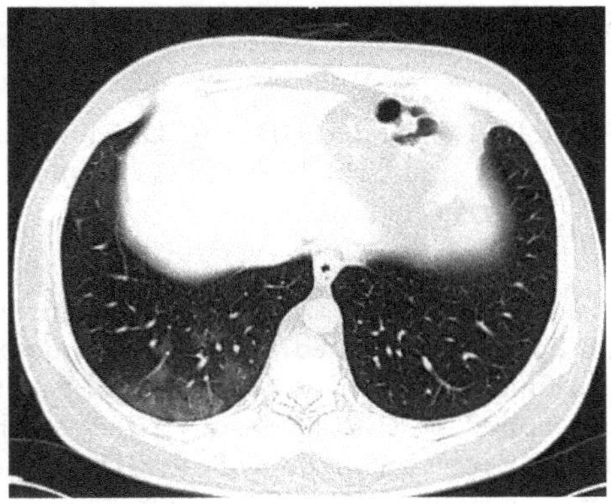

FIGURE 6: Beginning of GGO at the subclinical phase with non-frequent cough.

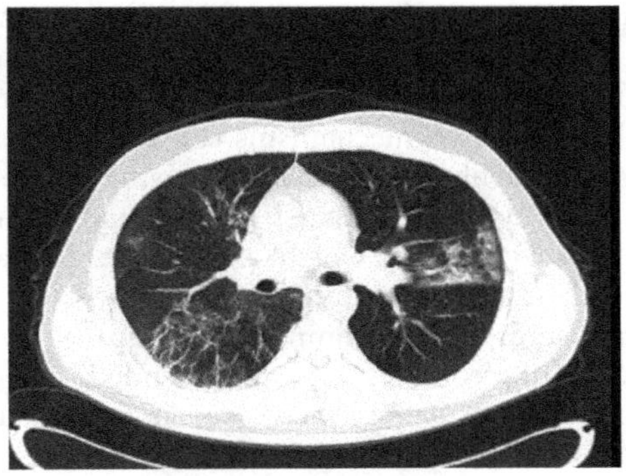

FIGURE 7: A middle age man after treatment and at 12th day of symptoms onset with fibrotic changes.

Chung et al. reported that the cases with the highest lung severity score at HRCT were admitted to the intensive care unit [17].

Data from 101 cases of COVID-19 pneumonia show that patients in the emergency group are more likely to have the following findings: architectural distortion, traction bronchiectasis, and higher CT involvement score [3].

Bilateral patchy consolidation and interstitial abnormalities on CT and CXR are reported to occur twice as frequently as in nonsevere patients [6]. This finding is generally expected in all pulmonary diseases with alveolar infections due to progression of the disease in critical cases.

A report of 62 patients with COVID-19 pneumonia comparing CT findings of the early phase (≤7 days after the onset of symptoms) to the advanced phase (8–14 days after the onset of symptoms) showed considerably increased prevalence of GGO plus a reticular pattern, fibrotic streaks, vacuolar sign, a subpleural transparent line, a subpleural line, bronchus distortion, air bronchogram, and pleural effusion. Meanwhile, GGOs diminished dramatically in advanced stages. These findings show a mixed pattern with both the interstitium and lung parenchyma patterns in the late stage [16].

The incidences of lymph node enlargement, pericardial effusion, and pleural effusion were higher in critical cases [3]. Li et al. described that "consolidation, linear opacities, crazy-paving pattern, bronchial wall thickening, high CT scores, and extrapulmonary lesions were features of severe/critical COVID-19 pneumonia" [9].

In children with critical status, similar chest CT findings were reported, but decreased CD16 + CD56 and Th/Ts, increased CD3, CD4, and CD8, IL-6 and IL-10, and increased IFN-γ were also reported [41].

4.7. Radiologic Findings and Outcomes. Predominantly diffused consolidations associated with ARDS are described as radiological findings in near-death studies of patients who eventually expired. ARDS is characterized as the final pathogenesis in severe pneumonia of COVID-19, and ARDS was reported in as many as 29% of admitted cases [51]. Radiologic findings in these cases are similar to ordinary ARDS [52, 53].

Fibrous tissue formation, which includes increased septal thickness and fibrotic stripes, is seen in improved patients, patients in the recovering phase, and in patients in the progressive stages, confirming significant parenchymal damage [43, 54]. Two mechanisms can explain the pathogenesis of these fibrotic fibers: underlying inflammatory processes and cytokine induced injuries and the external pressure from a ventilator, which expands the alveolar space, filling it with exudative material [55].

Further studies with comparing groups of ventilated versus nonventilated cases are recommended.

Although many patients have partial improvement in symptoms within two weeks, many do not respond to routine treatment and require intensive care. Lei et al. demonstrated that almost 54% of cases are refractory patients with male sex, anorexia, and no fever on admission, which predicted poor outcome [22]. This high rate of refractory patients may be due to the limited capacity of hospitals in epidemic conditions, where only patients with severe illnesses and the majority of COVID-19 pneumonia patients receive outpatient care. Finally, it seems that elderly patients with underlying diseases and severe radiological changes are most likely to fail to respond to treatment and progress to more severe stages [56].

Li et al. explained that "CT findings of consolidation, linear opacities, crazy-paving pattern, bronchial wall thickening, high CT scores, and extrapulmonary lesions were features of severe/critical COVID-19 pneumonia" [9]. These results partially contrast the prognostic radiological findings reported in patients with MERS (pleural effusion and higher CT lung and chest radiographic scores) [57]. This is the difference of being involved in the pathogenesis of the two diseases (MERS vs.SARS-CoV-2).

4.8. Radiologic Findings in COVID-19 and Non-COVID-19. A study on 19 cases with COVID-19 pneumonia and 15 cases with other types of pneumonia demonstrated that clinical symptoms were similar in these two groups. However, "78.95% of COVID-19 and 26.67% of non-NCOVID-19 patients had bilateral involvement, while 17 (89.47%) COVID-19 and 1 (6.67%) non-NCOVID-19 patients had multiple mottling and GGOs on chest CT images" [27]. Another similar study described that GGO (91% vs. 68%), peripheral distribution (80% vs. 57%), vascular thickening (59% vs. 22%), fine reticular opacity (56% vs. 22%), and reverse halo sign (11% vs. 1%) were significantly more common in COVID-19 cases compared to non-COVID-19 cases. Whereas air bronchogram (14% vs. 23%, $p = 0.014$), lymphadenopathy (2.7% vs. 10.2%), pleural thickening (15% vs. 33%), and pleural effusion (4 vs. 39%) are less common in COVID-19 cases [58].

Li and Xia reported similar findings in comparison of pneumonia in COVID-19 versus adenovirus cases, but more studies may be needed since their findings are based on a control group with a small sample size [59].

Predominant patterns of lung abnormalities in SARS cases include GGO (with or without superimposed linear opacities), consolidation, a reticular pattern, and a mixed pattern (consolidation, GGO, and a reticular pattern). During the 1st week, GGO with or without smooth interlobular septal thickening and dense opacities were the outstanding patterns. "GGO with superimposed irregular reticular opacities, a mixed pattern, and reticular opacities were noted from the 2nd week and peaked at or after the 4th week." After the 4th week, more than half of all cases had irregular linear opacities, with or without associated GGOs, and bronchial dilatation [60]. The aforementioned findings are partially similar to COVID-19 findings.

The frequency of chest CT findings in patients with positive results versus patients with negative results (non-COVID-19 pneumonia) was as follows: GGO, 100.0% vs. 90.9%; mixed GGO, 63.6% vs. 72.7%; consolidation, 54.5% vs. 77.3%; the median number of affected lung lobes, 5 vs. 3.5; and affected segments, 15 vs. 9. In patients with positive PCR, the air bronchogram reticular pattern was more frequent, but centrilobular nodules were uncommon [61].

Patchy and GGO opacities in middle and lower lobes with bronchial wall thickening and the nodular pattern have been confirmed to be more common in viral pneumonias. Nodularity is not frequent in these patients, and up to 40% of patients have the nodular pattern [62]. Also, halo appearance and round lung opacities can be seen in up to 33% of the chest CTs of symptomatic patients with COVID-19 [56]. Therefore, the above routine viral presentations inchest CT of COVID-19 are not expected.

5. Review on Biopsy Pathologic Findings

Diffuse alveolar damage as the main histopathologic pattern was found in pneumonia due to MERS. Type 2 pneumocytes and epithelial syncytial cells are the predominant target of viral antigens. Cytopathic effects of MERS contribute to respiratory symptoms. Detachment of type 2 pneumocytes and membrane blebbing (suggestive of apoptosis in favor of pneumocyte damage, in addition to other causes such as immune dysfunction) may be involved in the pathogenesis [63].

An autopsy report noted desquamation of pneumocytes, hyaline membrane formation, and pulmonary edema with hyaline membrane formation, indicating ARDS. "Interstitial mononuclear inflammatory infiltrates dominated by lymphocytes were seen in both lungs." Viral cytopathic-like changes without obvious intranuclear or intracytoplasmic viral inclusions were noted [64].

These findings are not very useful because they were performed in deceased patients that had died in the severe phase of respiratory failure of ARDS. Therefore, it is expected that routine findings of ARDS, like in other non-COVID-19 ARDS, were present.

However, in a unique study, Tian et al. reported pathologic findings of two cases of incidental COVID-19. The two cases underwent biopsy for their malignancy and were later found to have been infected with SARS-CoV-2. Because these specimens were collected in the early phase of the disease, these findings show a more realistic view of the pathological findings than the autopsy samples. They obtained the following findings in both cases: "edema and prominent proteinaceous exudates, vascular congestion, and inflammatory clusters with fibrinoid material and multinucleated giant cells." The findings noted reactive alveolar epithelial hyperplasia in one case and fibroblastic proliferation in another. No prominent neutrophil infiltration or large protein globules were reported. The aforementioned findings are usual in patients with SARS [65]. During this earlier phase, these observations are in favor of early organization and are seen in many acute inflammatory viral/nonviral injuries. Further studies regarding the progressive/intermediated phase are mandatory to assess the immune host response as a therapeutic target.

6. Correlation with Radiology Findings and Pathogenesis

GGO is defined as "hazy increased attenuation of the lung, but with preservation of bronchial and vascular margins, caused by partial filling of air spaces, interstitial thickening, partial collapse of alveoli, normal expiration, or increased capillary blood volume" [66]. Based on CT scans, 4 types of GGO may be recognized: type I as simple ground-glass-like shadow, type II as uneven density, type III as central high density with peripheral burring, and type IV as nodular GGO [67]. GGO lesions present as incomplete filling of the alveolar cavity with fluid or lung interstitial thickening. As expected, in COVID-19 cases, patchy GGO is noted due to alveolar cell injuries and inflammatory processes. However, this inflammation is not limited to pneumocytes, and depending on the immune response and severity of the inflammatory process, interstitial tissue, vessels, bronchioles, and even the pleural layer may be involved.

GGO with prominent vessels has been previously reported for tumorous GGO like bronchoalveolar adenocarcinoma, but many reports of COVID-19 reported these findings frequently, especially in periods of disease progression [68].

Vascular leaking and increased permeability in response to increased cytokines can be seen in early lung injuries (with GGO) and in the myocardial injuries also reported in COVID-19. In the progressive phase of the development of ARDS, "damage of epithelial cells and release of proteases from neutrophils decreases the VEGF level in the alveolar compartment, while serum VEGF is elevated" [69].

Patchy GGO was previously reported in the case of interstitial pneumonia, which is "characterized by a mononuclear inflammatory cellular infiltrate in the alveolar septa and the distal peribronchovascular interstitium. This interstitial inflammatory reaction is secondary to epithelial damage, with thickening in the peribronchial area and interlobular septa. The most common causes are viruses, *M. pneumoniae*, and *P. jirovecii*." Some cases develop into acute necrotic pneumonia, which overlaps with ARDS due to severe injuries of alveolar cells [70]. In the early stages of injury, many laboratory and imaging findings are consistent with an acute infectious pulmonary injury focused on the alveoli; however, the healing process in many of these patients is different than in almost all lung infections. This progressive process is more consistent with organizing pneumonia (OP).

In addition to GGOs in peripheral lower lobes as a routine CT manifestation, vascular thickening with pleural parallel sign (the most valuable characteristic), intralobular septal thickening, pleural effusion, and pneumatocele, and less commonly, halo/reversed halo sign were also seen in these cases (Figure 8). In the later period, it mainly manifested as organizing pneumonia and fibrosis [25]. In the study by Qin et al., 18F-FDG PET/CT was used for COVID-19 patients who had peripheral GGO and/or lung consolidations in more than two pulmonary lobes. "Lung lesions were characterized by a high 18F-FDG uptake, and there was evidence of lymph node involvement. Conversely, disseminated disease was absent, a finding suggesting that COVID-19 has pulmonary tropism." This finding is consistent with the hyperemic situation in this disease [71]. Therefore, assessing how VEGF and other cytokines affect vessel walls based on CT manifestations may be a target of further study.

Furthermore, Huang et al. commented on the role of interleukin- (IL-) 2, IL-7, granulocyte-colony stimulating factor, interferon-γ-inducible protein 10, monocyte chemoattractant protein 1, macrophage inflammatory protein 1-α, and tumor necrosis factor-α in ICU admitted cases of COVID-19 versus non-ICU cases [51]. These mediators have a role in immune system balance in pneumonia. There is an important balance between the inflammatory cytokines and the immunomedulatory cytokines. If either become abnormally elevated, secondary lung injury can occur due to the immune system hyperactivation or the progression of the infection [72]. This dysregulation of the immune system response is more frequent in the elderly, which is the population most at risk of critical stages of COVID-19 [73]. Likewise, the severity of disease in children with the undeveloped acquired immune system is more subtle.

This hyperinflammatory condition may be in line with secondary haemophagocytic lymphohistiocytosis (sHLH), which is most often triggered by viral infections. This syndrome is fulminant, and fatal hypercytokinaemia with multiorgan failure can result, which has been previously reported as one of the possible mechanisms of pathogenesis of the disease. Increased ferritin, decreased platelet counts, elevated procalcitonin, CRP, and ESR in the severe stage of COVID-19 are also consistent with this syndrome, and for this reason, steroids, IVIG, specific cytokine blockade (e.g.,

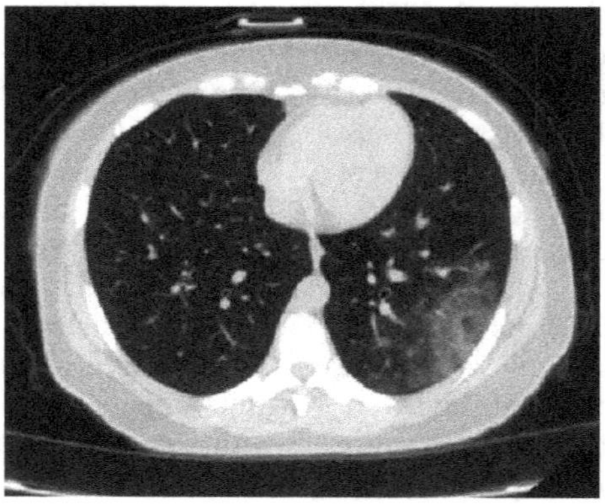

FIGURE 8: Halo sign in a case of PCR proved COVID-19.

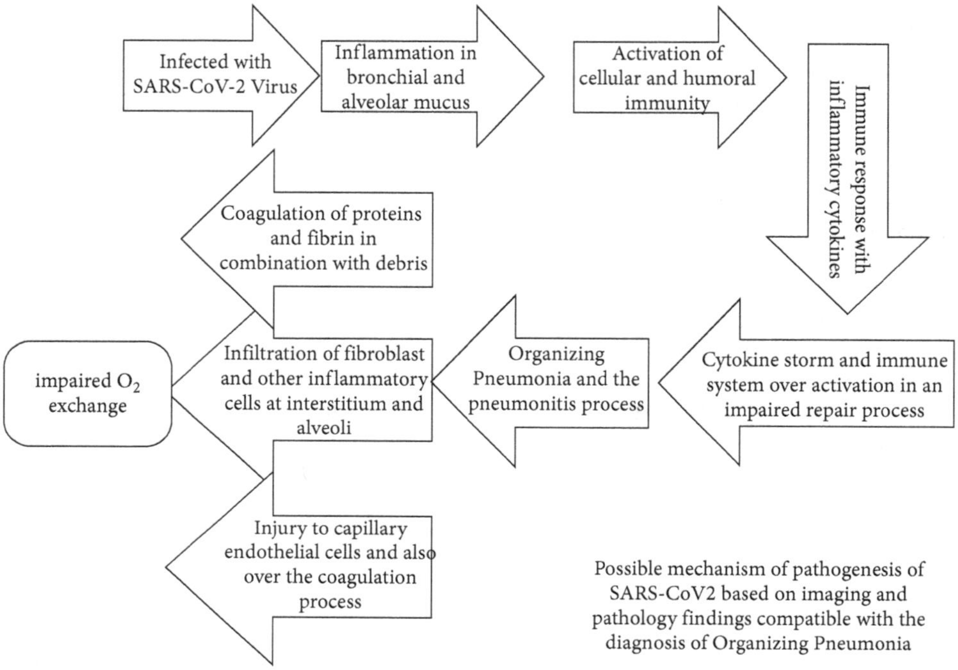

FIGURE 9: Diagram illustrating the main pathophysiological steps of COVID-19-related lung infection and damage (inflammatory and fibrotic).

baricitinib, anakinra, or tacilizumab), and JAK inhibition can be effective for these patients [74, 75].

In addition to GGO, mosaic attenuation patterns are a recognized finding in some viral infections, which was uncommonly reported in COVID-19. Hypoventilation of alveoli distal to bronchiolar obstruction (cicatricial scarring or inflammation of many bronchioles), which leads to secondary vasoconstriction (and, consequently, underperfused lung) is the main mechanism of mosaic attenuation patterns. This is different than the possible mechanism of COVID-19. This mechanism is based on two main pathologies, including vasospasm and narrowing of bronchioles, which seems to be absent in COVID-19. Bronchiolar obstruction and restriction, and therefore bronchiolitis obliterans organizing pneumonia (BOOP), are more common in other viral pneumonia and are not seen in COVID-19. Bronchial wall sparing or minimal involvements in COVID-19 indicate and suggest that treatments targeting small airway will be less effective in these patients [76]. More than OP, acute interstitial pneumonitis (AIP) is another possible pathogenesis of the middle phase of COVID-19. AIP reported as an entity encompasses a wide variety of etiologies that are often unidentified, in which some may be viral in origin [77].

7. Conclusion

In conclusion, our hypothesis states that after the early phase of pneumonia, some cases develop into an inflammatory/fibrotic phase of OP, and cases with underlying disorders develop into the severe form of OP with predominance of the inflammatory/toxic phase (Figure 9) (severe OP). On the other hand, some cases in the early phase present radiologic and laboratory results similar to acute interstitial pneumonitis (mixed condition of alveolar infection and its cytotoxicity and interstitial changes due to host reactive inflammation). We suggest that these cases are more susceptible for progression to the severe phase. The role of the innate immune system may be more prominent in these cases. Development to each phase is dependent on the host's immunologic reaction and response severity. Therefore, some cases had a positive response from corticosteroid and immunomedulatory medications, while it had no effect in other cases. Although imaging is known to be a predictor of outcomes, additional studies on the possible role of radiologic-pathologic correlations in the guidance of therapy may be needed.

Additional Points

We would like to discuss the diagnosis of SARS-COVID-19 and also underlying pulmonary abnormalities; evaluation of the severity and extent of the disease regarding architectural distortion; traction bronchiectasis; CT involvement score; interpretation of positive chest CT findings in some cases with negative results of PCR, especially during the first five days; avoiding unnecessary CT scans in patients with low probability for COVID-19 as a screening modality; distinguish unusual CT presentations from other causes according to clinical and laboratory findings; severity score determination of pulmonary involvement to distinguish critical cases from others; diagnosis of the complications of COVID-19; and the final possible pathogenesis related to the imaging findings.

Acknowledgments

The authors would like to thank Dr. Saadat from Baqiyatallah University of Medical Sciences, Tehran, Iran, for his comments.

References

[1] B. E. Young, S. W. X. Ong, S. Kalimuddin et al., "Epidemiologic features and clinical course of patients infected with SARS-CoV-2 in Singapore," *JAMA*, vol. 323, no. 15, 2020.

[2] J. P. Kanne, B. P. Little, J. H. Chung, B. M. Elicker, and L. H. Ketai, "Essentials for radiologists on COVID-19: an update—radiology scientific expert panel," *Radiology*, vol. 296, no. 2, pp. E113–E114, 2020.

[3] W. Zhao, Z. Zhong, X. Xie, Q. Yu, and J. Liu, "Relation between chest CT findings and clinical conditions of coronavirus disease (COVID-19) pneumonia: a multicenter study," *American Journal of Roentgenology*, vol. 214, no. 5, pp. 1072–1077, 2020.

[4] D. Caruso, M. Zerunian, M. Polici et al., "Chest CT features of COVID-19 in Rome, Italy," *Radiology*, vol. 296, no. 2, pp. E79–E85, 2020.

[5] A. M. Ajlan, R. A. Ahyad, L. G. Jamjoom, A. Alharthy, and T. A. Madani, "Middle East respiratory syndrome coronavirus (MERS-CoV) infection: chest CT findings," *American Journal of Roentgenology*, vol. 203, no. 4, pp. 782–787, 2014.

[6] W.-J. Guan, Z.-Y. Ni, Y. Hu et al., "Clinical characteristics of coronavirus disease 2019 in China," *New England Journal of Medicine*, vol. 382, pp. 1708–1720, 2020.

[7] P. Mo, Y. Xing, Y. Xiao et al., "Clinical characteristics of refractory COVID-19 pneumonia in Wuhan, China," *Clinical Infectious Diseases: An Official Publication of The Infectious Diseases Society of America*, 2020.

[8] S. Salehi, A. Abedi, S. Balakrishnan, and A. Gholamrezanezhad, "Coronavirus disease 2019 (COVID-19): a systematic review of imaging findings in 919 patients," *American Journal of Roentgenology*, vol. 215, no. 1, pp. 87–93, 2020.

[9] K. Li, J. Wu, F. Wu et al., "The clinical and chest CT features associated with severe and critical COVID-19 pneumonia," *Investigative Radiology*, vol. 55, no. 6, pp. 327–331, 2020.

[10] M. Watanabe, D. Caruso, D. Tuccinardi et al., "Visceral fat shows the strongest association with the need of intensive care in patients with COVID-19," *Metabolism*, vol. 111, p. 23, 2020.

[11] H. Hong, Y. Wang, H.-T. Chung, and C.-J. Chen, "Clinical characteristics of novel coronavirus disease 2019 (COVID-19) in newborns, infants and children," *Pediatrics & Neonatology*, vol. 61, no. 2, pp. 131-132, 2019.

[12] J. J. Zhang, X. Dong, Y. Y. Cao et al., "Clinical characteristics of 140 patients infected with SARS-CoV-2 in Wuhan, China," *Allergy*, vol. 75, no. 7, pp. 1730–1741, 2020.

[13] D. Caruso, T. Polidori, G. Guido et al., "Typical and atypical COVID-19 computed tomography findings," *World Journal of Clinical Cases*, vol. 8, no. 15, pp. 3177–3187, 2020.

[14] W. Yang, Q. Cao, L. Qin et al., "Clinical characteristics and imaging manifestations of the 2019 novel coronavirus disease (COVID-19): a multi-center study in Wenzhou city, Zhejiang, China," *Journal of Infection*, vol. 80, no. 4, pp. 388–393, 2020.

[15] Z. Y. Zu, M. D. Jiang, P. P. Xu et al., "Coronavirus disease 2019 (COVID-19): a perspective from China." *Radiology*, vol. 296, no. 2, 2020.

[16] S. Zhou, Y. Wang, T. Zhu, and L. Xia, "CT features of coronavirus disease 2019 (COVID-19) pneumonia in 62 patients in Wuhan, China," *American Journal of Roentgenology*, vol. 214, no. 6, pp. 1287–1294, 2020.

[17] M. Chung, A. Bernheim, X. Mei et al., "CT imaging features of 2019 novel coronavirus (2019-nCoV)," *Radiology*, vol. 295, no. 1, pp. 202–207, 2020.

[18] J. Wu, J. Liu, X. Zhao et al., "Clinical characteristics of imported cases of COVID-19 in Jiangsu province: a multicenter descriptive study," *Clinical Infectious Diseases: An Official Publication of the Infectious Diseases Society of America*, vol. 71, no. 15, pp. 706–712, 2020.

[19] X. Xu, C. Yu, J. Qu et al., "Imaging and clinical features of patients with 2019 novel coronavirus SARS-CoV-2," *European Journal of Nuclear Medicine and Molecular Imaging*, vol. 47, no. 5, pp. 1275–1280, 2020.

[20] M. Q. Zhang, X. H. Wang, Y. L. Chen et al., "Clinical features of 2019 novel coronavirus pneumonia in the early stage from a fever clinic in Beijing," *Zhonghua Jie He He Hu Xi Za Zhi*, vol. 43, no. 0, p. E013, 2020.

[21] Z. Ye, Y. Zhang, Y. Wang, Z. Huang, and B. Song, "Chest CT manifestations of new coronavirus disease 2019 (COVID-19):

a pictorial review," *European Radiology*, vol. 30, no. 10, pp. 4381–4389, 2020.
[22] J. Lei, J. Li, X. Li, and X. Qi, "CT imaging of the 2019 novel coronavirus (2019-nCoV) pneumonia," *Radiology*, vol. 295, no. 1, p. 18, 2020.
[23] C. Lin, Y. Ding, B. Xie et al., "Asymptomatic novel coronavirus pneumonia patient outside Wuhan: the value of CT images in the course of the disease," *Clinical Imaging*, vol. 63, pp. 7–9, 2020.
[24] F. Albarello, E. Pianura, F. Di Stefano et al., "2019-novel Coronavirus severe adult respiratory distress syndrome in two cases in Italy: an uncommon radiological presentation," *International Journal of Infectious Diseases*, vol. 93, pp. 192–197, 2020.
[25] J. Wu, C. L. Feng, X. Y. Xian et al., "Novel coronavirus pneumonia (COVID-19) CT distribution and sign features," *Zhonghua Jie He He Hu Xi Za Zhi*, vol. 43, no. 4, pp. 321–326, 2020.
[26] N. Chen, M. Zhou, X. Dong et al., "Epidemiological and clinical characteristics of 99 cases of 2019 novel coronavirus pneumonia in Wuhan, China: a descriptive study," *The Lancet*, vol. 395, no. 10223, pp. 507–513, 2020.
[27] X. Xie, Z. Zhong, W. Zhao, C. Zheng, F. Wang, and J. Liu, "Chest CT for typical 2019-nCoV pneumonia: relationship to negative RT-PCR testing," *Radiology*, vol. 296, no. 2, 2020.
[28] H. Shi, X. Han, N. Jiang, Y. Cao, O. Alwalid, J. Gu et al., "Radiological findings from 81 patients with COVID-19 pneumonia in Wuhan, China: a descriptive study," *The Lancet Infectious Diseases*, vol. 20, no. 4, pp. 425–434, 2020.
[29] Y. Pan, H. Guan, S. Zhou et al., "Initial CT findings and temporal changes in patients with the novel coronavirus pneumonia (2019-nCoV): a study of 63 patients in Wuhan, China," *European Radiology*, vol. 30, no. 6, pp. 3306–3309, 2020.
[30] A. Bernheim, X. Mei, M. Huang et al., "Chest CT findings in coronavirus disease-19 (COVID-19): relationship to duration of infection," *Radiology*, vol. 295, no. 3, 2020.
[31] F. Pan, T. Ye, P. Sun et al., "Time course of lung changes on chest CT during recovery from 2019 novel coronavirus (COVID-19) pneumonia," *Radiology*, vol. 295, no. 3, 2020.
[32] Y. Fang, H. Zhang, J. Xie et al., "Sensitivity of chest CT for COVID-19: comparison to RT-PCR," *Radiology*, vol. 296, no. 2, 2020.
[33] J. Rello, S. Tejada, C. Userovici, K. Arvaniti, J. Pugin, and G. Waterer, "Coronavirus disease 2019 (COVID-19): a critical care perspective beyond China," *Anaesthesia, Critical Care & Pain Medicine*, vol. 39, no. 2, pp. 167–169, 2020.
[34] Y. Wang, C. Dong, Y. Hu et al., "Temporal changes of CT findings in 90 patients with COVID-19 pneumonia: a longitudinal study," *Radiology*, vol. 296, no. 2, 2020.
[35] R. Han, L. Huang, H. Jiang, J. Dong, H. Peng, and D. Zhang, "Early clinical and CT manifestations of coronavirus disease 2019 (COVID-19) pneumonia," *American Journal of Roentgenology*, vol. 215, no. 2, pp. 338–343, 2020.
[36] Y. Zhu, Y.-L. Liu, Z.-P. Li et al., "Clinical and CT imaging features of 2019 novel coronavirus disease (COVID-19)," *Journal of Infection*, .
[37] K. Liu, Y. Chen, R. Lin, and K. Han, "Clinical feature of COVID-19 in elderly patients: a comparison with young and middle-aged patients," *Journal of Infection [Review]*, vol. 80, no. 6, pp. e14–e18, 2020.
[38] Z. W. Zhu, J. J. Tang, X. P. Chai et al., "Comparison of heart failure and 2019 novel coronavirus pneumonia in chest CT features and clinical characteristics," *Zhonghua Xin Xue Guan Bing Za Zhi*, vol. 48, no. 6, pp. 467–471, 2020.
[39] H. Liu, F. Liu, J. Li, T. Zhang, D. Wang, and W. Lan, "Clinical and CT imaging features of the COVID-19 pneumonia: focus on pregnant women and children," *Journal of Infection*, vol. 80, no. 5, pp. e7–e13, 2020.
[40] W. Li, H. Cui, K. Li, Y. Fang, and S. Li, "Chest computed tomography in children with COVID-19 respiratory infection," *Pediatric Radiology*, vol. 50, no. 6, pp. 796–799, 2020.
[41] D. Sun, H. Li, X.-X. Lu et al., "Clinical features of severe pediatric patients with coronavirus disease 2019 in Wuhan: a single center's observational study," *World Journal of Pediatrics*, vol. 16, no. 3, pp. 251–259, 2020.
[42] J. Wu, X. Wu, W. Zeng et al., "Chest CT findings in patients with corona virus disease 2019 and its relationship with clinical features," *Investigative Radiology*, vol. 55, no. 5, pp. 257–261, 2020.
[43] Y. Xiong, D. Sun, Y. Liu et al., "Clinical and high-resolution CT features of the COVID-19 infection: comparison of the initial and follow-up changes," *Investigative Radiology*, vol. 55, no. 6, pp. 332–339, 2020.
[44] G. Ye, Z. Pan, Y. Pan et al., "Clinical characteristics of severe acute respiratory syndrome coronavirus 2 reactivation," *Journal of Infection*, vol. 80, no. 5, pp. e14–e17, 2020.
[45] T. Ai, Z. Yang, H. Hou et al., "Correlation of chest CT and RT-PCR testing in coronavirus disease 2019 (COVID-19) in China: a report of 1014 cases," *Radiology*, vol. 296, no. 2, 2020.
[46] Y. H. Xu, J. H. Dong, W. M. An et al., "Clinical and computed tomographic imaging features of novel coronavirus pneumonia caused by SARS-CoV-2," *Journal of Infection*, vol. 80, pp. 394–400, 2020.
[47] D. Wang, B. Hu, C. Hu et al., "Clinical characteristics of 138 hospitalized patients with 2019 novel coronavirus-infected pneumonia in Wuhan, China," *JAMA*, vol. 323, no. 11, pp. 1061–1069, 2020.
[48] Z. Hu, C. Song, C. Xu et al., "Clinical characteristics of 24 asymptomatic infections with COVID-19 screened among close contacts in Nanjing, China," *Science China Life sciences*, vol. 63, no. 5, pp. 706–711, 2020.
[49] P. An, P. Song, K. Lian, and Y. Wang, "CT manifestations of novel coronavirus pneumonia: a case report," *Balkan Medical Journal*, vol. 37, no. 3, pp. 163–165, 2020.
[50] W. Zhu, K. Xie, H. Lu, L. Xu, S. Zhou, and S. Fang, "Initial clinical features of suspected coronavirus disease 2019 in two emergency departments outside of Hubei, China," *Journal of Medical Virology*, 2020.
[51] C. Huang, Y. Wang, X. Li et al., "Clinical features of patients infected with 2019 novel coronavirus in Wuhan, China," *The Lancet*, vol. 395, no. 10223, pp. 497–506, 2020.
[52] X. Yang, Y. Yu, J. Xu et al., "Clinical course and outcomes of critically ill patients with SARS-CoV-2 pneumonia in Wuhan, China: a single-centered, retrospective, observational study," *Lancet Respiratory Medicine*, vol. 8, no. 5, pp. 475–481, 2020.
[53] C. Wu, X. Chen, Y. Cai et al., "Risk factors associated with acute respiratory distress syndrome and death in patients with coronavirus disease 2019 pneumonia in Wuhan, China," *JAMA Internal Medicine*, vol. 180, no. 7, pp. 934–943, 2020.
[54] J. Wei, H. Xu, J. Xiong et al., "Novel coronavirus (COVID-19) pneumonia: serial computed tomography findings," *Korean Journal of Radiology. [Case Reports]*, vol. 21, no. 4, pp. 501–504, 2019.

[55] D. S. Faffe and W. A. Zin, "Lung parenchymal mechanics in health and disease," *Physiological Reviews*, vol. 89, no. 3, pp. 759–775, 2009.

[56] F. Kay and S. Abbara, "The many faces of COVID-19: spectrum of imaging manifestations," *Radiology: Cardiothoracic Imaging*, vol. 2, no. 1, 2020.

[57] K. M. Das, E. Y. Lee, M. A. Enani et al., "CT correlation with outcomes in 15 patients with acute Middle East respiratory syndrome coronavirus," *American Journal of Roentgenology*, vol. 204, no. 4, pp. 736–742, 2015.

[58] H. X. Bai, B. Hsieh, Z. Xiong et al., "Performance of radiologists in differentiating COVID-19 from viral pneumonia on chest CT," *Radiology*, vol. 296, no. 2, pp. E46–E54.

[59] Y. Li and L. Xia, "Coronavirus disease 2019 (COVID-19): role of chest CT in diagnosis and management," *American Journal of Roentgenology*, vol. 214, no. 6, pp. 1280–1286, 2020.

[60] G. C. Ooi, P. L. Khong, N. L. Müller et al., "Severe acute respiratory syndrome: temporal lung changes at thin-section CT in 30 patients," *Radiology*, vol. 230, no. 3, pp. 836–844, 2004.

[61] Z. Cheng, Y. Lu, Q. Cao et al., "Clinical features and chest CT manifestations of coronavirus disease 2019 (COVID-19) in a single-center study in shanghai, China," *American Journal of Roentgenology*, vol. 215, no. 1, pp. 121–126, 2020.

[62] S. H. Yoon, K. H. Lee, J. Y. Kim et al., "Chest radiographic and CT findings of the 2019 novel coronavirus disease (COVID-19): analysis of nine patients treated in Korea," *Korean Journal of Radiology*, vol. 21, no. 4, pp. 494–500, 2020.

[63] D. L. Ng, F. Al Hosani, M. K. Keating et al., "Clinicopathologic, immunohistochemical, and ultrastructural findings of a fatal case of Middle East respiratory syndrome coronavirus infection in the United Arab Emirates," *The American Journal of Pathology*, vol. 186, no. 3, pp. 652–658, 2016.

[64] Z. Xu, L. Shi, Y. Wang et al., "Pathological findings of COVID-19 associated with acute respiratory distress syndrome," *Lancet Respiratory Medicine [Case Reports]*, vol. 8, no. 4, pp. 420–422, 2020.

[65] S. Tian, W. Hu, L. Niu, H. Liu, H. Xu, and S.-Y. Xiao, "Pulmonary pathology of early-phase 2019 novel coronavirus (COVID-19) pneumonia in two patients with lung cancer," *Journal of Thoracic Oncology*, vol. 15, no. 5, pp. 700–704, 2019.

[66] J. H. Austin, N. L. Müller, P. J. Friedman et al., "Glossary of terms for CT of the lungs: recommendations of the nomenclature committee of the fleischner society," *Radiology*, vol. 200, no. 2, pp. 327–331, 1996.

[67] H. Yu, S. Liu, C. Zhang et al., "Computed tomography and pathology evaluation of lung ground-glass opacity," *Experimental and Therapeutic Medicine*, vol. 16, no. 6, pp. 5305–5309, 2018.

[68] G. Liu, M. Li, G. Li et al., "Assessing the blood supply status of the focal ground-glass opacity in lungs using spectral computed tomography," *Korean Journal of Radiology*, vol. 19, no. 1, pp. 130–138, 2018.

[69] Á. Papp, Z. Bene, I. Gáspár et al., "Decreased VEGF level is associated with elevated ferritin concentration in bronchoalveolar lavage fluid of children with interstitial lung diseases," *Respiration*, vol. 90, no. 6, pp. 443–450, 2015.

[70] C. Beigelman-Aubry, C. Godet, and E. Caumes, "Lung infections: the radiologist's perspective," *Diagnostic and Interventional Imaging*, vol. 93, no. 6, pp. 431–440, 2012.

[71] C. Qin, F. Liu, T. C. Yen, and X. Lan, "(18) F-FDG PET/CT findings of COVID-19: a series of four highly suspected cases," *European Journal of Nuclear Medicine and Molecular Imaging*, vol. 47, no. 5, pp. 1281–1286, 2020.

[72] A. R. Kerr, J. J. Irvine, J. J. Search et al., "Role of inflammatory mediators in resistance and susceptibility to pneumococcal infection," *Infection and Immunity*, vol. 70, no. 3, pp. 1547–1557, 2002.

[73] A. R. Boyd and C. J. Orihuela, "Dysregulated inflammation as a risk factor for pneumonia in the elderly," *Aging and Disease*, vol. 2, no. 6, pp. 487–500, 2011.

[74] P. Mehta, D. F. McAuley, M. Brown, E. Sanchez, R. S. Tattersall, and J. J. Mansonvol. 395, no. 10229, pp. 1033-1034, 2020.

[75] P. Richardson, I. Griffin, C. Tucker et al., "Baricitinib as potential treatment for 2019-nCoV acute respiratory disease," *The Lancet*, vol. 395, no. 10223, pp. e30–e31, 2020.

[76] T. Franquet, "Imaging of pulmonary viral pneumonia," *Radiology*, vol. 260, no. 1, pp. 18–39, 2011.

[77] O. Galante, Y. S. Avni, L. Fuchs, O. A. Ferster, and Y. Almog, "Coronavirus NL63-induced adult respiratory distress syndrome," *American Journal of Respiratory and Critical Care Medicine*, vol. 193, no. 1, pp. 100-101, 2016.

6

Image Quality and Dose Comparison of Single-Energy CT (SECT) and Dual-Energy CT (DECT)

Ramin Ghasemi Shayan, Maryam Oladghaffari, Fakhrosadat Sajjadian, and Mona Fazel Ghaziyani

Radiology Department, Tabriz University of Medical Sciences, Tabriz 51368, Iran

Correspondence should be addressed to Mona Fazel Ghaziyani; fazel.mona@gmail.com

Academic Editor: Paul Sijens

CT and its comprehensive usage have become one of the most indispensable components in medical field especially in the diagnosis of several diseases. SECT and DECT have developed CT diagnostic potentials in several means. In this review article we have discussed the basic principles of single-energy and dual-energy computed tomography and their important physical differences which can cause better diagnostic evaluation. Moreover, different organs diagnostic evaluations through single-energy and dual-energy computed tomography have been discussed. Conventional or single-energy CT (SECT) uses a single polychromatic X-ray beam (ranging from 70 to 140 kVp with a standard of 120 kVp) emitted from a single source and received by a single detector. The concept of dual-energy computed tomography (DECT) is almost as old as the CT technology itself; DECT initially required substantially higher radiation doses (nearly two times higher than those employed in single-energy CT) and presented problems associated with spatial misregistration of the two different kV image datasets between the two separate acquisitions. The basic principles of single-energy and dual-energy computed tomography and their important physical differences can cause better diagnostic evaluation. Moreover, different organs diagnostic evaluations through single-energy and dual-energy computed tomography have been discussed. According to diverse data and statistics it is controversial to definitely indicate the accurate comparison of image quality and dose amount.

1. Introduction

Computerized tomography (CT) has been hailed as a revolutionary diagnostic imaging tool in medicine ever since its introduction in the early 1970s [1]. The arrival of 64-slice CT systems has further validated CT imaging of the heart in clinical routine and also the achieved examination times of 5–10 s lead to short breath hold times, even for patients with dyspnea [2, 3]. There are diverse differences between conventional radiography and computerized tomography. Computerized Tomography (CT) improves upon conventional 2D radiography by producing 3D cross-sectional images of an object from flat X-ray images. The increasing speed of CT along with developments in low-contrast detectability and image quality have allowed the technique to be much more vigorous and this, in turn, has enabled CT to become a majority in medical care throughout the world [4]. Unlike X-ray radiography, the detectors of the CT scanner do not produce an image; they measure the transmission of a thin beam (1–10 mm) of X-rays through a full scan of the body. The image of that section is taken from different angles which allows retrieving the information on the depth (in the third dimension). Conventional or single-energy CT (SECT) uses a single polychromatic X-ray beam (ranging from 70 to 140 kVp with a standard of 120 kVp) emitted from a single source and received by a single detector [5]. The contrast of the image which is caused by this process depends on alterations in photon attenuation of the numerous materials that organize the human body (i.e., soft tissue, air, calcium, and fat) [5]. In SECT, components having diverse fundamental conformations can be characterized by the same CT numbers, making the differentiation and organization of dissimilar types of tissues extremely puzzling. However, the allocation of the scale of grays to each pixel signifies the attenuation of X-rays by the constructions in the tomographic slice [6]. Tissue composition and photon energy level are intrinsic factors and components which can affect the attenuation level of X-ray [5]. Therefore, tissue attenuation can be manipulated by changing photon energy levels which is the fundamental factor of image composition in dual-energy CT [5]. The concept of dual-energy CT was primarily nominated in 1973 [7, 8] and reemerged in the field of clinical radiology with the current technical advances in CT. Although the concept of dual-energy computed tomography (DECT) is almost as old as the CT technology itself, DECT initially required substantially higher radiation doses (nearly two times higher than that employed in single-energy CT) and presented problems associated with spatial misregistration of the two different kV image datasets between the two separate acquisitions [9, 10]. In this regard, dual-energy CT introduced as a first generation dual-source CT system which can develop material variation by using two different X-ray energy spectra [7, 11]. Moreover, two energy levels (typically 80 and 140 kVp) are used to obtain images that can be administered to produce additional datasets and attenuation measurements obtained at a second energy allow the decomposition of a mixture of two or three materials into its constituent materials. Dual-energy CT expands the diagnostic performance and assurance of CT by increasing iodine contrast-to-noise ratio and providing material-specific information [7]. In this regard, the technical diversities and clinical applications of dual-energy CT are ceaselessly on the rise [7, 12]. Overall, rather than increasing image quality and better diagnosis in dual-energy CT, dose reduction is of paramount importance.

This review attempts to discuss the basic and fundamental factors of image formation in single- and dual-energy CT and to compare the image quality and dose in various clinical organs.

2. Basic Principles of Image Formation

2.1. General Basics According to X-Ray Spectra and Attenuation Coefficient. X-ray photons principally interrelate with matter via the photoelectric effect and Compton scattering producing the diagnostic images used in medicine today. When an atom undertakes the photoelectric effect, the electron from that respected K-shell otherwise referred to as the inner shell is evicted via the incident photon. As that electron is excited, unoccupied space is filled by a neighboring electron, freeing energy as a photoelectron. According to single-energy CT, the attenuation coefficient is counted as the measure of how easily a material can be entered by an X-ray beam. It enumerates how much the beam is "attenuated" (i.e., weakened) by the material it is passing through. A small attenuation coefficient designates that the material in question is relatively translucent, while a larger value indicates greater degrees of opacity. The attenuation coefficient is dependent upon the type of material and the energy of the radiation. Generally, for electromagnetic radiation, the higher the energy of the incident photons and the less dense the material in question, the lower the corresponding attenuation coefficient. In short, when a photon has sufficient energy to overcome the electron's binding energy in the K-shell, that atom undergoes the photoelectric effect. Each substance owns a unique K-shell binding energy, known as the K-edge. There is a significant spike in attenuation that results just beyond the energy of the K-edge; this peak is unique to every material and holds valuable information about the substance's composition. To separate attenuation coefficients into two basis-material components and generate basis-material density images, we must remember that the CT number of water is not energy dependent. Thus CT numbers of soft tissues (with Z (eff) values comparable to those of water) remain almost constant when varying the X-ray beam energy. DECT is based on the principle that the attenuation of tissues (reflected by their CT attenuation number in Hounsfield units [HUs]) depends not only on their density but also on their atomic number Z, as well as on the energy of the photon beam. To get the best material characterization, DECT should be performed in these conditions [13]:

(1) Using two monochromatic (only one X-ray energy) beams with very different energy levels

(2) Acquiring both datasets simultaneously

(3) Getting images with the same quantity of photons on the detectors

2.2. Major Steps in Production of Image. The most sophisticated subjects in dual-energy CT is related to image formation and production during the three fundamental steps: data acquisition, image reconstruction, and image display storage and communication.

2.2.1. Data Acquisition. Currently all systems are based on the rotation of the object and different CT data attainment methods have been advanced essentially [14]. Alternatively, this can be attained by rotating the detector and the source of X-rays around the object, but mathematically both methods are equal [14]. To enhance the scan speed fan beam type or even cone beam geometry and multirow or flat panel detectors which obtain more than one slice during a single rotation are used [14]. The dual CT acquisition system has exceptional technical approaches. Since this early work, a number of technical approaches have been industrialized for obtaining the dual-energy dataset such as sequential acquisition, rapid switching of X-ray tube potential, dual-source CT, and multilayer detector.

Two datasets at diverse tube voltages which are entitled sequential acquisition are an approach that necessitates the least hardware effort [12]. Sequential acquisition can be accomplished either as two subsequent helical scans or as a sequence with subsequent rotations at alternating tube voltages and stepwise table feed [12]. Rapid switching of X-ray tube potential has a significant clinical application which is engrossed on bone densitometry measurements [15]. An indispensable problem which stops the increasing of tube current is the low tube potential measurements which restricts attaining comparable noise levels both low and high to your potential datasets also its alteration in noise limited extension of the technique beyond bone densitometry applications [16]. Dual-source computed tomography (DSCT) is one of the latest innovations in multislice CT technology, which is composed of two X-ray tubes and two corresponding detectors. The gantry rotation time is 0.33 s; the temporal resolution of 83 ms is faster than the other MSCT before [17]. This setup requires nearly twofold investments in hardware but offers important advantages for DECT: the voltage, current, and filter can be chosen autonomously for both tubes to attain an optimal spectral contrast with enough transmission and the least overlap and also the data are developed instantaneously by both orthogonal systems [12]. A fourth mechanism for obtaining dual-energy CT projection data is to use a single high tube potential beam and layered or "sandwich" scintillation detectors. The low-energy data are collected from the front or inmost detector layer, while the high-energy data are collected from the back or outmost detector layer [16].

2.2.2. Image Reconstruction. Image reconstruction involves the use of the attenuation readings collected all around the patient and sent to the computer for processing. The major task of the computer in CT is to reconstruct a digital image using special algorithms to systematically build up the image. One of the more commonplace reconstruction algorithms used in CT is the filtered backprojection algorithm [14, 18, 19]. For optimal clinical benefit, images generated from dual-energy CT datasets should provide structural information similar to that provided by conventional single-energy CT scans; in addition, they can provide material-specific information [20].

To obtain material-specific information, the dual-energy datasets are processed either after the reconstruction of high- and low-energy images (in image-domain decomposition) or before images are reconstructed from high- and low-energy sinograms (in data-domain or projection space decomposition) [20, 21]. There are generally two approaches to extract dual-energy information from projection data. A straightforward method is to subtract equivalent projections and apply filtered backprojection to reconstruct the difference as spectral information and another way is to, first, reconstruct standard CT images consisting of voxels in Hounsfield units and then to use postprocessing algorithms to extract specific spectral information from the difference between the corresponding voxels [12]. Currently, the more commonly used approach is the latter, with the image reconstruction system providing low- and high-kilovoltage images and a series of weighted average images [12].

In addition to reconstruction methods a novel scheme based on measurement of DECT data has been advanced in order to attain clinically satisfactory DECT images from low-mAs acquisitions. In this scheme, enthused by the success of edge-preserving nonlocal means (NLM) filtering in CT imaging and the inherent features underlying DECT images, i.e., global correlation and nonlocal similarity, an averaged image induced NLM-based (aviNLM) regularization is combined into the penalized weighted least-squares (PWLS) framework [22]. More prominently, it provides the best qualitative outcomes with the premium details and the fewest noise-induced artifacts, due to the aviNLM regularization learned from DECT images [22].

Also, to suppress momentous statistical noise in the noisy and inadequate sinograms, an adaptive sinogram restoration (ASR) method is first suggested with attention of the statistical property of sinogram data, and then to additionally obtain a high-quality image, an entire deviation based projection onto convex sets (TV-POCS) method is implemented with a slight alteration [23]. For easiness, the current reconstruction strategy was termed as "ASR-TV-POCS." Experimental outcomes have confirmed that the current ASR-TV-POCS method can attain promising improvements over other current methods in terms of the noise reduction, contrast-to-noise ratio, and edge detail conservation [23].

Moreover, an innovative adaptive-weighted total variation (AwTV) minimization model for low-dose CT image reconstruction from sparse-view projection measurements needs to be introduced [24]. By presenting an anisotropic diffusion-based adaptive weight to reserve the edge info in the conventional TV minimization paradigm, the gain in modifying the oversmoothing on the edges in the conventional TV minimization was detected by comparing the presentation of the presented AwTV-POCS implementation with the established TV-POCS algorithm [24].

2.2.3. Material Identification. The most major clinical contribution is from iodine and water; new algorithms permit the separation and characterization of supplementary material datasets that have shown multiple potential applications [25]. Various material-specific images gained from a single contrast-enhanced DECT acquisition permit radiation dose reduction by decreasing the need to implement multiphase attainment while providing the essential info for the diagnostic task [25]. The variation of iodine can be observed as a most auspicious application, which can be expected to expand the valuation of vascular malady in CT angiography [11]. Also, an uptake of iodinated contrast material can be determined in a single phase examination more precisely and can develop tissue categorization [11].

2.2.4. Image Display Storage and Communication. PACS has been extensively used in most of large-scale hospitals to obtain and store archived images from medical imaging modalities (including CT, MR, CR, DX, and any other DICOM devices, except US) and dispense them to DICOM devices [26, 27]. DICOM data saved in PACS servers will not deform images. The images can be stored for long periods of time and can be recovered anytime in any computer where PACS client has been set up and also surgeons trained in a few hours can process DICOM by PACS like radiologists and are able to get more beneficial information [26]. There are no differences in the display of dual-energy CT images and all the steps are similar to other CT modalities.

2.3. Detector Technology. In SECT most manufacturers share a common detector enterprise; that is, the compressed design has three indispensable layers: conversion of X-ray to light (scintillator), light to current (photodiode), and a substrate to provide the mechanical and electrical infrastructure [28]. Current DECT methodologies either rely on completely separate X-ray sources and corresponding detectors or rely on reading out the projection data at dissimilar time points [12]. Two-layer or "sandwich" detectors with different spectral compassions could offer spectral information in single-source systems but to date have not been employed in clinical scanners [12]. In the future, cadmium-based semiconductors, such as CdZnTe, may serve as semiconductors for photon-counting detectors, which resolve the energy of each individual photon, a method already used in nondestructive material testing and luggage scanners at airports. However, this detector technology cannot yet manage with the high photon flux and cannot supply the high image quality obligatory for clinical CT [12].

2.4. Radiation. Although the consequences of preliminary studies showed that dual-energy CT produce higher radiation doses in comparison with single-energy CT [29], many succeeding clinical studies of dual-source dual-energy CT have revealed that dual-energy CT exposes patients to radiation doses similarly to those received during conventional single-energy CT [20, 30, 31]. The outcomes of the more recent studies on dual-energy CT achieved with fast kilovoltage substituting have proved aforementioned result [20].

2.5. Clinical Applications of Dual-Energy CT. Dual-energy CT uses can largely be divided into exploration of material-nonspecific and material-specific energy-dependent information [7]. Both assessments can be qualitative or quantitative and the former contains virtual monoenergetic imaging, effective atomic map, and electron density map [7]. Dual-energy CT offers thrilling applications and possibilities that are previously inaccessible with conventional single-energy CT. The potential assistances of DECT comprise increased lesion detection and classification, improved oncologic staging and assessment of treatment reaction, and reduced artifacts, all at comparable or even reduced radiation doses [5].

Assessing the quality and dose variance between SECT and DECT plays a key role in detecting abnormalities. There are diverse clinical applications of dual-energy CT which are being discussed in the following topics, emphasizing the image quality aspects such as CNR, SNR, and dose underpinned by statistical data and diagrams.

2.5.1. Head and Neck. Head and neck are two of the most indispensable and intrinsic diagnostic parts of the body because of its complicated anatomy and numerous physiological processes. Due to an examination (patients mean age 58 ± 17 years) diverse image parameters have been compared between dual-energy and single-energy CT which are going to be discussed below (Figure 1). The CTDIvol and

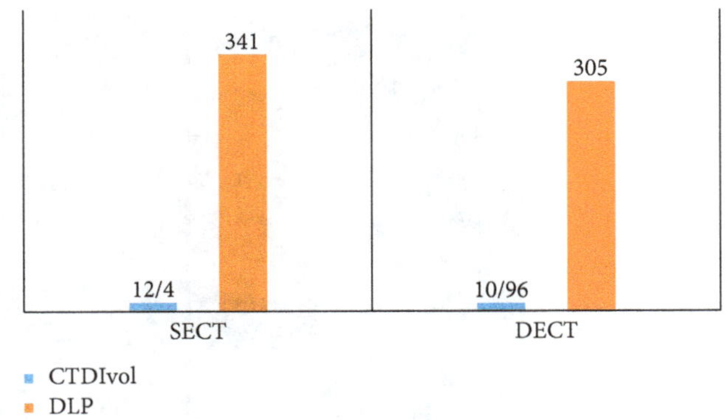

FIGURE 1: CTDIvol and DLP comparison. The comparison of CTDIvol and DLP factor between patients with the mean age 58 ± 17 years through DECT and SECT in head and neck. All numbers are mean ± SD mGy [32].

DLP were significantly lower by 12% and 10%, respectively, in DECT compared with SECT protocols, with no significant differences in noise level, attenuation measurements. In addition to, the subjective image quality between the 2 protocols has no significant differences in image noise, sharpness, or overall image quality observed between DE and SECT of head and nose [32]. As it can be realized from the comparison of axial contrast-enhanced images of neck, one is DECT and the other is SECT which has been done at 120 kv. Dose rate is slightly lower in DECT (Figure 2).

Also the similar exam has been done on pediatrics for a 10 year-old child-based phantom in order to examine and compare the CTDIvol of SECT and DECT. The two radiologists who autonomously studied the series of phantom images reported seeing no significant alteration in image quality when images of dual-energy scans were compared with those of single-energy scans [33]. Also CTDIv measurement through organs of a 10-years-old patient is different in both SECT and DECT (Figure 3). It is of note that the amount of dose in SECT is significantly more than DECT [33]. According to diagram CTDIvol of SECT head is 26.01 mSv while in DECT head we reach to the result of 24.33 mSv.

2.6. Hepatic Imaging. Liver or hepatic imaging is one of the vital examinations in diagnostic radiology. In contrast to other studies, filtration is the main factor in image dose and quality in hepatic imaging. For DE protocols without added filtration, the blended images have lower CNR than the SE images collected at the optimal kVp without considering the patient size. Furthermore, if tin filtration is applied to the high-energy spectrum, for precontrast scans, the composite CNR of the DE blended image can recover noticeably and surpasses the CNR of SE images without tin filtration [34]. An optimized SE protocol produces up to 5% higher CNR for a range of clinical tasks and a clinical study have observed that 120 kVp SE scans have better image quality than blended DE images which do not have a fundamental CNR advantage over enhanced SE images (Figure 4) [34]. According to Figure 5, three factors (CNR, SNR, and CTDIv) have been examined in liver and a remarkable

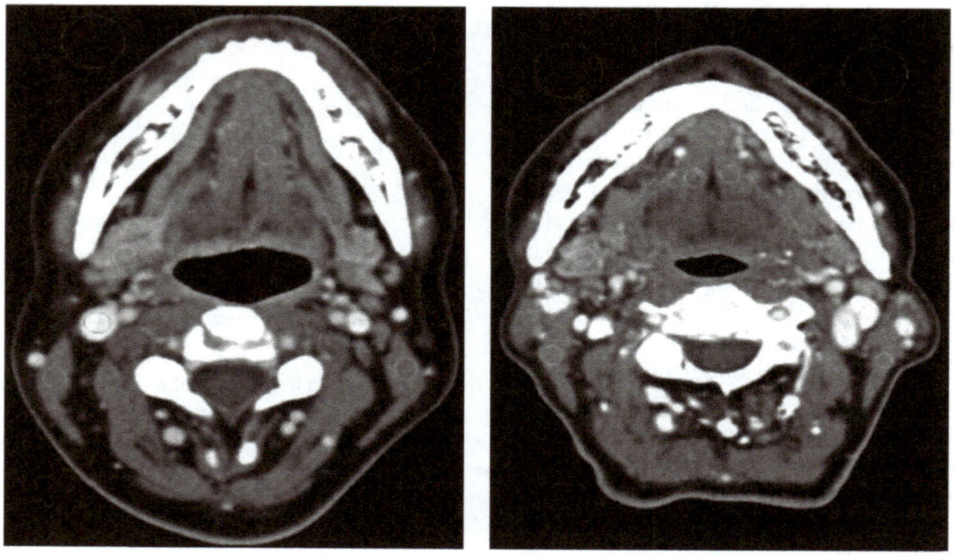

(a) (b)

Figure 2: Axial contrast-enhanced images of neck. DE WA images; (a) SE image (b). Both in 120 kv [32].

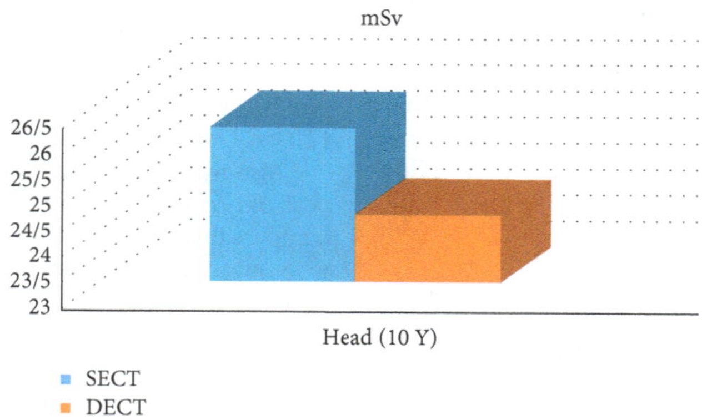

Figure 3: Measurement of CTDIv. CTDIv measurement through head of a 10-year-old patient in both SECT and DECT [33].

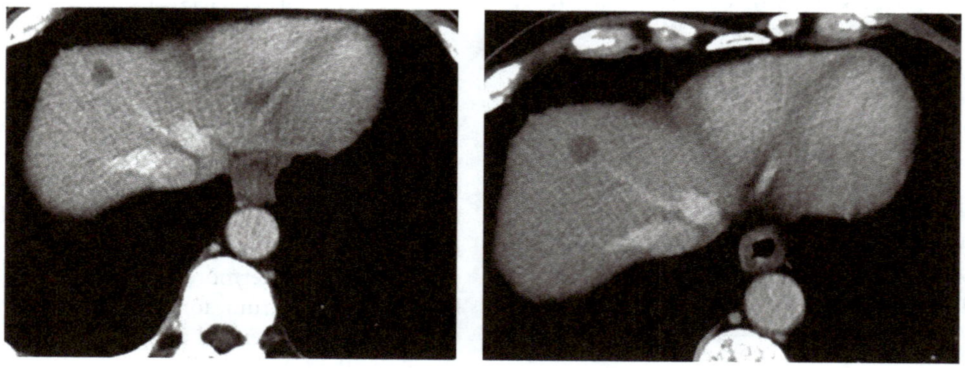

(a) (b)

Figure 4: Liver metastasis from gastric carcinoma. SECT scan. (a) CTDIvol = 10.00. (b) DECT scan obtained 57 days after (a) for both mean kv is 90 [34].

reduction in all factors is obvious in DECT. As it can be seen in Figure 5, CNR and SNR are 23.55, 19.33 and 13.81, 11.75, respectively, in SECT and DECT in hepatic and CTDIvol in SECT is 12.61 mSv while it is 9.81 mSv in DECT. In short explanation CNR, SNR, and CTDIvol in SECT of hepatic are more than DECT of hepatic.

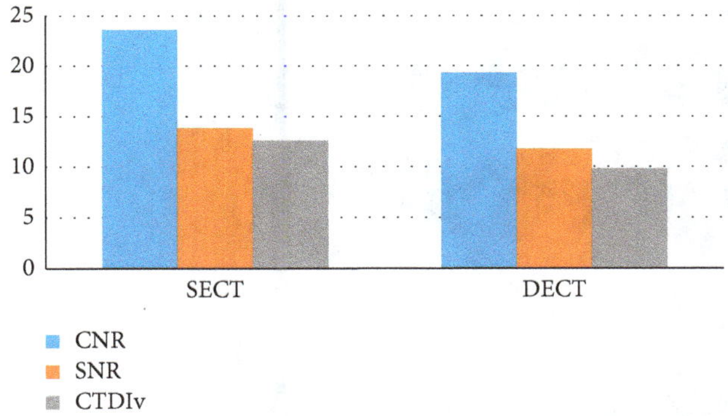

Figure 5: CNR, SNR, and CTDIv. Comparison of CNR, SNR, and CTDIv (mSv) in both SECT and DECT in liver [34].

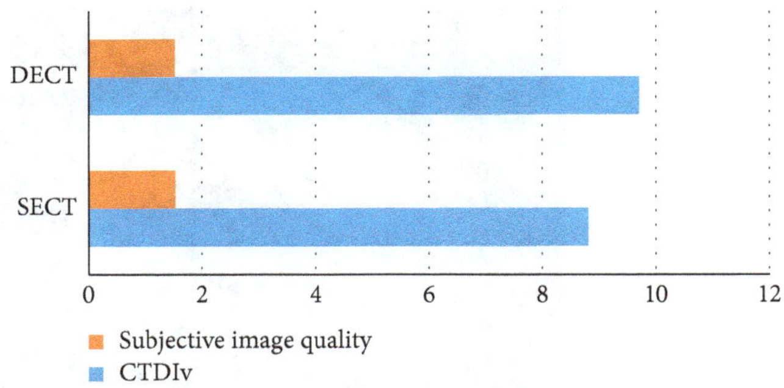

Figure 6: CNR, SNR, and CTDIv. Comparison of CNR, SNR, and CTDIv (mSv) in both SECT and DECT in abdomen [36].

2.7. Abdominal Imaging. The role of dual-energy CT is becoming progressively predominant in abdominal imaging due to the obtainability of scanners and growing field of research. This role of DE in abdominal imaging has been significant in acute bowel ischemia. The addition of iodine maps and 40 keV monoenergetic images to standard single-energy CT images was found to increase reader confidence and precision in diagnosing acute bowel ischemia. Ischemic segments have been found to have lower densities and iodine concentrations in comparison of nonischemic segments [35]. A broad comparison of CNR, SNR, and CTDIv in both single- and dual-energy CT of the abdomen is shown in the diameter below [36]. All the parameters included just mean of CTDIv and subjective image quality. It is necessary to indicate that there are two different ways of measuring image quality, featuring a subjective and an objective approach. According to Figure 6 the factor of subjective image quality of abdominal imaging in DECT is 1.52 and in SECT is 1.53 and also CTDIvol in SECT of abdominal imaging is 8.8 mSv and in DECT is 9.7 mSv. These results indicate that subjective image quality in SECT is more than DECT and also CTDIvol in SECT is less than DECT. Here is a comparison of DECT and SECT of abdomen which is done at 120 kV. As it is transparent, CNR and SNR are better in DECT of abdomen rather than SECT of abdomen (Figure 7).

To compare the CTDIvol of SECT and DECT, a study has been done on pediatrics for a 10-year-old child phantom (Figure 8) [33].

2.8. Urinary Imaging. Dual-energy CT has a number of clinical applications in the assessment of the urinary system particularly in the realm of artifact reduction and material composition.

(a) Renal stone composition:

Renal calculi are composed of different substances such as uric acid, calcium phosphate, calcium oxalate, cystine, and brushite. Clinical administration diverges by stone type. Dual-energy CT uses progressive postprocessing techniques to determine the composition of the calculi accurately [37–39]. For example, if a stone is principally fabricated of uric acid, patients can endure standard urinary alkalinization rather than have an interventional process [40].

(b) Pseudoenhancement of renal cysts:

Virtual monoenergetic images ranging from 80 to 90 keV created from dual-energy datasets can be fashioned to overcome beam hardening and partial volume of indeterminate renal masses. This can be done retrospectively and act as a convenient utensil when calculating for pseudoenhancement of renal cysts [15, 41].

2.9. Virtual Noncontrast Imaging. Virtual noncontrast imaging is an image postprocessing technique used to create "noncontrast" images of contrast-enhanced scans via the subtraction of iodine. It is an imaging technique unique to dual-energy CT. Clinical applications of this method have been bolded in differentiation of hemorrhage from iodinated contrast. Contrast staining of the brain parenchyma after iodinated contrast can lead to interpretation issues, especially when the density of contrast is similar to that of blood. Virtual noncontrast imaging is a precise [42] method in differentiating intracranial hemorrhage from iodinated contrast staining following interventional processes such as endovascular clot retrieval. A complete comparison of image quality between single-energy CT urinary and dual-energy CT virtual noncontrast by utilizing new (Somatom definition) and old scanner (Somatom definition flash) has been done for which the results are shown below. By consuming old scanner system, the image quality of urinary (SECT) is more than virtual noncontrast (DECT). Therefore by consuming new scanner system the image quality of virtual noncontrast (DECT) has been enhanced sensationally in comparison of urinary (SECT) [43]. The image quality comparison of DECT virtual noncontrast and SECT urinary is shown in Figure 9, and the factor in image quality of DECT VNC is 53 which is noticeably more than urinary SECT (47). Moreover, comparison of image quality between SECT urinary and DECT VNC shows that image quality in DECT virtual noncontrast is greater than SECT urinary (Figure 10).

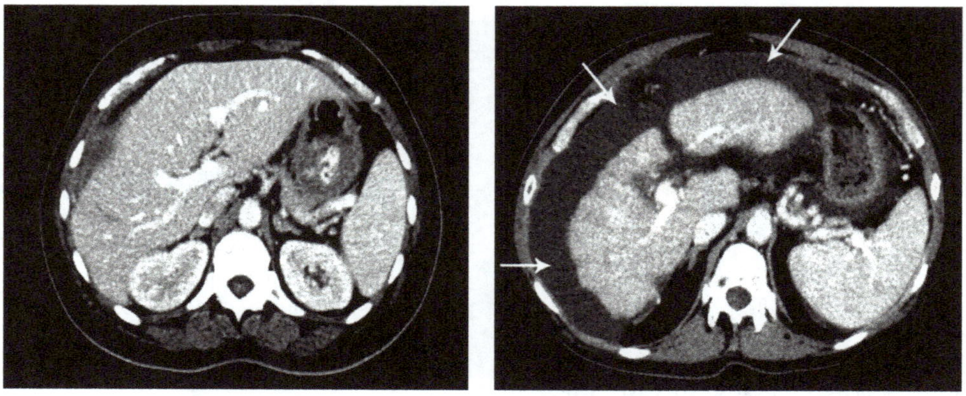

(a) (b)

FIGURE 7: DECT and SECT of abdomen. Abdominal 120 kV second generation. (a) Effective dose adjusted for standard 40 cm acquisition length was 6.5 mSv. Images from a second-generation dual-energy CT (DECT) study in a 58-year-old male with a BMI of 26.5 kg/m^2 demonstrating extensive ascites (arrows). (b) Adjusted effective dose was 7.0 mSv [36].

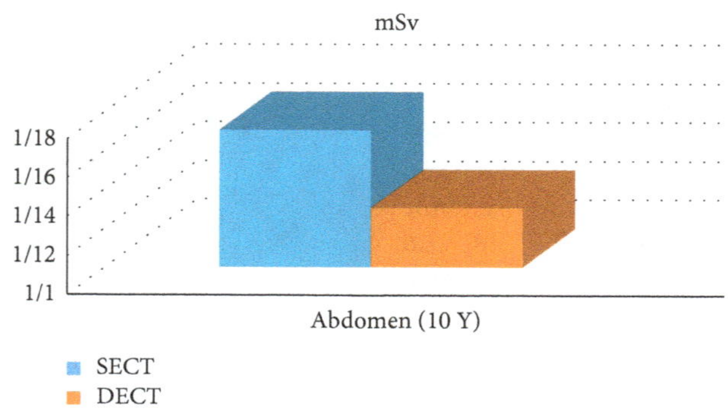

FIGURE 8: Measurement of CTDIv. CTDIv measurement through abdomen of a 10-year-old patient in both SECT and DECT [33].

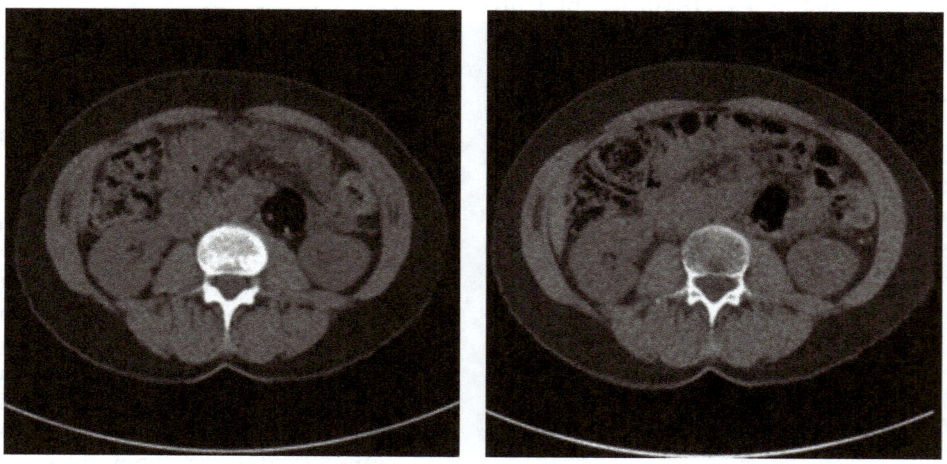

(a) (b)

FIGURE 9: SECT and virtual noncontrast comparison. Single-energy image series before administration of intravenous contrast media. (a) A virtual noncontrast series from the dual-energy contrast-enhanced images. (b) kv used in this examination is 120 [43].

2.10. CT Angiography. One of the most alluring uses of dual-energy CT is direct CT angiography. In this method, the dual-energy algorithm classifies and eradicates bone, permitting direct imagining of iodinated vessels [16]. On the most recent dual-source CT system, the field of view of the second X-ray source restricts dual-energy bone removal to a

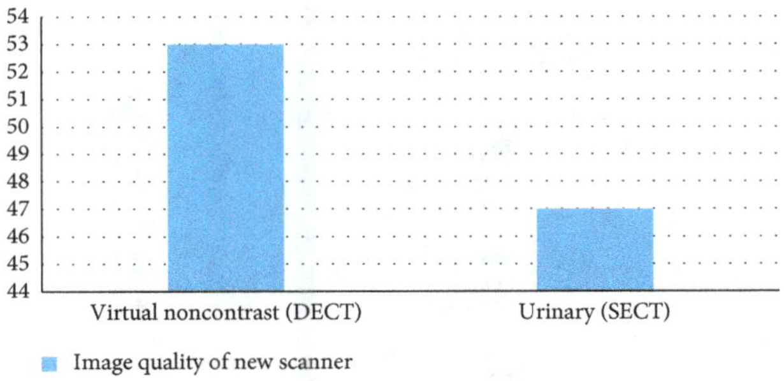

Figure 10: Comparison of image quality between SECT urinary and DECT VNC. It is clear that image quality in DECT virtual noncontrast is greater than SECT urinary [43].

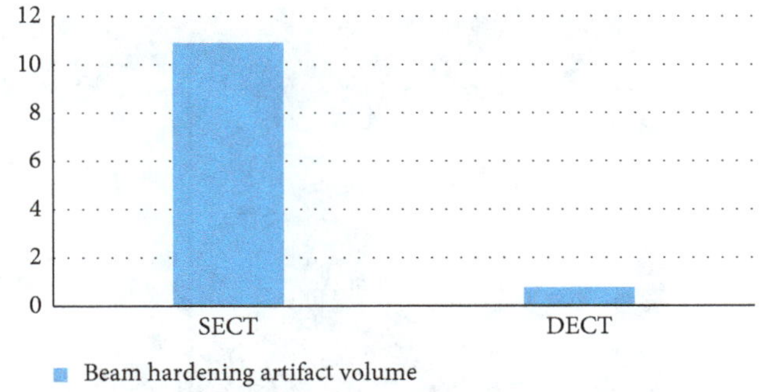

Figure 11: Image quality of DECT and SECT through beam hardening artifact volume. Image quality comparison of surgical group who are undergoing intracranial aneurysm repair with the factor of beam hardening artifact volume and its scale is ml [44].

35 cm field of view; single-energy bone elimination algorithms are used outside the 35 cm field of view on that system [16]. The dual-energy technique of CTA has markedly simplified bone removal on cerebrovascular, abdominal, and peripheral run-off studies, replacing a laborious and time-consuming manual chore by an easy step that takes less than a minute to perform on a workstation for image analysis and postprocessing. In addition, based on a newly developed software algorithms, the dual-energy technique allows the automated removal of calcified plaque from the vessel. This permits readily detecting and displaying narrowed segments of the arterial tree otherwise obscured by overlying calcifications without time-consuming manual postprocessing. This technique is particularly helpful in patients with advanced atherosclerosis, when conventional CT angiograms are difficult to interpret. Overall, dual-energy imaging with facilitated bone and plaque removal overcomes limitations of standard CT, improves diagnostic confidence of CT angiographic imaging of the entire vascular territory, and is expected to improve patient care. There are diverse applications of single-energy and dual-energy CT angiography through diverse organs of body. Comparison of image quality and radiation dose in SECT and DECT are shown on Figures 11 and 12. The comparative factor of image quality is beam hardening and the factor of radiation dose is DLP [44] (all these numbers are related to the surgical group who are undergoing intracranial aneurysm repair). In terms of image quality, it is apparent that the factor of beam hardening in SECT (10.91) is noticeably more than DECT (0.77). Here is a comparison of DECT and SECT of brain in both coronal and axial planes. As it is clear, beam hardening artifact is shown in SECT (Figure 13).

Also the DLP factor in surgical group who are undergoing intracranial aneurysm repair in SECT is 925 mGy and in DECT is 534 mGy which shows remarkable DLP in SECT.

2.11. Cardiac Imaging. Coronary computed tomographic (CT) angiography provides angiographic images of coronary stenosis but is a poor predictor of the physiologic importance of any given stenosis. The addition of functional imaging with other modalities such as echo, magnetic resonance imaging which has been compared with DECT in Figure 14, and nuclear medicine is required for patient risk stratification and treatment planning. Dual-energy CT in combination with CT angiography may supplant the need for multiple modality imaging by virtue of its ability to provide for improved plaque characterization and analysis of downstream myocardial perfusion and myocardial viability. Primary proof on the valuation of myocardial ischemia and infarction by DECT as an addition to coronary CT angiography recommend that DECT is an auspicious step toward wide-ranging assessment of coronary heart malady with a single noninvasive modality. However, considerable research examinations will be obligatory before DECT can be considered for repetitive clinical application [46]. Finally, the motion artifacts significantly reduce image quality. However, due to the rapid scanning of dual-energy CT and fast KV switching CT, the motion artifacts are effectively avoided.

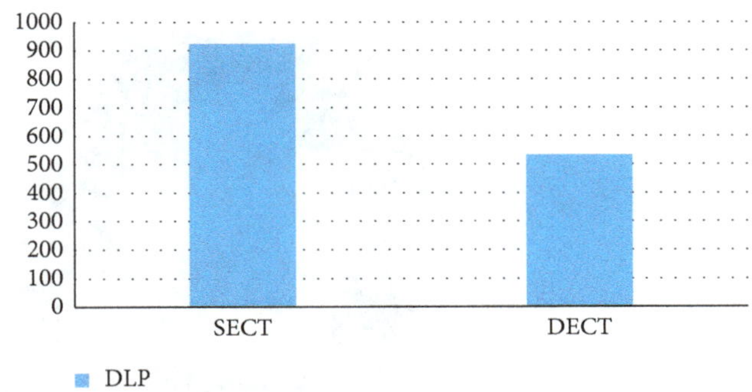

Figure 12: Comparison of DLP in SECT and DECT. Radiation dose comparison of surgical group who are undergoing intracranial aneurysm repair with the factor of DLP and its scale is mGy [44].

3. Conclusion

CT and its comprehensive usage have become one of the most indispensable components in medical field especially in the diagnosis of several diseases. SECT and DECT have developed CT diagnostic potentials in several means. In this review article we have discussed the basic principles of single-energy and dual-energy computed tomography and

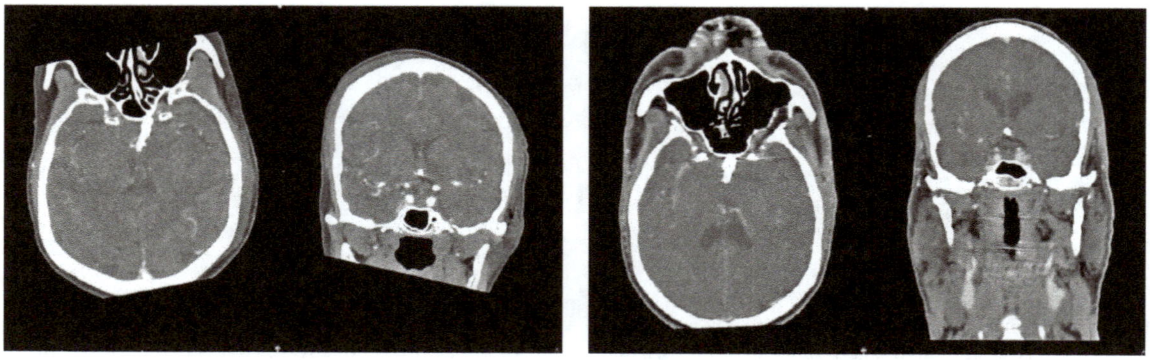

Figure 13: DE-CTA and SE-CTA. Axial and coronal DE-CTA (a) and SE-CTA (b) kv is 100/Sn140 and mAs is 111 [44].

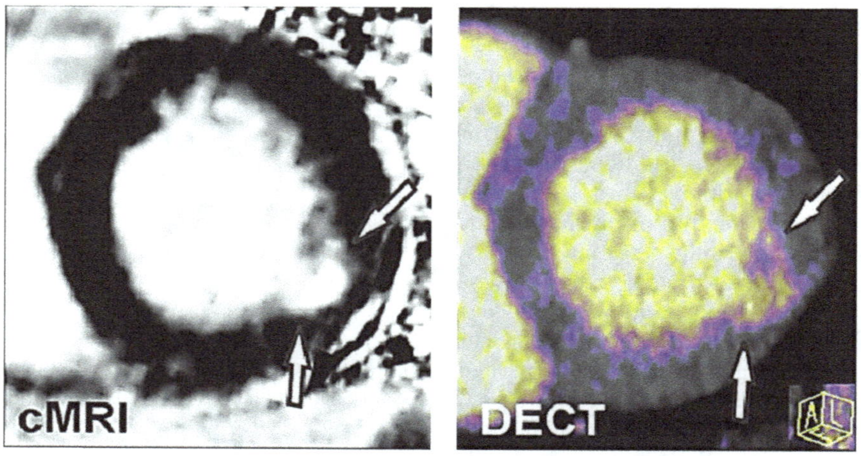

Figure 14: Cardiac magnetic resonance imaging (cMRI) and dual-energy computed tomography (DECT) imaging of myocardial infarction. Iodine color map reconstructed from a DECT image demonstrates good agreement when compared with delayed enhancement cMRI of a subject with prior myocardial infarction of the lateral wall. Similar to cMRI, DECT offers the potential to assess myocardial infarction as well as myocardial salvage through the use of pre- and postcontrast techniques [45].

their important physical differences which can cause better diagnostic evaluation. Moreover, different organs diagnostic evaluations through single-energy and dual-energy computed tomography have discussed. According to diverse data and statistics it is controversial to definitely indicate the accurate comparison of image quality and dose amount. In more items single-energy computed tomography has shown better image quality rather than to dual-energy computed tomography also in more items and organs single-energy computer tomography has shown greater CT dose index volume in comparison to dual-energy computed tomography.

Abbreviations

SECT: Single-energy computed tomography
DECT: Dual-energy computed tomography
DSCT: Dual-source computed tomography
CTDIv: Computed tomography dose index volume
DLP: Dose length product
SNR: Signal-to-noise ratio
CNR: Contrast-to-noise ratio
SE-CTA: Single-energy computed tomography angiography
DE-CTA: Dual-energy computed tomography angiography.

Disclosure

This article does not contain any studies with animals or humans performed by any of the authors.

Authors' Contributions

The main idea of the article was from Mr. Ramin Ghasemi Shayan, and literature search and data analyses were performed by all the authors. Dr. Mona Fazel Ghaziyani drafted and critically revised the work.

References

[1] E. Seeram, "Computed tomography: physical principles and recent technical advances," *Journal of Medical Imaging and Radiation Sciences*, vol. 41, no. 2, pp. 87–109, 2010.

[2] G. L. Raff, M. J. Gallagher, W. W. O'Neill, and J. A. Goldstein, "Diagnostic accuracy of noninvasive coronary angiography using 64-slice spiral computed tomography," *Journal of the American College of Cardiology*, vol. 46, no. 3, pp. 552–557, 2005.

[3] M. Petersilka, H. Bruder, B. Krauss, K. Stierstorfer, and T. G. Flohr, "Technical principles of dual source CT," *European Journal of Radiology*, vol. 68, no. 3, pp. 362–368, 2008.

[4] N. J. Pelc, "Recent and future directions in CT imaging," *Annals of Biomedical Engineering*, vol. 42, no. 2, pp. 260–268, 2014.

[5] J. Grajo, M. Patino, A. Prochowski, and D. Sahani, "Dual energy in practice: basic principles and applications," *Applied Radiology*, vol. 45, no. 7, p. 12, 2016.

[6] J. T. Hathcock and R. L. Stickle, "Principles and concepts of computed tomography," *Veterinary Clinics of North America: Small Animal Practice*, vol. 23, no. 2, pp. 399–415, 1993.

[7] H. W. Goo and J. M. Goo, "Dual-energy CT: new horizon in medical imaging," *Korean Journal of Radiology*, vol. 18, no. 4, pp. 555–569, 2017.

[8] G. N. Hounsfield, "Computerized transverse axial scanning (tomography): part 1. description of system," *The British Journal of Radiology*, vol. 46, no. 552, pp. 1016–1022, 1973.

[9] R. Canellas, S. Digumarthy, A. Tabari et al., "Radiation dose reduction in chest dual-energy computed tomography: effect on image quality and diagnostic information," *Radiologia Brasileira*, vol. 51, no. 6, pp. 377–384, 2018.

[10] W. Kan, A. Wiley Jr., G. Wirtanen et al., "High Z elements in human sarcomata: assessment by multienergy CT and neutron activation analysis," *American Journal of Roentgenology*, vol. 135, no. 1, pp. 123–129, 1980.

[11] T. R. C. Johnson, B. Krauss, M. Sedlmair et al., "Material differentiation by dual energy CT: initial experience," *European Radiology*, vol. 17, no. 6, pp. 1510–1517, 2007.

[12] T. R. C. Johnson, "Dual-energy CT: general principles," *American Journal of Roentgenology*, vol. 199, no. 5, pp. S3–S8, 2012.

[13] P. Omoumi, F. R. Verdun, R. Guggenberger, G. Andreisek, and F. Becce, "Dual-energy CT: basic principles, technical approaches, and applications in musculoskeletal imaging," *Seminars in Musculoskeletal Radiology*, vol. 19, no. 5, pp. 438–445, 2015.

[14] T. Fuchs, T. Schön, and R. Hanke, "Translational computed tomography: a new data acquisition," in *Proceedings of 2nd International Symposium on NTD in Aerospace 2010*, pp. 22–24, Hamburg, Germany, November 2010.

[15] A. Mileto, R. C. Nelson, E. Samei et al., "Impact of dual-energy multi-detector row CT with virtual monochromatic imaging on renal cyst pseudoenhancement: in vitro and in vivo study," *Radiology*, vol. 272, no. 3, pp. 767–776, 2014.

[16] C. H. McCollough, S. Leng, L. Yu, and J. G. Fletcher, "Dual- and multi-energy CT: principles, technical approaches, and clinical applications," *Radiology*, vol. 276, no. 3, pp. 637–653, 2015.

[17] Z. Lei, J. Gu, Q. Fu et al., "The diagnostic evaluation of dual-source CT (DSCT) in the diagnosis of coronary artery stenoses," *Pakistan Journal of Medical Sciences*, vol. 29, no. 1, pp. 107–111, 2013.

[18] L. W. Goldman, "Principles of CT and CT technology," *Journal of Nuclear Medicine Technology*, vol. 35, no. 3, pp. 115–128, 2007.

[19] E. Seeram, *Computed Tomography: Physical Principles, Clinical Applications, and Quality Control*, Saunders/Elsevier, Philadelphia, PA, USA, 2013.

[20] R. K. Kaza, J. F. Platt, R. H. Cohan, E. M. Caoili, M. M. Al-Hawary, and A. Wasnik, "Dual-energy CT with single- and dual-source scanners: current applications in evaluating the genitourinary tract," *RadioGraphics*, vol. 32, no. 2, pp. 353–369, 2012.

[21] C. H. McCollough, B. Schmidt, X. Liu, L. Yu, and S. Leng, "Dual-energy algorithms and postprocessing techniques," in *Dual Energy CT in Clinical Practice*, T. Johnson, C. Fink, S. O. Schönberg et al., Eds., pp. 43–51, Springer, Berlin, Germany, 2011.

[22] H. Zhang, D. Zeng, J. Lin et al., "Iterative reconstruction for dual energy CT with an average image-induced nonlocal means regularization," *Physics in Medicine & Biology*, vol. 62, no. 13, pp. 5556–5574, 2017.

[23] Y. Gao, Z. Bian, J. Huang et al., "Low-dose X-ray computed tomography image reconstruction with a combined low-mAs and sparse-view protocol," *Optics Express*, vol. 22, no. 12, pp. 15190–15210, 2014.

[24] Y. Liu, J. Ma, Y. Fan, and Z. Liang, "Adaptive-weighted total variation minimization for sparse data toward low-dose X-ray computed tomography image reconstruction," *Physics in Medicine and Biology*, vol. 57, no. 23, pp. 7923–7956, 2012.

[25] M. Patino, A. Prochowski, M. D. Agrawal et al., "Material separation using dual-energy CT: current and emerging applications," *RadioGraphics*, vol. 36, no. 4, pp. 1087–1105, 2016.

[26] H. P. Xue, X. W. Liu, J. Tian et al., "Application of computed tomography processed by picture archiving and communication systems in the diagnosis of acute achilles tendon rupture," *BioMed Research International*, vol. 2016, Article ID 6043638, 8 pages, 2016.

[27] W. S. Tzeng, K. M. Kuo, H. W. Lin, and T. Y. Chen, "A socio-technical assessment of the success of picture archiving and communication systems: the radiology technologist's perspective," *BMC Medical Informatics and Decision Making*, vol. 13, no. 1, p. 109, 2013.

[28] E. Shefer, A. Altman, R. Behling et al., "State of the art of CT detectors and sources: a literature review," *Current Radiology Reports*, vol. 1, no. 1, pp. 76–91, 2013.

[29] L. M. Ho, T. T. Yoshizumi, L. M. Hurwitz et al., "Dual energy versus single energy MDCT: measurement of radiation dose using adult abdominal imaging protocols," *Academic Radiology*, vol. 16, no. 11, pp. 1400–1407, 2009.

[30] L. Yu, A. N. Primak, X. Liu, and C. H. McCollough, "Image quality optimization and evaluation of linearly mixed images in dual-source, dual-energy CT," *Medical Physics*, vol. 36, no. 3, pp. 1019–1024, 2009.

[31] C. Thomas, O. Patschan, D. Ketelsen et al., "Dual-energy CT for the characterization of urinary calculi: in vitro and in vivo evaluation of a low-dose scanning protocol," *European Radiology*, vol. 19, no. 6, pp. 1553–1559, 2009.

[32] A. M. Tawfik, J. M. Kerl, A. A. Razek et al., "Image quality and radiation dose of dual-energy CT of the head and neck compared with a standard 120-kVp acquisition," *American Journal of Neuroradiology*, vol. 32, no. 11, pp. 1994–1999, 2011.

[33] X. Zhu, W. P. McCullough, P. Mecca, S. Servaes, and K. Darge, "Dual-energy compared to single-energy CT in pediatric imaging: a phantom study for DECT clinical guidance," *Pediatric Radiology*, vol. 46, no. 12, pp. 1671–1679, 2016.

[34] Y. Yao, J. M. Ng, A. J. Megibow, and N. J. Pelc, "Image quality comparison between single energy and dual energy CT protocols for hepatic imaging," *Medical Physics*, vol. 43, no. 8, pp. 4877–4890, 2016.

[35] M. A. Mazzei, F. Gentili, and L. Volterrani, "Dual-energy CT iodine mapping and 40-keV monoenergetic applications in the diagnosis of acute bowel ischemia: a necessary clarification," *American Journal of Roentgenology*, vol. 212, no. 3, pp. W93–W94, 2019.

[36] J. L. Wichmann, A. D. Hardie, U. J. Schoepf et al., "Single- and dual-energy CT of the abdomen: comparison of radiation dose and image quality of 2nd and 3rd generation dual-source CT," *European Radiology*, vol. 27, no. 2, pp. 642–650, 2017.

[37] R. Guggenberger, R. Gnannt, J. Hodler et al., "Diagnostic performance of dual-energy CT for the detection of traumatic bone marrow lesions in the ankle: comparison with MR imaging," *Radiology*, vol. 264, no. 1, pp. 164–173, 2012.

[38] P. Stolzmann, H. Scheffel, K. Rentsch et al., "Dual-energy computed tomography for the differentiation of uric acid stones: ex vivo performance evaluation," *Urological Research*, vol. 36, no. 3-4, pp. 133–138, 2008.

[39] S. Leng, A. Huang, J. M. Cardona, X. Duan, J. C. Williams, and C. H. McCollough, "Dual-energy CT for quantification of urinary stone composition in mixed stones: a phantom study," *American Journal of Roentgenology*, vol. 207, no. 2, pp. 321–329, 2016.

[40] J. A. McAteer and A. P. Evan, "The acute and long-term adverse effects of shock wave lithotripsy," *Seminars in Nephrology*, vol. 28, no. 2, pp. 200–213, 2008.

[41] Z. J. Wang, F. V. Coakley, Y. Fu et al., "Renal cyst pseudoenhancement at multidetector CT: what are the effects of number of detectors and peak tube voltage?" *Radiology*, vol. 248, no. 3, pp. 910–916, 2008.

[42] C. M. Phan, A. J. Yoo, J. A. Hirsch, R. G. Nogueira, and R. Gupta, "Differentiation of hemorrhage from iodinated contrast in different intracranial compartments using dual-energy head CT," *American Journal of Neuroradiology*, vol. 33, no. 6, pp. 1088–1094, 2012.

[43] M. Lundin, M. Liden, A. Magnuson et al., "Virtual non-contrast dual-energy CT compared to single-energy CT of the urinary tract: a prospective study," *Acta Radiologica*, vol. 53, no. 6, pp. 689–694, 2012.

[44] A. Abdulazim, C. Rubbert, D. Reichelt et al., "Dual- versus single-energy CT-angiography imaging for patients undergoing intracranial aneurysm repair," *Cerebrovascular Diseases*, vol. 43, no. 5-6, pp. 272–282, 2017.

[45] W. Wince, P. Suranyi, and U. Schoepf, "Contemporary cardiovascular imaging methods for the assessment of at-risk myocardium," *Journal of the American Heart Association*, vol. 3, no. 5, 2014.

[46] R. Vliegenthart, G. J. Pelgrim, U. Ebersberger, G. W. Rowe, M. Oudkerk, and U. J. Schoepf, "Dual-energy CT of the heart," *American Journal of Roentgenology*, vol. 199, no. 5, pp. S54–S63, 2012.

7

Prevalence, Spectrum and Outcomes of Single Coronary Artery Detected on Coronary Computed Tomography Angiography (CCTA)

Rashid Al Umairi[1] **and Maryam Al-khouri**[2]

[1]*Department of Radiology, The Royal Hospital, Muscat, Oman*
[2]*Oman Medical Specialty Board, Muscat, Oman*

Correspondence should be addressed to Rashid Al Umairi; alumairi1@yahoo.com

Academic Editor: Paul Sijens

Background. Single coronary artery (SCA) is a rare congenital anomaly in which there is an isolated coronary artery that arises from a single coronary ostium and provides coronary blood supply to the entire myocardium. SCA is classified into different types based on the origin, branching pattern, and course. Although the majority of patients with SCA are asymptomatic, some patients can present with life-threatening symptoms. *Aim*. To examine the prevalence, anatomical distribution, and outcome of the single coronary artery anomaly detected on coronary computed tomography angiography (CCTA) in a single center in Oman. *Methods*. Retrospectively, we reviewed 4,445 patients who underwent coronary computed tomography angiography between September 2012 and August 2018 at the National Heart Center, Muscat, Oman. We identified patients with a single coronary artery, and we evaluated the origin, course, and outcome of SCA. *Results*. We found 12 patients with single coronary artery among 4,445 patients with a mean age of 56.4 years (age range: 34 to 71 years; male : female ratio: 5 : 7). The most common class was RIII-C seen in 4 patients. Other SCA included RII-C, RII-A, and RII-S, two in each class. One patient had RI and one had LII-P. Two patients had coronary artery bypass graft. No major adverse cardiac events were reported over a mean follow-up of 25.3 months. *Conclusion*. Single coronary artery (SCA) is a rare congenital anomaly classified into different types. In our study, the prevalence of SCA was 0.27% that is higher than the figures from previous reports.

1. Introduction

Single coronary artery (SCA) is a congenital anomaly that is usually discovered incidentally and has an estimated incidence ranging between 0.024% and 0.066% among patients undergoing routine coronary artery catheterization [1]. SCA can be either an isolated anomaly or associated with other congenital abnormalities such as coronary artery fistula and bicuspid aortic valve [2–4]. Based on the site of origin and anatomical distribution of the branches, Lipton et al. classified SCA into two main categories: "R," right type, and "L," left type. These two types were further divided into I, II, and III subtypes according to the anatomical courses of the branches [5]. Although conventional coronary angiography is the gold standard procedure for coronary artery assessment, it is an invasive procedure and has limited ability in demonstrating the anatomy of complex coronary artery anomalies. In contrast, CCTA is a noninvasive test and has the ability to show complex coronary artery anatomy [6]. The aim of this study is to discuss the prevalence, anatomical distribution, and outcome of singe coronary artery anomaly detected on coronary computed tomography angiography (CCTA) in a single center in Oman.

2. Patients and Methods

The Scientific Research Committee of The Royal Hospital, Muscat, Oman, approved this retrospective single institution study and waived informed consent.

2.1. Patient Selection. This study included 4,445 consecutive patients who underwent CCTA at the National Heart Center, Muscat, Oman, from September 2012 to August 2018. The indications for performing CCTA were chest pain to exclude coronary artery disease, assessment of coronary artery grafts or stents, cardiomyopathy, evaluation of congenital heart disease, evaluation of syncope, and precardiac surgery assessment. Exclusion criteria for CCTA were a history of prior allergy to iodinated contrast material, impaired renal function (estimated glomerular filtration rate less than 45 mL/min/1.73 m^2), inability to follow the breathing instruction, uncontrolled heart rate, cardiac arrhythmia, and severe coronary calcification in calcium score scan.

Prior to the scan, electrocardiogram (ECG), heart rate, and blood pressure of all patients were checked. Procedure preparation included administration of 25–100 mg of atenolol orally to all patients with a baseline heart rate >70 beats/min to lower the heart rate. Sublingual nitroglycerine (0.8 mg) was administered to all patients 1 minute prior to the injection of the contrast unless it was contraindicated. Scanning was performed using a dual-source 256-slice (2 × 128) CT scanner (SOMATOM Definition Flash, Siemens, Erlangen, Germany) with rotation time 280 ms and a dual-source 384-slice (2 × 192) CT scanner (SOMATOM Force, Siemens, Erlangen, Germany) with rotation time 250 ms. All scans started with topogram, followed by a prospective ECG-gated nonenhanced CT scan at 75% of RR interval. The CCTA scan was performed by injecting 60 to 75 mL of contrast followed by 30 mL of saline solution at a rate of 6 mL/s. In the contrast-enhanced scan, ECG-gated prospective or retrospective scan with a slice thickness of 0.6 mm was acquired during breath holding in inspiration. The scan parameters were adjusted automatically or manually to acquire the best quality with the least radiation dose.

Data from the scanners were sent to separate image-processing working stations (syngo.via, Siemens, Berlin, Germany), and coronary arteries were assessed for atherosclerotic disease, anomalous origin, course, and termination. The single coronary artery is defined as an isolated coronary artery arising from a single coronary ostium in the absence of a second coronary ostium. Patients with a single coronary artery were selected, and images were again analyzed. SCA was categorized into different categories based on modified Lipton's classification.

3. Results

We identified 12 patients with a single coronary artery with a prevalence of 0.27% (Table 1). Their mean age was 56.4 years (age range: 34 to 71 years; male : female ratio: 5 : 7). Of the 12 patients with SCA, only one patient had SCA originating from the left coronary sinus (Figure 1) and 11 had SCA originating from the right coronary sinus (Figures 2–6). Four patients had a dual LAD variant (Cases 1, 3, 6, and 9). None of the patient had any other congenital cardiac anomalies.

Chest pain was the most common symptom reported in ten patients. Eight patients had a history of shortness of breath on exertion, and five patients had a history of palpitation. The baseline clinical characteristics of the patients are shown in Table 1.

Four patients had myocardial perfusion imaging, two were negative for myocardial ischemia, one had an inconclusive test, and one had mild ischemia in the LAD territory (Case 8). One patient had an exercise treadmill test, and it was inconclusive (Case 11).

Coronary angiography was performed in nine patients which confirms the diagnosis of SCA. Three of them had no atherosclerosis (Cases 5, 6, and 11), two had mild (25–49%) coronary artery narrowing (Cases 4 and 8), and four had severe (≥70%) coronary artery stenosis (Cases 2, 3, 7, and 10). Two patients had coronary artery bypass graft because of severe coronary artery stenosis. The other patients with atherosclerotic disease were treated conservatively.

The mean time of follow-up was 23.3 months. None of the 12 patients had major adverse cardiovascular events during follow-up.

4. Discussion

Single coronary artery (SCA) is defined as an isolated coronary artery that arises from a single coronary ostium and provides blood supply to the entire myocardium [1]. SCA is usually detected incidentally while imaging the heart for other reasons, and it has a prevalence ranging between 0.024 and 0.098% among patients undergoing coronary computed tomography angiography [7–12]. The prevalence of SCA among our population was 0.27% that is higher than that previously reported. SCA can either be isolated or coexist with other cardiac congenital anomalies including transposition of great vessels, coronary arteriovenous fistula [2, 3, 13], tetralogy of Fallot, truncus arteriosus [14], interventricular septal defect, patent ductus arteriosus, bicuspid aortic valve, and patent foramen ovale [15–17]. None of our patients had other congenital cardiac anomalies. However, 4 of our patients had a dual LAD variant with the long and short LADs supplying the normal course of the LAD [18].

In the literatures, there are different classification systems of SCA based on necropsy findings and conventional coronary angiography. In 1979, Lipton et al. suggested a classification system in which they incorporated two prior classification systems that were suggested by Smith in 1950 and Ogden and Goodyer in 1970 [5, 19]. According to Lipton's classification, SCA is divided into two main types: "R," right type, and "L," left type, to indicate the origin of the SCA from the right or the left coronary sinus, respectively [5]. SCA is further divided into three subtypes based on the anatomical course of SCA. Type I in which there is a single coronary artery arising from either the right or the left coronary sinus is RCA, and then it continues in the left atrioventricular groove as LCX before it terminates as LAD, or as LM that gives LCX and LAD; the RCA formed is a continuation of the LCX. In type II, a single coronary artery

TABLE 1: Baseline clinical characteristics of the patients with coronary artery anomalies.

Mean age (years)		56.4
Gender (M : F)		5 : 7
Risk factors	Hypertension	6
	Diabetes	5
	Dyslipidemia	5
	Smoking	3
Known CAD		2
Presenting symptoms	Chest pain	10
	Shortness of breath	8
	Palpitation	4
Intervention		2
Mean follow-up (months)		25.3

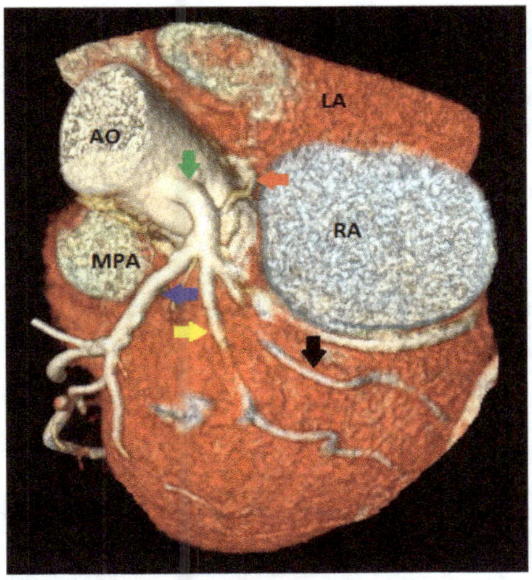

FIGURE 1: Case 3: 3D volume-rendered coronary image showing a single coronary artery arising from the left coronary sinus (LCS). The right coronary artery (RCA) (red arrow) arises from the proximal left main coronary artery, and then it courses posterior to the aorta (retroaortic course) before it reaches the right interventricular groove. The left main coronary artery trifurcates and gives the left anterior descending artery (blue arrow), the ramus intermedius (yellow arrow), and the left circumflex artery (black arrow). AO: aorta; LA: left atrium; RA: right atrium; MPA: main pulmonary artery.

arises from either the right or the left coronary sinus, and from the proximal segment of this single coronary artery, an anomalous artery arises that crosses the base of the heart before it resumes its inherited course. In type III, the LCX and LAD have separate origins from the proximal RCA [5]. Based on the relationship of the SCA to the aorta and the main pulmonary artery, Lipton et al. categorized SCA into three categories: category A in which the anomalous artery passes anterior to the main pulmonary artery, category B in which the anomalous artery passes between the ascending aorta and the main pulmonary artery, and category P in which the anomalous artery passes posterior to the ascending aorta [5]. In 1990, Yamanaka and Hobbs modified the classification proposed by Yamanaka and Hobbs and added two new groups S and C indicating transseptal and combined courses, respectively [20]. More recently, in 2005, Rigatelli et al. proposed a new classification system based on the clinical significance of the single coronary anomaly and categorized SCA into four different classes. Class I is considered a benign type, class II is associated with fixed myocardial ischemia, class III is related to sudden cardiac death, and class IV is associated with superimposed coronary artery disease [21]. In our survey, we had a variety of SCA subtypes with RIII-C as the most frequent type (Table 2).

Most of the patients with SCA are asymptomatic or might present with nonspecific symptoms; however, patients with some variants of SCA can present with typical chest pain, myocardial infarction, syncope, ventricular tachycardia, and sudden cardiac death [5, 15]. SCA with an interarterial anomalous artery has been strongly linked with sudden death and myocardial ischemia especially among young competitive athletes [15]. This is more common among patients with anomalous coronary artery arising from the right coronary sinus and coursing to the left between the aorta and the main pulmonary artery [22]. Although the exact mechanism is not fully understood, it is assumed that as the aorta and the main pulmonary artery become dilated during exercise, they squeeze the apparent artery [23]. Therefore, identification of patients with an SCA that has an interarterial course and is differentiated from the subpulmonic transseptal course is crucial for management.

SCA can be diagnosed by different diagnostic modalities including conventional coronary angiography, coronary computed tomography angiography, and cardiac MRI. Conventional coronary angiography is the gold standard for assessment of the coronary artery; however, it is an invasive procedure and has a risk of complications [6]. Moreover, even with multiple projections and angiographic views, delineation of the anatomy of the complex cases can be difficult [24]. On the contrary, coronary computed tomography angiography (CCTA) is a noninvasive diagnostic tool with high temporal and spatial resolution that has emerged as a gold standard for detection and characterization of coronary artery anomalies [6, 25, 26]. CCTA can precisely delineate the course of the anomalous artery and provide 3-dimensional information about the relation of the anomalous artery to other cardiovascular structures, namely, cardiac chambers and major arteries [13, 27]. However, despite the advances in CT technology to reduce radiation exposure, CCTA is still an ionizing examination. Cardiovascular MRI, on the contrary, is a nonionizing test that can be used to detect SCA and delineate the anatomy of the anomalous coronary artery along with the viability assessment of the myocardium; however, it has a lower temporal and spatial resolution compared to the CCTA. Moreover, MRI is less available than other diagnostic modalities and contraindicated in patients with pacemakers [28]. All our patients with SCA were diagnosed by CCTA, by which we were able to precisely delineate the origin and the course of the anomalous artery.

The presence of atherosclerotic disease in patients with coronary artery anomaly has a clinical implication, particularly when the decision is to be made between percutaneous

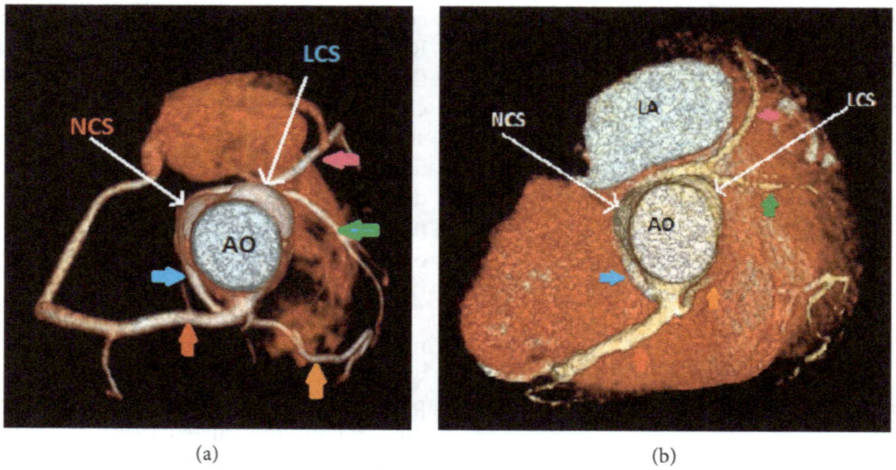

FIGURE 2: Case 1 (a) and case 9 (b): 3D volume-rendered coronary image showing a single coronary artery arising from the right coronary sinus (RCS) with a dual left anterior descending artery (LAD) variant. The right coronary artery (red arrow) has a normal course. The left main coronary artery (blue arrow) arises from the proximal RCA, and then it has a retroaortic course to the left before it gives the short segment of the LAD (green arrow) and the left circumflex artery (pink arrow). The long segment of the dual LAD variant arises from the proximal RCA, and it has a prepulmonic course in case 1 and transseptal course in case 9 before it reaches the distal anterior interventricular groove (orange arrow). AO: aorta; LCS: left coronary sinus; NCS: none coronary sinus; LA left atrium.

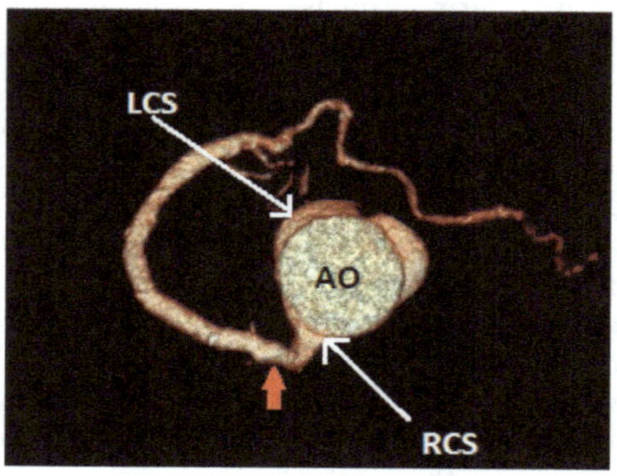

FIGURE 3: Case 2: 3D volume-rendered coronary image showing a single coronary artery (red arrow) arising from the right coronary sinus (RCS). The right coronary artery courses within the right atrioventricular groove before it continues within the left atrioventricular groove as the left circumflex artery. AO: aorta; LCS: left coronary sinus.

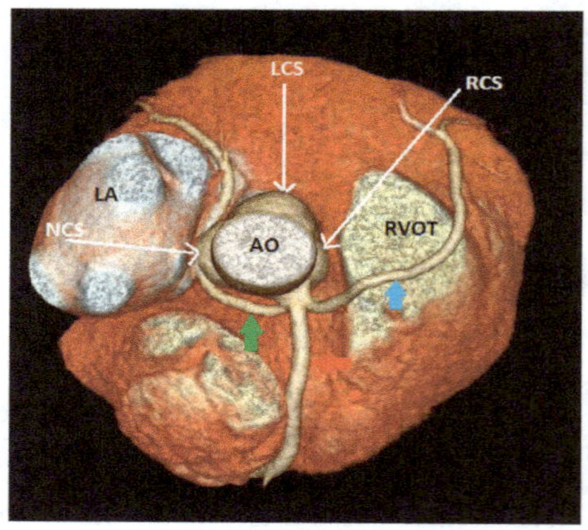

FIGURE 4: Case 3: 3D volume-rendered coronary image showing a single coronary artery arising from the right coronary sinus (RCS). The right coronary artery (RCA) (red arrow) has a normal course. The left anterior descending artery (blue arrow) arises from the proximal RCA and then courses to the left anterior to the right ventricular outflow tract (RVOT). The left circumflex artery arises from the proximal RCA, and then it has a retroaortic course before it reaches the left atrioventricular groove. AO: aorta; LCS: left coronary sinus; NCS: none coronary sinus; LA: left atrium.

coronary intervention (PCI) and coronary artery bypass graft (CABG). Moreover, awareness of presence of coronary artery anomalies and their anomalous course prior to CABG is crucial to avoid potential surgical complications as unrecognized anomalous artery can be excluded from perfusion during cardiopulmonary bypass or might be unintentionally damaged [15].

Given the vast variety of anatomical courses of SCA, the multidisciplinary approach involving interventional cardiologists and cardiothoracic surgeons should be considered to decide on the best treatment options. In the majority of asymptomatic patients with no atherosclerotic disease, usually, no invasive intervention is recommended [29]. Invasive interventions including PCI with stent placement and surgical intervention are preserved for symptomatic patients and patients with a malignant course of the anomalous artery [30, 31]. Surgical interventions include reimplantation of the anomalous artery to the aorta, osteoplasty, coronary artery bypass grafting (CABG) of the anomalous artery, and pulmonary artery translocation [32]. Two of our patients had signification coronary artery disease and underwent CABG.

5. Conclusion

The prevalence of SCA among our population is higher than that reported in other parts of the world. SCA is divided into different subtypes based on the course of the anomalous

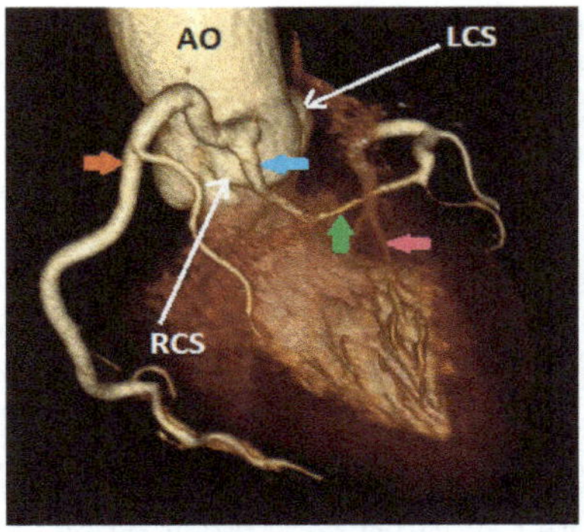

FIGURE 5: Case 4: 3D volume-rendered coronary image showing a single coronary artery arising from the right coronary sinus (RCS). The right coronary artery (red arrow) has a normal course. The left main coronary artery (blue arrow) arises from the proximal RCA and then courses to the left through the septal myocardium (transseptal) before it emerges in the proximal left interventricular groove and gives rise to the left anterior descending artery and left circumflex artery (pink arrow). There is significant narrowing of the transseptal segment of the left main coronary artery (green arrow). AO: aorta; LCS: left coronary sinus.

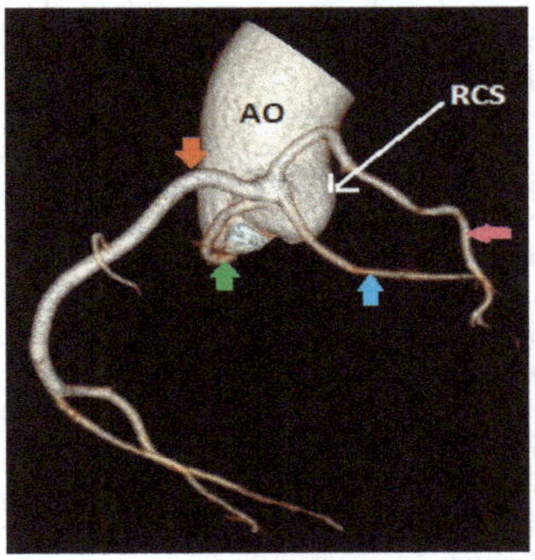

FIGURE 6: Case 6: 3D volume-rendered coronary image showing a single coronary artery arising from the right coronary sinus (RCS) with a dual left anterior descending artery (LAD) variant. The right coronary artery (red arrow) has a normal course. The left circumflex artery (green arrow) arises from the proximal RCA, and then it has a retroaortic course before it reaches the left interventricular groove. The short segment of the LAD courses through the septum myocardium before it reaches the proximal interventricular groove (blue arrow). The long segment of the LAD (pink arrow) has a prepulmonic course before it reaches the distal interventricular groove. AO: aorta.

TABLE 2

	Classification	Invasive angiography	Myocardial perfusion	Exercise treadmill test	Stress echocardiogram
Case 1	RII-C	—	Inconclusive	—	−ve
Case 2	RI	Yes	−ve	—	−ve
Case 3	RII-C	Yes	—	—	Global hypokinesia
Case 4	RIII-C	—	—	—	Inferior wall hypokinesia
Case 5	RII-S	Yes	—	—	Lateral wall hypokinesia
Case 6	RIII-C	—	—	—	−ve
Case 7	RII-A	Yes	—	—	Wall motion abnormalities
Case 8	LII-P	—	Mild ischemia in LAD territory	—	—
Case 9	RIII-C	—	—	—	−ve
Case 10	RII-A	Yes	—	—	Hypokinesia
Case 11	RIII-C	Yes	−ve	Inconclusive	—
Case 12	RII-S	—	—	—	−ve

artery. Awareness of these types is essential as it has an implication for planning patient management. Coronary computed tomography angiography has an important role in diagnosis of different classes of SCA.

References

[1] W. Desmet, J. Vanhaecke, M. Vrolix et al., "Isolated single coronary artery: a review of 50 000 consecutive coronary angiographies," *European Heart Journal*, vol. 13, no. 12, pp. 1637–1640, 1992.

[2] A. A. El-Menyar, K. M. Das, and J. Al-Suwaidi, "Anomalous origin of the three coronary arteries from the right aortic sinus Valsalva: role of MDCT coronary angiography," *The International Journal of Cardiovascular Imaging*, vol. 22, no. 5, pp. 723–729, 2006.

[3] R. Bolognesi, D. Tsialtas, F. Barbaresi, and C. Manca, "Single coronary artery-right ventricular fistula with a partially thrombosed large aneurysm of its proximal tract in a 66- year-old man," *European Heart Journal*, vol. 15, no. 12, pp. 1720–1724, 1994.

[4] A. I. Larsen, S. Ørn, S. Barvik, and D. W. T. Nilsen, "Anomalies of the coronary arteries originating from the right sinus of Valsalva. (1) single coronary artery originating from the right sinus associated with fusion of the left and the non coronary cusp and atrophy of the left coronary ostium (2) three separate coronary arteries originating from the right sinus of Valsalva," *International Journal of Cardiology*, vol. 115, no. 2, pp. e86–e89, 2007.

[5] M. J. Lipton, W. H. Barry, I. Obrez, J. F. Silverman, and L. Wexler, "Isolated single coronary artery: diagnosis, angiographic classification, and clinical significance," *Radiology*, vol. 130, no. 1, pp. 39–47, 1979.

[6] R. S. Al Umairi, F. Al Kindi, and F. Al Busaidi, "Anomalous origin of the left coronary artery from the pulmonary artery: the role of multislice computed tomography (MSCT)," *Oman Medical Journal*, vol. 31, no. 5, pp. 387–389, 2016.

[7] F. Zukic, M. Miljko, S. Vegar-Zubovic, A. Behmen, and A. K. Arapovic, "Prevalence of coronary artery anomalies detected by coronary CT angiography in Canton Sarajevo, Bosnia and Herzegovina," *Psychiatria Danubina*, vol. 29, no. 4, pp. 830–834, 2017.

[8] O. A. Smettei, S. Sayed, and R. M. Abazid, "The prevalence of coronary artery anomalies in Qassim province detected by cardiac computed tomography angiography," *Journal of the Saudi Heart Association*, vol. 29, no. 2, pp. 84–89, 2017.

[9] C. N. Sirasapalli, J. Christopher, and V. Ravilla, "Prevalence and spectrum of coronary artery anomalies in 8021 patients: a single center study in south India," *Indian Heart Journal*, vol. 70, no. 6, pp. 852–856, 2018.

[10] C. Gräni, D. C. Benz, C. Schmied et al., "Prevalence and characteristics of coronary artery anomalies detected by coronary computed tomography angiography in 5634 consecutive patients in a single centre in Switzerland," *Swiss Medical Weekly*, vol. 146, article w14294, 2016.

[11] C. Graidis, D. Dimitriadis, V. Karasavvidis et al., "Prevalence and characteristics of coronary artery anomalies in an adult population undergoing multidetector-row computed tomography for the evaluation of coronary artery disease," *BMC Cardiovascular Disorders*, vol. 15, no. 1, p. 112, 2015.

[12] S. Fujimoto, T. Kondo, T. Orihara et al., "Prevalence of anomalous origin of coronary artery detected by multi-detector computed tomography at one center," *Journal of Cardiology*, vol. 57, no. 1, pp. 69–76, 2011.

[13] K. H. Soon, J. Selvanayagam, K. W. Bell et al., "Giant single coronary system with coronary cameral fistula diagnosed on MSCT," *International Journal of Cardiology*, vol. 106, no. 2, pp. 276–278, 2006.

[14] S. Shrivastava, J. C. Mohan, S. Mukhopadhyay, M. Rajani, and R. Tandon, "Coronary artery anomalies in tetralogy of Fallot," *CardioVascular and Interventional Radiology*, vol. 10, no. 4, pp. 215–218, 1987.

[15] S. A. Said, W. G. De Voogt, S. Bulut et al., "Coronary artery disease in congenital single coronary artery in adults: a Dutch case series," *World Journal of Cardiology*, vol. 6, no. 4, pp. 196–204, 2014.

[16] J. A. Poynter, W. G. Williams, S. McIntyre et al., "Anomalous aortic origin of a coronary artery: a report from the congenital heart surgeons society registry," *World Journal for Pediatric and Congenital Heart Surgery*, vol. 5, no. 1, pp. 22–30, 2014.

[17] E. Ermis, S. Demirelli, A. F. Korkmaz, B. D. Sahin, and A. Kantarci, "An isolated single L-II type coronary artery anomaly: a rare coronary anomaly," *Intractable & Rare Diseases Research*, vol. 4, no. 4, pp. 203–206, 2015.

[18] R. S. Al-Umairi, F. A. Al-Kindi, and S. A. Al-Tai, "A new variant of dual left anterior descending artery anomaly: type XI," *Sultan Qaboos University Medical Journal [SQUMJ]*, vol. 18, no. 3, pp. 386–388, 2018.

[19] A. Canbay, O. Ozcan, S. Aydoğdu, and E. Diker, "Single coronary artery anomaly: a report of three cases," *Turk Kardiyoloji Dernegi Arsivi: Turk Kardiyoloji Derneginin Yayin Organidir*, vol. 36, no. 7, pp. 473–475, 2008.

[20] O. Yamanaka and R. E. Hobbs, "Coronary artery anomalies in 126,595 patients undergoing coronary arteriography," *Catheterization and Cardiovascular Diagnosis*, vol. 21, no. 1, pp. 28–40, 1990.

[21] G. Rigatelli, G. Docali, P. Rossi, A. Bandello, and G. Rigatelli, "Validation of a clinical-significance-based classification of coronary artery anomalies," *Angiology*, vol. 56, no. 1, pp. 25–34, 2005.

[22] A. J. Taylor, K. M. Rogan, and R. Virmani, "Sudden cardiac death associated with isolated congenital coronary artery anomalies," *Journal of the American College of Cardiology*, vol. 20, no. 3, pp. 640–647, 1992.

[23] H. Evrengul, E. E. Ozcan, H. Turhan, and A. Ozturk, "Single coronary artery originating from the right sinus of Valsalva and hypoplastic left anterior descending artery: an extremely rare combination of congenital coronary artery anomalies," *Experimental & Clinical Cardiology*, vol. 17, no. 4, pp. 243-244, 2012.

[24] N. H. Bunce, C. H. Lorenz, J. Keegan et al., "Coronary artery anomalies: assessment with free-breathing three-dimensional coronary MR angiography," *Radiology*, vol. 227, no. 1, pp. 201–208, 2003.

[25] J. Datta, C. S. White, R. C. Gilkeson et al., "Anomalous coronary arteries in adults: depiction at multi-detector row CT angiography," *Radiology*, vol. 235, no. 3, pp. 812–818, 2005.

[26] E. Venturini and L. Magni, "Single coronary artery from the right sinus of Valsalva," *Heart International*, vol. 6, no. 1, article hi.2011.e5, 2011.

[27] N. Aldana-Sepulveda, C. S. Restrepo, and E. Kimura-Hayama, "Single coronary artery: spectrum of imaging findings with multidetector CT," *Journal of Cardiovascular Computed Tomography*, vol. 7, no. 6, pp. 391–399, 2013.

[28] S. Mavrogeni, K. Spargias, S. Karagiannis et al., "Anomalous origin of right coronary artery: magnetic resonance angiography

and viability study," *International Journal of Cardiology*, vol. 109, no. 2, pp. 195–200, 2006.

[29] A. Elbadawi, B. Baig, I. Y. Elgendy et al., "Single coronary artery anomaly: a case report and review of literature," *Cardiology and Therapy*, vol. 7, no. 1, pp. 119–123, 2018.

[30] L.-F. Hong, S.-H. Luo, and J.-J. Li, "Percutaneous coronary intervention with anomalous origin of right coronary artery: case reports and literature review," *Journal of Geriatric Cardiology*, vol. 10, no. 2, pp. 205–209, 2013.

[31] S.-H. Cho, H.-C. Joo, K.-J. Yoo, and Y.-N. Youn, "Anomalous origin of right coronary artery from left coronary sinus: surgical management and clinical result," *The Thoracic and Cardiovascular Surgeon*, vol. 63, no. 5, pp. 360–366, 2015.

[32] C. S. Ong, C. S. Cameron, and M. L. Jacobs, "Surgical management of anomalous coronary arteries," *Annals of Cardiothoracic Surgery*, vol. 7, no. 5, pp. 604–610, 2018.

8

Proportion of Variant Anatomy of the Circle of Willis and Association with Vascular Anomalies on Cerebral CT Angiography

Roy Munialo Machasio,[1] **Rose Nyabanda,**[2] **and Timothy Musila Mutala**[1]

[1] *University of Nairobi, Department of Diagnostic Imaging and Radiation Medicine, Kenya*
[2] *Kenyatta National Hospital, Kenya*

Correspondence should be addressed to Roy Munialo Machasio; rmachasio@gmail.com

Academic Editor: Paul Sijens

Background and Purpose. There is a wide variation in the anatomy of the CW in different individuals and population groups. The purpose of this study was to determine the proportion of variant anatomy of the circle of Willis (CW) and associated anomalies in patients with suspected cerebrovascular disease referred for cerebral computed tomography angiography (CTA) in two tertiary hospitals in Kenya. *Methodology.* This was a cross-sectional descriptive study conducted on 94 patients referred for cerebral CTA at the Kenyatta and Nairobi hospitals from August 2017 to February 2018. MIP and 3D reformatted images were analyzed by two senior radiologists to determine the final configuration of the CW and presence of vascular pathology. Vessels with diameters <0.8 mm were considered to be absent or hypoplastic. Chen et al. classification was used to determine the final configuration of CW. *Results.* Complete CW was seen in 37.2% (37.7% vs. 36.6% in males and females, respectively, p=0.909). Type A variant was the commonest anterior variant at 78.7%. Type E variant was the dominant posterior variant at 41.5%. Fetal PCA was demonstrated in 25.5%, unilateral > bilateral fetal PCA. Aneurysms were seen in 24.5% of patients. ACoA aneurysms were commonest at 43.6%. AVMs were seen in 8.5% of patients. Azygous ACA, fenestration, and duplication of vessels and persistent TA were not demonstrated. There is no significant association between aneurysms/AVMs and CW configuration. *Conclusion.* The findings in this study demonstrate slight differences in the CW configuration. A higher proportion of complete anterior CW was seen in female patients. Type A anterior and type E posterior circulation variants were the commonest in both males and females. No significant association was demonstrated between CW configuration and occurrence of aneurysms/AVMs in this study. Various methods of classification of CW configuration have been proposed with no standardized method to date, thus the need for consensus building between neuroanatomists, neurologists, neurosurgeons, and neuroradiologists for ease of comparison between similar future studies on the CW.

1. Introduction

The circle of Willis (CW) is an important anastomotic arterial polygon at the base of the brain that connects the carotid and vertebrobasilar systems [1–3]. It is an essential route for collateral supply of blood to the brain in cases of occlusion in either system [4, 5]. CW variants include fenestration, duplication, hypoplasia, or agenesis [6]. These variants influence the cerebral blood flow hemodynamics with influence on vascular territories, pathophysiology of cerebral arterial remodeling, aneurysm formation/rupture, and stroke development [7–11]. A complete CW configuration has also been associated with reduced risk of intracranial hemorrhage following intravenous thrombolysis in patients with ischaemic stroke [12]. Persistent embryonic carotid-vertebrobasilar anastomosis such as hypoglossal, proatlantal, otic, and persistent trigeminal arteries are extremely rare occurring in about 0.1%-0.6% of the general population [13]. CT angiography (CTA) is a fast reliable noninvasive method for evaluation of the circle of Willis as well as other intracranial arteries and aneurysms with high sensitivity and specificity comparable to gold standard catheter angiography [14].

TABLE 1: Percentage distribution of complete vs incomplete CW in males vs female patients.

GENDER	PERCENTAGE DISTRIBUTION OF CW CONFIGURATION	
	COMPLETE	INCOMPLETE
MALE	37.7% (n = 20)	62.3% (n = 33)
FEMALE	36.6% (n = 15)	63.4% (n = 26)
COMBINED(MALE AND FEMALE)	37.2% (n = 35)	62.8% (n = 59)

Various methods have been proposed for classification of the morphology of the CW due to complex anterior and posterior circulation variations [1, 15–17]. Chen et al. classified variations in both anterior and posterior CW from A-J [18, 19]. For the purposes of this study, Chen et al. classification was used due to its simplicity as compared to the other methods.

The goal of the current study was to establish the proportion of variant anatomy of the CW and associated anomalies in patients with suspected cerebrovascular disease referred for cerebral CTA in two tertiary hospitals in Kenya.

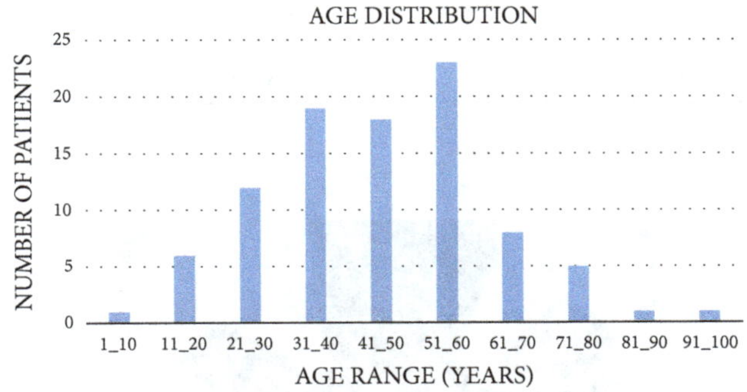

FIGURE 1: Age distribution of patients referred for cerebral CTA.

2. Materials and Methods

This was a cross-sectional descriptive study carried out on patients referred for cerebral CTA at Kenyatta National Hospital and Nairobi Hospital, both located in Nairobi County, Kenya.

CT image acquisition was done by SIEMENS SOMATOM definition AS +128 and PHILLIP'S BRILLIANCE 64 SLICE at Kenyatta and Nairobi hospitals, respectively.

Nonenhanced scans were acquired first to demonstrate hemorrhage or calcification.

80 mls of LOCM (300mg/ml) via pump injector at injection rate of 5mls/second through an antecubital vein cannula (at least gauge 20) with a delay time of 7 seconds was used for acquisition of images in adult patients at Kenyatta National Hospital.

20 mls saline push before contrast administration, followed by 60 mls of LOCM at an injection rate of 4-5 mls/s via pump injector and 30 mls of saline chase with a scan delay time of 4.2 seconds, was used at Nairobi Hospital.

For young children and infants, a 22- or 24-gauge IV catheter was used and LOCM used at an injection rate of 2 mls/second.

A total of 94 patients (53 males and 41 females) referred for cerebral CTA at Kenyatta National Hospital and Nairobi Hospital from August 2017 to February 2018 were included. MIP and 3D cerebral CTA images were analyzed for anatomic variants and pathology. A cut-off value 0.8 mm vessel diameter was used. Any vessel less than 0.8 mm was considered hypoplastic/absent. Final configuration and pathology were confirmed by 2 senior radiologists. Patient's age, gender, anatomic variants of the circle of Willis, and presence of aneurysms and AVMs were recorded in the patient data sheet.

Statistical analysis using SPSS version 20.0 was done to determine association between the variants with aneurysms and arteriovenous malformations. P value was set at 0.05.

3. Results

Male patients accounted for 56.4% while 43.6% were female patients with and approx. male to female ratio of 1:1.

The age distribution of patients referred for cerebral CTA is depicted in Figure 1.

Majority of patients were referred for cerebral CTA due to clinically suspected intracranial hemorrhage accounting for 30.85%. Other clinical indications included suspected AVMs, aneurysms, cerebral sinus thrombosis, stroke, trauma, and tumor.

4. Proportion of Complete vs. Incomplete Circle of Willis

A complete CW was seen in 37.2% of the patients with no statistically significant difference between males and females (p=0.9) as shown in Table 1.

Figure 2 depicts a patient with complete circle of Willis in our study.

5. Anterior and Posterior Circulation Variants

Type A variant accounted for 78.7% of the anterior circulation variants and was significantly higher in females than male patients (p=0.016) as demonstrated in Table 2.

Figure 3 demonstrates a patient with combined type A anterior and type E posterior circulation variants.

Type E posterior circulation variant was the commonest seen accounting for 41.5% of the posterior circulation variants (Table 3).

TABLE 2: Anterior circulation variant percentage distribution.

ANTERIOR CW	FREQUENCY (IN BOTH MALE AND FEMALES)	FREQUENCY IN MALES	FREQUENCY IN FEMALES
TYPEA	78.7% (n=74)	69.8% (n=37)	90.2% (n=37)
TYPE B	0% (n=0)		
TYPE C	1.1% (n=1)		
TYPE D	4.3% (n=4)		
TYPE E	0% (n=0)		
TYPE F	0% (n=0)		
TYPE G	4.3% (n=4)		
TYPE H	11.7% (n=11)		
TYPE I	0% (n=0)		
TYPE J	0% (n=0)		

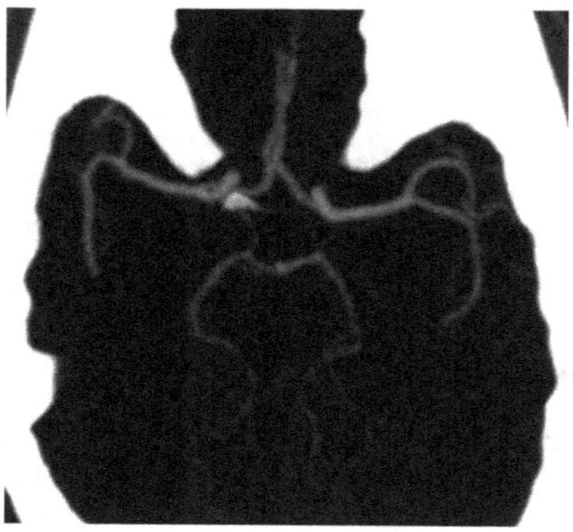

FIGURE 2: Axial cerebral CTA MIP image showing a complete CW configuration.

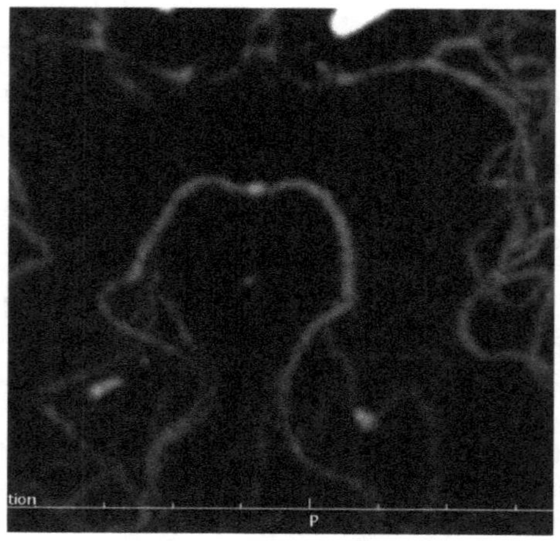

FIGURE 3: Axial MIP image showing combined type A anterior circulation variant and type E posterior circulation variant.

TABLE 3: Proportion of posterior circulation variants.

POSTERIOR CW	FREQUENCY
TYPE A	27.7% (26)
TYPE B	4.3% (4)
TYPE C	7.4% (7)
TYPE D	4.3% (4)
TYPE E	41.5% (39)
TYPE F	2.1% (2)
TYPE G	7.4% (7)
TYPE H	0% (0)
TYPE I	0% (0)
TYPE J	5.3% (5)

6. Complete Anterior Circulation Variants (TYPES A-F)

A complete anterior CW configuration was seen in 84%. The proportion of this configuration was significantly higher in females than males (92.7% vs. 77.4%, p=0.044).

7. Complete Posterior Circulation Variants (TYPES A-C)

A complete posterior CW configuration was seen in 39.4% (39.6% vs. 39% in males and females, respectively, p=0.953).

7.1. Adult Configuration of the Posterior Cerebral Arteries. There was a significantly higher proportion of adult PCA configuration in females than males (95%vs 81% p=0.044).

8. Fetal PCA

Fetal PCA (Figure 4) was seen in 25.5% (28.3% vs. 22.0% in males and females, respectively, p=0.484).

9. Presence of Aneurysms and Location

Aneurysms were seen in 24.5% of the patients referred for cerebral CTA (Table 4).

Figure 5 demonstrates a saccular aneurysm involving the ACoA.

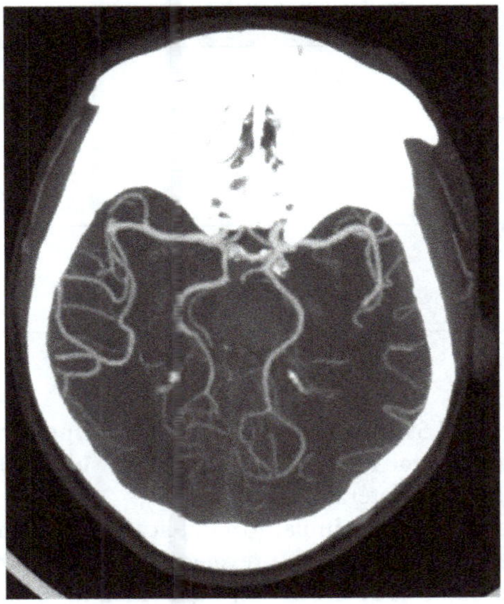

Figure 4: Axial cerebral CTA image showing bilateral fetal PCA with right P1 segment aplasia.

Table 4: Distribution of intracranial aneurysms.

Location of aneurysms		
ACOA	10	43.60%
MCA	5	21.70%
ICA	5	21.70%
Other vessels than	3	13.00%

10. Association of CW Configuration and Aneurysms

There was no association between CW configuration and presence of aneurysms as shown in Table 5.

11. Presence of Cerebral Arteriovenous Malformations

AVMs were seen in 8 (8.5%) of patients undergoing cerebral CTA (Figure 6). No association was found between CW configuration and presence of AVM (P=0.987).

Fenestrations, duplications, azygous ACA, and persistent TA were not observed in this study.

12. Discussion

Previous anatomic, CTA, and MRA studies have demonstrated significant variations in the configuration of the CW in various population groups.

The purpose of this study was to determine the proportion of variant anatomy of the circle of Willis (CW) and associated anomalies in patients with suspected cerebrovascular disease referred for cerebral CTA in 2 tertiary Kenyan hospitals. No similar studies on the CW configuration have been done in Kenya.

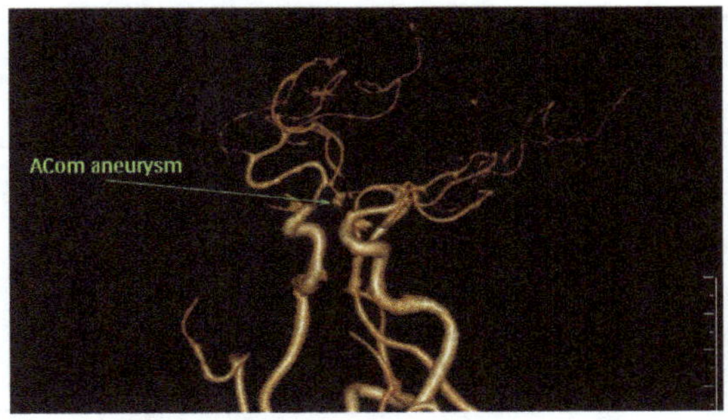

Figure 5: 3D cerebral CTA showing a saccular aneurysm at the ACoA.

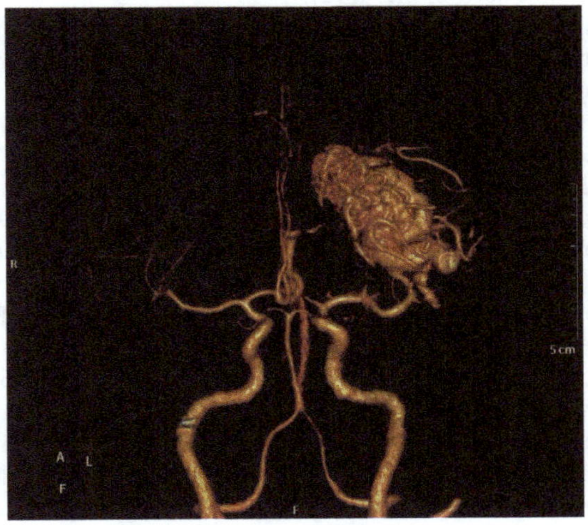

Figure 6: 3D cerebral CTA image showing an AVM with feeding artery arising from the left MCA.

Variations in the CW configuration have been associated with cerebrovascular diseases [20, 21].

Various methods have been proposed for classification of variant anatomy of CW. The classification of CW configuration in this study is based on the Chen et al. classification which classified anterior and posterior variants into 10 groups (A-J) [18, 19].

The proportion of patients with complete CW configuration was 37.2% (n=35). This was slightly higher in males than females: 37.7% vs. 36.6%. The findings in the current study are consistent with previous studies which have demonstrated a prevalence of between 12.24%-60% [19, 22]. An MRA-TOF study by Chuanya Qiu et al. on 2246 healthy Chinese male population showed a lower prevalence of complete CW at 12.24% [4]. In contrast, an Egyptian MRA-TOF study by Mohammed Abdelatif et al. on 180 patients with no manifestations of cerebrovascular disease showed a higher prevalence of complete CW in 46.7% [23]. In our study, patients with cerebrovascular diseases referred for cerebral CTA were included unlike the above two MRA-TOF studies which were conducted on patients with no manifestations of cerebrovascular disease. The findings in the current study could thus be attributed to the difference in the study

Table 5: Presence and number of aneurysms in complete and incomplete CW.

Characteristics	Total	Circle of WILLS anatomy		P value
		Incomplete	Complete	
Presence of Aneurysm				
No	71(75.5%)	43(72.9%)	28(80.0%)	0.438
Yes	23(24.5%)	16(27.1%)	7(20.0%)	
Number of Aneurysms				
1 Aneurysm	18(78.3%)	12(75.0%)	6(85.7%)	0.567
More than 1 Aneurysm	5(21.7%)	4(25.0%)	1(14.3%)	

population, technique used, racial differences, and the lower sample size used in this study.

An incomplete CW configuration was seen in 62.8% of patients, 62.3% in males versus 63.4% in females. Previous studies have demonstrated a correlation between an incomplete CW and stroke severity and prognosis [10, 24].

According to the Chen et al., classification type A-F anterior variants are considered to be complete [18]. In our study, a complete anterior CW was seen in 84% (n=79). A complete anterior CW was significantly higher in female than male patients (92.7% vs. 77.4%, p=0.04). The prevalence of complete anterior CW in this study was higher than an MRA-TOF study by Sherif Mohamed Zaki et al. on 100 patents with no evidence of cerebrovascular disease which showed a prevalence of 66% [25]. The finding in our study was also higher than an MRA-TOF study by Shartri J et al. on 513 adults without cerebrovascular disease which demonstrated a complete anterior CW in 64.3% [26]. The higher prevalence of a complete anterior CW in our study could be due to higher spatial resolution of CTA as compared to MRA, sample size differences, and racial differences.

The commonest anterior circulation variant was type A variant accounting for 78.7% (n=74). This configuration was seen in 69.8% (n=37) and 90.2% (n=37) of males and females, respectively. This finding is similar to studies done by Naveen SR et al. and Dr. Arjun Bhaddur et al. which showed type A variant being the most common anterior circulation variant [27, 28].

Type E posterior variant has been associated with increased risk of ischaemic stroke [8]. This variant is of importance to surgeons and neurologists in the evaluation of patients with intracranial tumors, traumatic injuries, and cardiovascular complications [29].

In our study, type E posterior circulation variant was the commonest posterior circulation variant accounting for 41.5%. This study finding is similar to findings on an MRA-TOF study by Reddy Ravikanth et al. which demonstrated a predominance of type E posterior circulation at 53% [30].

A cerebral CTA study done by Zhang Ning Jin et al. on Chinese population with family history of stroke showed dominance of type E posterior variant with a prevalence of 52.3% [4], which is higher than the current study. The slight difference in prevalence of type E posterior variant could be due to racial and sample size differences.

In the current study, fetal PCA was seen in 30.9% (n=29). Complete PCA was demonstrated in 6.4% while partial PCA was seen in 24.5%. Unilateral fetal PCA was more common than bilateral fetal PCA. 12.8% were right sided, 10.6% left sided, and 5.6% bilateral fetal PCA.

These findings are similar to a publication by Dimmick SJ Faulder et al. which show a prevalence of 15%-32% for fetal PCA with bilateral fPCA at 8%, right sided at 10%, and left sided fPCA at 10% [13]. Fetal PCA has been found to increase the extent and severity of anterior circulation stroke as well as aneurysm formation [11, 31].

In the current study, aneurysms were seen in 24.5% (n=23) of patients referred for cerebral CTA. 69.6% of the aneurysms were located in the anterior CW while 4.3% were located in the posterior CW. 78.3% of patients had one aneurysm while 21.7% had more than 1 aneurysm.

26.1% (n=6) were located in other vessels other than the CW. The prevalence of aneurysms in this study is lower than that in an earlier Kenyan study by Chepsiror et al. based on conventional angiography which showed a higher prevalence of aneurysms at 40.9% and anterior circulation aneurysms at 95.2% [32]. The study by Chepsiror et al. was done on 88 patients with suspected cerebrovascular disease who were referred for conventional angiography in the two tertiary hospitals in Kenya. The difference in general prevalence of aneurysms in the two studies could be due to the higher sensitivity of conventional angiography for aneurysm detection.

In the current study, ACoA aneurysms were the commonest at 43.6% (n=10).

21.7% were located in the MCA, 21.7% were located in the ICA, and 13% were seen in other vessels than the CW. These findings are similar to a multimodality study on size and location of ruptured intracranial aneurysms by Young Gyun et al. which showed that a majority of aneurysms were located in the ACoA [33]. These study findings are, however, in contrast to a conventional angiographic study on pattern of cerebrovascular disease in Kenyatta and Nairobi hospitals done by Chepsiror et al. which showed 30.6% at ICA-PCoA, ACoA 22.2%, and MCA bifurcation 13% [32].

AVMs were seen in 8.5% (n=8) in the current study.

62.5% (n=5) had incomplete CW while 37.5% (n=3) had a complete CW configuration.

These study findings are similar to an earlier Kenyan conventional angiographic study by Chepsiror et al. which showed a prevalence of 8% [32].

Association between duplication and fenestration of intracranial arteries with aneurysmal formation has been documented in previous studies [13, 34]. Fenestration and duplication of CW were not observed in our study. Previous publication by Dimmick SJ Faulder et al. has shown a low prevalence for duplications and fenestrations in angiographic studies of 0.058% [13]. A similarly low prevalence of anterior circulation fenestration at 0.48% was demonstrated in a study by Roger M et al. on 411 patients undergoing cerebral CTA [35].

In the study by Roger M et al., patients with intracranial pathology such as subarachnoid hemorrhage, stroke, tumor, and aneurysms were excluded from the study. In a previous Kenyan cadaveric study by Hassan Said et al. on 36 adult brains, fenestration and duplication of ACoA were seen in 26% and 13%, respectively [36]. Another study by Dhanalakshmi V et al. on 50 adult cadaveric brains showed a relatively lower prevalence of duplications and fenestration of the ACoA at 8% and 4%, respectively [37]. The absence of fenestration and duplication in our study could be due to the general low incidence of duplications and fenestrations on angiographic studies, low sample size, and the unexplained discrepancy between angiographic and cadaveric studies.

Persistent trigeminal artery was not demonstrated in the current study. There is a general low prevalence of persistent trigeminal artery at 0.1-0.6% of all cerebral angiograms [38]. The absence of this variant could be explained based on the low prevalence in the general population and the low sample size used in this study.

In our study, no case of azygous anterior cerebral artery was identified. In a previous publication on aneurysms of the azygous anterior cerebral artery by Rajesh Kumar et al., prevalence of azygous ACA was quoted at <1% with a range of 0.21%-3.73% [39]. The finding in our study could be attributed to the low prevalence of azygous ACA in the general population and the lower sample size.

In the current study no association was found between the CW configuration and presence of aneurysms (p=0.567). These findings are similar to a retrospective cerebral CTA study by P. Brzegowy et al. which showed no association between anatomic variations of the MCA and CW with aneurysms [40].

There was no significant correlation between CW configuration and occurrence of AVMs (P=0.987).

13. Conclusion

The findings in this study demonstrate slight differences in the CW configuration. A higher proportion of complete anterior CW was seen in female patients. Type A anterior and type E posterior circulation variants were the commonest in both males and females. No significant association was demonstrated between CW configuration and occurrence of aneurysms/AVMs in this study. Various methods of classification of CW configuration have been proposed with no standardized method to date, thus the need for consensus building between neuroanatomists, neurologists, neurosurgeons, and neuroradiologists for ease of comparison between similar future studies on the CW.

Disclosure

This manuscript was submitted to the University of Nairobi as part of fulfillment for master's degree in diagnostic radiology.

References

[1] S. Kathuria, L. Gregg, J. Chen, and D. Gandhi, "Normal cerebral arterial development and variations," *Seminars in Ultrasound, CT and MRI*, vol. 32, no. 3, pp. 242–251, 2011.

[2] J. Rosner and F. Lui, "Neuroanatomy, Circle of Willis," in *StatPearls*, StatPearls Publishing, Treasure Island, FL, USA, 2019.

[3] T. Takakuwa, T. Koike, T. Muranaka, C. Uwabe, and S. Yamada, "Formation of the circle of Willis during human embryonic development," *Congenital Anomalies*, vol. 56, no. 5, pp. 233–236, 2016.

[4] C. Qiu, Y. Zhang, C. Xue, S. Jiang, and W. Zhang, "MRA study on variation of the circle of Willis in healthy Chinese male adults," *BioMed Research International*, vol. 2015, Article ID 976340, 8 pages, 2015.

[5] B. M. Carlson, *Human Embryology and Developmental Biology*, Elsevier/Saunders, Philadelphia, Penn, USA, 5th edition, 2014.

[6] K. Menshawi, J. P. Mohr, and J. Gutierrez, "A functional perspective on the embryology and anatomy of the cerebral blood supply," *Journal of Stroke*, vol. 17, no. 2, pp. 144–158, 2015.

[7] M. A. Lazzaro, B. Ouyang, and M. Chen, "The role of circle of Willis anomalies in cerebral aneurysm rupture," *Journal of NeuroInterventional Surgery*, vol. 4, no. 1, pp. 22–26, 2011.

[8] T. van Seeters, J. Hendrikse, G. J. Biessels et al., "Completeness of the circle of Willis and risk of ischemic stroke in patients without cerebrovascular disease," *Neuroradiology*, vol. 57, no. 12, pp. 1247–1251, 2015.

[9] M. Polguj, M. Majos, M. Topol, and A. Majos, "An asymmetrical fenestration of the basilar artery coexisting with two aneurysms in a patient with Subarachnoid haemorrhage: Case report and review of the literature," *Folia Morphologica (Poland)*, vol. 73, no. 2, pp. 229–233, 2014.

[10] H. Zhou, J. Sun, X. Ji et al., "Correlation between the integrity of the circle of willis and the severity of initial noncardiac cerebral infarction and clinical prognosis," *Medicine*, vol. 95, no. 10, p. e2892, 2016.

[11] Z. He and Y. Wan, "Is fetal-type posterior cerebral artery a risk factor for intracranial aneurysm as analyzed by multislice CT angiography?" *Experimental and Therapeutic Medicine*, vol. 15, no. 1, pp. 838–846, 2018.

[12] Y.-M. Chuang, L. Chan, Y.-J. Lai et al., "Configuration of the Circle of Willis is associated with less symptomatic intracerebral hemorrhage in ischemic stroke patients treated with intravenous thrombolysis," *Journal of Critical Care*, vol. 28, no. 2, pp. 166–172, 2013.

[13] S. J. Dimmick and K. C. Faulder, "Normal variants of the cerebral circulation at multidetector CT angiography," *RadioGraphics*, vol. 29, no. 4, pp. 1027–1043, 2009.

[14] Z. L. Yang, Q. Q. Ni, U. J. Schoepf et al., "Small intracranial aneurysms: Diagnostic accuracy of CT angiography," *Radiology*, vol. 285, no. 3, pp. 941–952, 2017.

[15] H. P. Dorcas, "The development of the cranial arteries in the human embryo," *Contributions to Embryology*, vol. 32, no. 212, pp. 205–262, 1948.

[16] A. Zurada and J. S. Gielecki, "A novel formula for the classification of blood vessels according to symmetry, asymmetry and hypoplasia," *Folia Morphologica*, vol. 66, no. 4, pp. 339–345, 2007.

[17] M. J. Krabbe-Hartkamp, J. Van Der Grond, F.-E. De Leeuw et al., "Circle of Willis: morphologic variation on three-dimensional time-of- flight MR angiograms," *Radiology*, vol. 207, no. 1, pp. 103–112, 1998.

[18] Q. Li, J. Li, F. Lv, K. Li, T. Luo, and P. Xie, "A multidetector CT angiography study of variations in the circle of Willis in a Chinese population," *Journal of Clinical Neuroscience*, vol. 18, no. 3, pp. 379–383, 2011.

[19] H.-W. Chen, P.-S. Yen, C.-C. Lee et al., "Magnetic resonance angiographic evaluation of circle of Willis in general population: a morphologic study in 507 cases," *Chinese Journal of Radiology-Taipei*, vol. 29, no. 5, pp. 223–229, 2004.

[20] J. A. Ogeng'o, P. M. Mwachaka, D. E. Odhiambo et al., "Geometric features of vertebrobasilar arterial system in adult black kenyans," *International Journal of Morphology*, vol. 36, no. 2, pp. 544–550, 2018.

[21] Z. Liu, Y. Cai, G.-Z. Chen, G.-M. Lu, and Z.-Y. Li, "Anatomical variations in circle of willis and intracranial aneurysm formation," *Molecular & Cellular Biomechanics*, vol. 14, pp. 19–31, 2017.

[22] M. J. Krabbe-Hartkamp, J. Van Der Grond, K. J. Van Everdingen, B. Hillen, and W. P. T. M. Mali, "Circle of Willis collateral flow investigated by magnetic resonance angiography," *Stroke*, vol. 30, no. 12, pp. 2671–2678, 1999.

[23] M. A. Maaly and A. A. Ismail, "Three dimensional magnetic resonance angiography of the circle of Willis: anatomical variations in general Egyptian population," *The Egyptian Journal of Radiology & Nuclear Medicine*, vol. 42, no. 3-4, pp. 405–412, 2011.

[24] C. Zhou, C. Yuan, R. Li, W. Wang, C. Li, and X. Zhao, "Association between incomplete circle of willis and carotid vulnerable atherosclerotic plaques," *Arteriosclerosis, Thrombosis, and Vascular Biology*, vol. 38, no. 11, pp. 2744–2749, 2018.

[25] S. M. Zaki, M. H. Shaaban, W. A. Abd Al Galeel, and A. A. El Husseiny, "Configuration of the circle of Willis and its two parts among Egyptian: a magnetic resonance angiographic study," *Folia Morphologica*, 2019.

[26] J. Shatri, S. Cerkezi, V. Ademi, V. Reci, and S. Bexheti, "Anatomical variations and dimensions of arteries in the anterior part of the circle of Willis," *Folia Morphologica*, 2018.

[27] S. R. Naveen, V. Bhat, and G. A. Karthik, "Magnetic resonance angiographic evaluation of circle of Willis: A morphologic study in a tertiary hospital set up," *Annals of Indian Academy of Neurology*, vol. 18, no. 4, pp. 391–397, 2015.

[28] Arjun Bahaddur and G. Chandan, "Anatomic variants of circle of willis in South Indian population:a study by using magnetic resonance angiography," *International Journal of Science Research*, 2013.

[29] E. S. Sussman, C. P. Kellner, J. L. Mergeche et al., "Radiographic absence of the posterior communicating arteries and the prediction of cognitive dysfunction after carotid endarterectomy: Clinical article," *Journal of Neurosurgery*, vol. 121, no. 3, pp. 593–598, 2014.

[30] R. Ravikanth and B. Philip, "Magnetic resonance angiography determined variations in the circle of Willis: Analysis of a large series from a single center," *Tzu Chi Medical Journal*, vol. 31, no. 1, p. 52, 2019.

[31] S. L. Lambert, F. J. Williams, Z. Z. Oganisyan, L. A. Branch, and E. C. Mader, "Fetal-type variants of the posterior cerebral artery and concurrent infarction in the major arterial territories of the cerebral hemisphere," *Journal of Investigative Medicine High Impact Case Reports*, vol. 4, no. 3, Article ID 2324709616665409, 2016.

[32] D. K. Chepsiror, *The pattern of radiological findings seen in four-vessel cerebral angiography done at the KNH and Nairobi Hospital [Thesis]*, University of Nairobi, Nairobi, Kenya, 2006.

[33] Y.-G. Jeong, Y.-T. Jung, M.-S. Kim, C.-K. Eun, and S.-H. Jang, "Size and location of ruptured intracranial aneurysms," *Journal of Korean Neurosurgical Society*, vol. 45, no. 1, pp. 11–15, 2009.

[34] W. P. Sanders, P. A. Sorek, and B. A. Mehta, "Fenestration of intracranial arteries with special attention to associated aneurysms and other anomalies," *American Journal of Neuroradiology*, vol. 14, no. 3, pp. 675–680, 1993.

[35] R. M. Krzyżewski, K. A. Tomaszewski, M. Kochana, M. Kopeć, W. Klimek-Piotrowska, and J. A. Walocha, "Anatomical variations of the anterior communicating artery complex: gender relationship," *Surgical and Radiologic Anatomy*, vol. 37, no. 1, pp. 81–86, 2014.

[36] S. H. Hassan Profs, P. Kitunguu, and J. A. Ogengo, "Variant anatomy of the anterior cerebral artery in Adult Kenyans," *African Journal of Neurological Sciences*, vol. 27, pp. 97–105, 2008.

[37] D. Lakshmi, S. Kumar, S. T. Kumar, and K. A. kumar, "Anterior communicating artery: a cadaveric study," *International Journal of Anatomy and Research*, vol. 7, pp. 6261–6264, 2019.

[38] A. Tomalczyk, Z. Kaurzel, W. Szubert, and P. Oszukowski, "Arteria trigemina primitiva - radiological report of three cases and review of literature," *Folia Morphologica (Poland)*, vol. 76, no. 4, pp. 757–761, 2017.

[39] R. Ghanta, M. Kesanakurthy, and V. Vemuri, "Aneurysm of azygos anterior cerebral artery: A report of two cases," *Asian Journal of Neurosurgery*, vol. 11, no. 3, p. 312, 2016.

[40] P. Brzegowy, J. Polak, J. Wnuk, B. Łasocha, J. Walocha, and T. J. Popiela, "Middle cerebral artery anatomical variations and aneurysms: A retrospective study based on computed tomography angiography findings," *Folia Morphologica (Poland)*, vol. 77, no. 3, pp. 434–440, 2018.

9

Contribution of Computed Tomography Scan to the Diagnosis of Spinal Tuberculosis in 14 Cases in Assaba, Mauritania

Boushab Mohamed Boushab,[1] **Noukhoum Kone**,[2] **and Leonardo K. Basco**[3,4]

[1]*Department of Internal Medicine and Infectious Diseases, Kiffa Regional Hospital, Assaba, Mauritania*
[2]*Department of Neurosurgery, Kiffa Regional Hospital, Assaba, Mauritania*
[3]*Aix-Marseille Univ, IRD, AP-HM, SSA, VITROME, Marseille, France*
[4]*IHU-Méditerranée Infection, Marseille, France*

Correspondence should be addressed to Boushab Mohamed Boushab; bboushab@gmail.com

Academic Editor: Paul Sijens

Background. The incidence of tuberculosis has increased in recent years in both developed and developing countries. *Objective.* This retrospective study aimed to review all cases of spinal tuberculosis diagnosed at the Department of Internal Medicine and Infectious Diseases in Kiffa Regional Hospital and assess the role of computed tomography (CT) scan in establishing definite diagnosis. *Patients and Methods.* Data were collected from clinical records of patients admitted to the hospital for rachialgia between August 2016 and July 2018. *Results.* Fourteen (12.2%) adults with spinal tuberculosis were found among 115 patients with all forms of tuberculosis during the study period. The mean (± standard deviation) age of our patients was 47.5 ± 22.0 years old with male:female (8/6) sex ratio of 1.3. The mean duration of evolution of the disease was 15 months. The presenting signs and symptoms included rachialgia in most patients (93%), associated with segmental spinal stiffness (50%) and/or neurological complications (50%). Diagnosis was established on the basis of clinical history, clinical examination, standard vertebral column radiography, and CT scan. Vertebral imaging showed a clear predominance of lumbar lesions (57%), followed by dorsal (36%) and cervical (7%) involvement. The evolution under treatment was favorable, with the exception of two cases of medullary compression. *Conclusion.* Spinal tuberculosis is the most common form of osteoarticular tuberculosis. It affects predominantly lumbar and dorsal vertebrae. In the absence of histological confirmation, the presence of back pain associated with major radiological signs of spondylosis disc disease seems to justify the use of CT scan to confirm the diagnosis of this pathology.

1. Introduction

Tuberculosis (TB) is a public health problem worldwide [1]. Spinal tuberculosis, also known as "Pott's disease," is one of the complications affecting about 1 to 2% of all cases of tuberculosis [2–4]. The coexistence of human immunodeficiency virus (HIV), which is endemic in many regions where TB is commonly encountered, adds to the burden and complexity of clinical management [2]. Among different forms of skeletal TB, the spine is most common affected site [5–7], followed by the hip and knees. The exact incidence and prevalence of spinal tuberculosis in most parts of the world are unknown. In countries with a high burden of pulmonary TB, the incidence of spinal TB is expected to be proportionately high. Spinal TB is a serious complication due to the possibility of permanent neurological damage [7].

Computed tomography (CT) scan has become a major contributor to confirm diagnosis, assess the degree of injury, and search for complications of spinal TB [8]. There is no previous study on the description of clinical aspects of spinal TB in Mauritania. The aims of the present study were to determine the prevalence of spinal TB, describe typical radiological aspects found in our patients, and evaluate the importance of CT scan in establishing a reliable diagnosis of spinal TB in a Mauritanian setting.

2. Materials and Methods

This is a retrospective analysis of 115 TB patients admitted in the Department of Internal Medicine and Infectious Diseases of Kiffa Regional Hospital over a period of 2 years (August

2016 - July 2018). The diagnosis of spinal TB was based on a set of clinical, radiological, and therapeutic observations (i.e., a satisfactory evolution under antituberculosis treatment). Diagnosis was not established on the basis of bacteriological or histological examinations due to the lack of a technical platform. However, vertebral CT scan was performed in all patients with suspected spinal TB. Quadruple antituberculosis treatment administered to all patients consisted of the combination regimen: rifampicin (10 mg/kg/day), isoniazid (5 mg/kg/day), ethambutol (20 mg/kg/day), and pyrazinamide (30 mg/kg/day), for two months, followed by dual therapy with rifampicin and isoniazid at the same doses for 10 months. Treatment was started in all patients with radiological confirmation of diagnosis of spinal TB. A favorable response to the treatment was defined as the recovery of the body weight, disappearance of pain and fever, and evidence of radiological improvement. Each patient was seen at least 2 times after completing the full anti-TB treatment course.

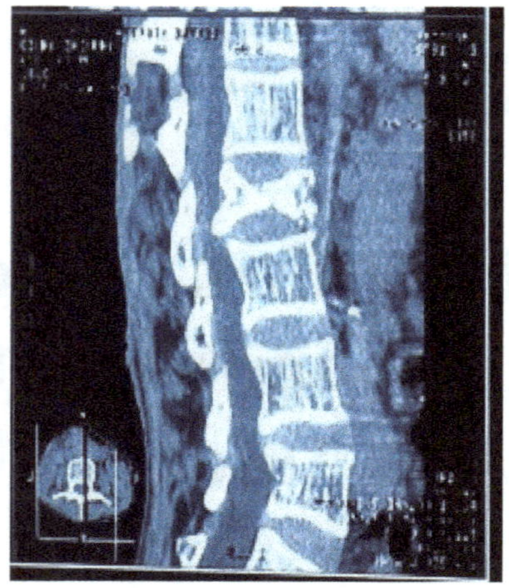

Figure 1: A 45-year-old paraplegic patient with tuberculous spondylitis and osteolysis of L2.

3. Results

During the 2-year study period, 14 (12.2%) cases of spinal tuberculosis were diagnosed among 115 patients with all forms of TB. The mean (± standard deviation [SD]) age of 14 patients was 47.5 ± 22.0 years old. The sex ratio (M/F) was 1.3. Many of the patients (8/14, 57%) came from suburban areas, and 6 of 14 (43%) were jobless. Pulmonary or extrapulmonary (but not spinal) TB was diagnosed prior to consultation in our hospital in 5 (36%) patients. Three patients had a concomitant chronic disease: noninsulin-dependent diabetes, rheumatoid arthritis, or gout. The mean (± SD) time to diagnosis from the appearance of first clinical signs attributable to discovertebral infection was 13.8 ± 4.0 months.

The presenting signs and symptoms were inflammatory rachialgia (13/14 patients; 93%) associated with segmental spinal stiffness (7/14; 50%) or deterioration of the general state and signs of spinal compression (7/14; 50%). CT scan was performed in all 14 patients and confirmed the diagnosis of spinal TB. It showed perilesional osteocondensation (14/14; 100%) and sequestrum (5/14; 36%). According to the topography of the lesions, there was a clear predominance of lumbar lesions (8/14; 57%) (Figure 1), followed by dorsal (5/14; 36%) (Figure 2) and cervical lesions (1/14; 7%) (Figure 3).

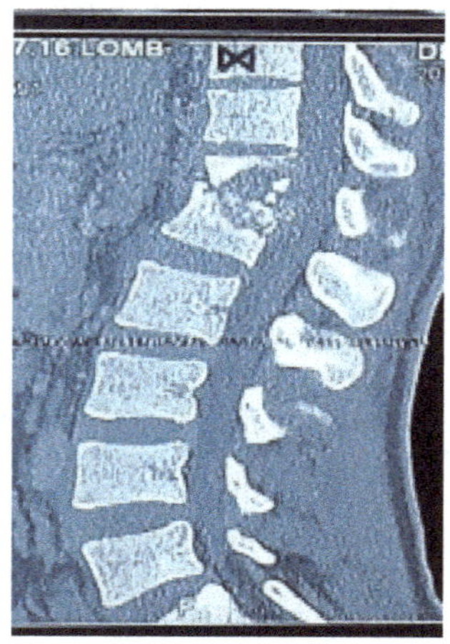

Figure 2: A 60-year-old paraplegic patient with tuberculous spondylitis and osteolysis of D12-L1 and 40° kyphosis.

A quadruple anti-TB treatment was prescribed for the first two months, followed by isoniazid and rifampicin bitherapy for at least the next 10 months. A corset immobilization was indicated in six patients who were at risk. In two patients who presented with neurological complications related to spinal epiduritis, corticosteroid treatment associated with anti-TB chemotherapy resulted in clinical amelioration. During the clinical course of one patient, abscess developed in thoracic spine D11-L2 but was treated successfully with antibiotics (ciprofloxacin 500 mg twice daily for two months). Spinal TB was cured in this patient.

Of 14 patients with spinal TB included in the present study, 11 (79%) recovered without sequelae after 12 months of treatment, 1 patient required surgical intervention (Figure 4), and 2 patients died (Table 1).

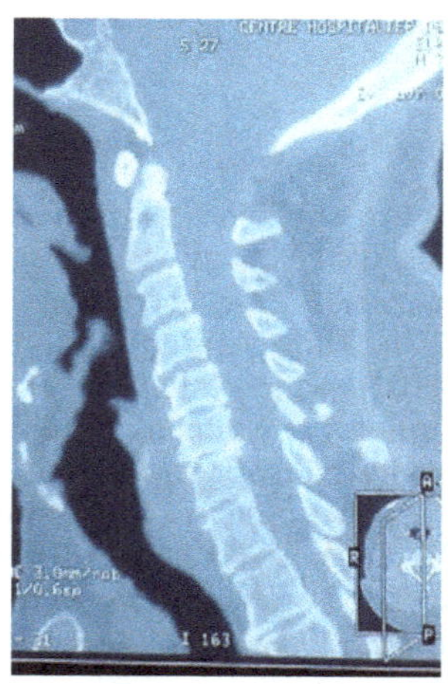

Figure 3: A 57-year-old patient with tuberculous cervical spondylitis and osteophytosis of C4-C5-C6.

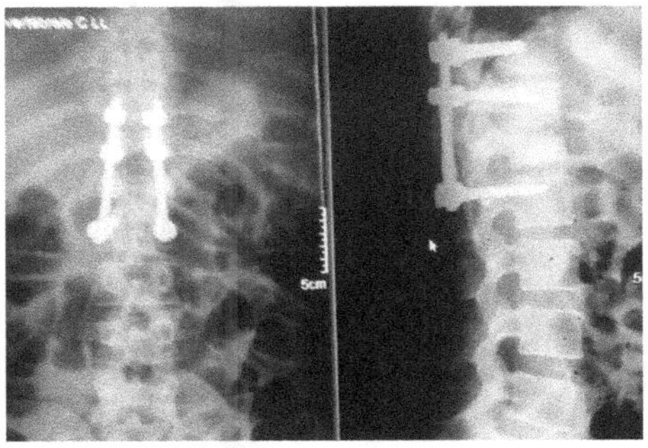

FIGURE 4: After incision of abscess followed by excision of necrotic tissue, corpectomy and fixation of D11-L2 disc using a plating system were performed.

4. Discussion

Spinal TB is commonly observed in developing countries where TB is highly prevalent and is also increasingly observed in developed countries [2, 3]. Although skeletal TB occurs mostly in the spine, followed by the hip, knees, and foot, or ankle, the epidemiology of extrapulmonary TB and in particular musculoskeletal TB remains largely unknown in areas of high prevalence of TB [4]. The average age of our patients at the time of diagnosis was 47.5 years, which was similar to other studies conducted in Africa that reported age of adult patients with musculoskeletal TB ranging from 40 to 60 years [7, 9–11]. A slight male predominance of the disease has often been reported in the literature [8, 12]. As noted by other authors, patients with spinal TB were of lower social class [8, 13], and many of them did not present earlier with signs of pulmonary TB [10]. Several risk factors have been reported, including diabetes, nephropathy, and recent spine surgery [7]. In our study, some patients had diabetes, rheumatoid arthritis, or gout.

The clinical presentation, insidious evolution of signs and symptoms, and the absence of prominent general signs are generally responsible for a diagnostic delay ranging from 1 to 26 months [6, 8, 14]. In our series, the average delay was 13.8 months, which was due to the frequent use of traditional medicine for initial therapy, poor access to health facilities, and poverty. The majority of patients were afebrile during the first visit, and routine laboratory examinations were not helpful in establishing the diagnosis. Inflammatory rachialgia with segmental spinal stiffness was the major presenting symptoms. However, the total absence of an inflammatory syndrome does not exclude the diagnosis of spinal TB since 12 to 50% of patients may have no biological signs of inflammation [15]. Half of our patients had neurological complications, similar to the reports from other authors, i.e., 20 to 50% [7, 8, 16]. The neurological deficit depends on the extension of the infectious process, compression, and epidural extension [17].

Standard radiography suggested spinal TB in our patients. However, standard vertebral X-ray may be normal even in the presence of spinal TB [18]. In such cases, CT scan is a valuable diagnostic tool, especially in detecting abscess within the vertebral canal. Bone destruction is well visualized in CT scan. The association of bone lesions with sequestrum and peritoneal abscess containing bone fragments is, in some patients, pathognomonic of TB [7, 19]. The presence of a bone sequestrum, osteosclerosis, and epidural or soft tissue abscess is an important element in orienting the diagnosis [19, 20].

The distribution of lesions along the spinal column observed in our series, with the thoracolumbar area being most affected, has also been reported by other authors in adult patients [6–8, 21, 22]. This finding is explained by the spread of TB from the initial pulmonary focus via vertebral, intercostal, and lumbar arteries [23]. Cervical involvement is rare, accounting for about 5% of spinal TB [7, 24]. Cervical involvement was observed in one patient in our study. Usually, pain associated with spinal TB affects 2 vertebral segments: cervicolumbar, dorsolumbar, or cervicodorsal segments [25]. Concomitant involvement of all 3 spinal segments is rare, and only 3 cases have so far been reported in the literature [26]. Spinal TB in most of our patients (93%) was characterized by a single location. Other authors have also found a single location in more than 70% of cases [8, 27].

In our study, the diagnosis of spinal TB was made on the basis of clinical and radiological evidences, including CT scan, confirmed by a favorable therapeutic response to anti-TB therapy. However, in developed countries with a modern medical diagnostic laboratory and surgical practice, definitive diagnostic methods of spinal TB are based on bacteriological examinations to detect, cultivate, and isolate *Mycobacterium tuberculosis* if an abscess can be accessed for biopsy or if biopsy is performed preoperatively. These procedures were not performed in our study due to inadequate laboratory facilities. Instead, CT was performed when indicated as it is more sensitive than standard radiography to diagnose spondylodiscitis. In health facilities without sophisticated medical laboratory for bacteriological culture, CT imaging is probably the best available diagnostic method. If available, magnetic resonance imaging is even more accurate and sensitive than CT.

A well-managed anti-TB treatment for a period of 12 to 18 months is usually sufficient to achieve cure. The average duration of treatment of our patients was 12 months. In addition to drug treatment, surgical treatment was necessary in one of our patients. Because there are surgical risks and medical treatment alone may be adequate to cure spinal TB, surgical indications were based on the following: the failure of a well-conducted medical treatment, in which case surgery is the only alternative for the paraplegic patient; paraplegia with significant bone destruction and/or vertebral instability; acute compression due to bulky abscess and fistula or mechanical compression by sequestrum; or paraplegia with kyphosis that requires correction or prevention of aggravation. The rate of surgical intervention (1/14 patients; 7%) in our study was low because this type of surgery is reserved for patients with no other alternatives in the context of very limited resources in our country, including the technical platform, availability of intensive care units, the experience of surgeons and anesthesiologists, medical costs, and the overall risk benefit assessment of the patient [28]. In other studies performed in developing countries, a similar

TABLE 1: Characteristics of 14 patients with spinal tuberculosis included in our study.

Characteristics	Case 1	Case 2	Case 3	Case 4	Case 5	Case 6	Case 7	Case 8	Case 9	Case 10	Case 11	Case 12	Case 13	Case 14
Age (yr)	12	15	20	60	68	61	45	37	82	26	50	65	65	60
Sex[1]	M	M	M	F	F	F	F	F	M	M	F	F	M	F
Pulmonary TB	Yes	Yes	No	Yes	No	Yes	No	No	No	Yes	No	No	No	No
Concomitant disease				Diabetes	Gout	RA[2]					AH[3]			
Time to diagnosis (months)	12	21	9	18	17	22	13	14	17	12	9	12	9	9
Presenting symptoms														
Spinal stiffness	Yes	Yes	No	No	Yes	No	Yes	Yes	Yes	Yes	No	No	No	No
Rachialgia	Yes	Yes	Yes	No	Yes	Yes	Yes	Yes	Yes	Yes	Yes	Yes	Yes	Yes
Spinal compression	No	No	Yes	No	Yes	Yes	No	No	Yes	Yes	Yes	Yes	No	No
Location of the lesion[4]	D5	L4-L5	D10-D12	L2	D3-D5	D12-L1	L4	L4-L5	L2-L3	L4-L5	C4-C6	L4-L5	L3-L4	D11-L2
Surgical treatment	No	No	No	No	No	No	No	No	No	No	No	No	No	Yes
Corset immobilization	No	No	Yes	No	Yes	No	No	No	Yes	No	Yes	Yes	No	Yes
Outcome	cured	cured	cured	cured	cured	cured	cured	cured	deceased	cured	deceased	cured	cured	Yes

1M, Male; F, Female;
2RA: Rheumatoid Arthritis;
3AH: arterial hypertension;
4D, dorsal vertebrae; L, lumbar vertebrae; C, Cervical vertebrae.
In all 14 patients, spinal TB was confirmed by CT scan, and the standard anti-TB treatment was administered.

low rate of surgical treatment for spinal TB was observed [5, 7, 9, 13, 23, 25, 28].

The role of surgery in treating spinal TB has been controversial over the past decades, and there is no standard recommended surgical procedure for spinal TB [23]. Although a routine use of surgery is not advocated by most medical practitioners, in case of nerve compression leading to neurological deficit, surgery is definitely beneficial to patients for a more rapid recovery and shorter duration of use of the corset. In our patient, a stable fixation was achieved using screws and an osteosynthesis plate spanning the posterior pedicular D11-L2. Similar successful results were obtained by other authors [13, 18, 25]. A more sophisticated surgical treatment practiced in advanced countries involves a double anterior approach followed by posterior intervention, which provides additional plaster and allows early ambulation. Despite successful surgical operations that may lead to less kyphosis, more rapid pain relief, and bone fusion, until more evidence for immediate and long-term benefits is available after surgical interventions, a more conservative approach based on anti-TB medical treatment and case-to-case assessment for possible advantages of surgical procedures is probably more appropriate in developing countries.

Drug treatment of spinal TB is based on anti-TB treatment which should be maintained for at least 12 months [1, 5, 14, 16, 24, 28–30]. In addition to drug treatment, immobilization can reduce pain and limit sequelae. Six patients in our series had been immobilized, which improved case management in all these cases.

Commonly observed complications of spinal TB include kyphosis, neurological deficit (motor and sensory impairment), spinal deformity, and abscess. The risk of kyphosis can be limited by using braces to protect the spine. Neurological deficit and spinal deformity can be improved and corrected in most cases with effective anti-TB therapy. Likewise, abscess, when present, usually resolves with effective anti-TB therapy.

5. Conclusion

Spinal TB is still common in Mauritania. The insidious clinical picture often leads to a delay in diagnosis and complications. Modern imaging techniques, including CT scan, are helpful in confirming the diagnosis of spinal TB. Early diagnosis and prompt and appropriate treatment can considerably improve the prognosis of spinal TB. Moreover, control of TB during its early stages can prevent spinal TB.

Acknowledgments

We would like to thank the physicians at the Kiffa Regional Hospital for their technical assistance in diagnosis and investigations.

References

[1] World Health Organization, *Global Tuberculosis Report 2014*, WHO, Geneva, Switzerland, 2015.

[2] R. N. Dunn and M. Ben Husien, "Spinal tuberculosis," *The Bone & Joint Journal*, vol. 100-B, no. 4, pp. 425–431, 2018.

[3] C. Ben Taarit, S. Turki, and H. Maïz, "La tuberculose ostéoarticulaire en Tunisie : étude rétrospective de 180 cas," *Médecine et Maladies Infectieuses*, vol. 33, no. 4, pp. 210–214, 2003.

[4] M. F. G. Held, S. Hoppe, M. Laubscher et al., "Epidemiology of musculoskeletal tuberculosis in an area with high disease prevalence," *Asian Spine Journal*, vol. 11, no. 3, pp. 405–411, 2017.

[5] M. P. Gautam, P. Karki, S. Rijal, and R. Singh, "Pott's spine and paraplegia," *J Nepal Med Assoc*, vol. 44, pp. 106–115, 2005.

[6] H. Annabi, M. Abdelkafi, and M. Trabelsi, "La tuberculose ostéo-articulaire," *Tun Orthop.*, vol. 1, no. 1, pp. 7–17, 2008.

[7] B. Fedoul, K. Chakour, and M. El Faiz Chaoui, "Le mal de Pott: à propos de 82 cas," *Pan African Medical Journal*, vol. 8, no. 1, p. 22, 2011.

[8] M. Gbané-Koné, B. Ouattara, M. Diomandé et al., "Apport de la tomodensitométrie dans le diagnostic de la tuberculose vertébrale à propos de 496 cas à Abidjan," *Pan African Medical Journal*, vol. 20, p. 201, 2015.

[9] I. S. Johansen, S. L. Nielsen, M. Hove et al., "Characteristics and clinical outcome of bone and joint tuberculosis from 1994 to 2011: a retrospective register-based study in Denmark," *Clinical Infectious Diseases*, vol. 61, no. 4, pp. 554–562, 2015.

[10] D. N'Dri Oka, M.-A. N'Dri-Yoboue, G. Varlet, A. Haidara, and V. Ba Zeze, "Spinal tuberculosis. Epidemiologic and diagnostic aspects: A study of 28 clinical observations," *Cahiers/Santé*, vol. 14, no. 2, pp. 81–84, 2004.

[11] J. D. Colmenero, M. E. Jiménez-Mejías, J. M. Reguera, J. Palomino-Nicás, J. D. Ruiz-Mesa, J. Márquez-Rivas et al., "Tuberculous vertebral osteomyelitis in the new millennium: still a diagnostic and therapeutic challenge," *European Journal of Clinical Microbiology & Infectious Diseases*, vol. 23, no. 6, pp. 477–483, 2004.

[12] Y. Toloba, S. Diallo, Y. Maiga et al., "Spinal tuberculosis (Pott's disease): epidemiological, clinical, radiological and evolutionary aspects at the University Hospital of Point G," *Le Mali Médical*, vol. 26, no. 2, pp. 8–11, 2011.

[13] V. Narayan, N. Mohammed, A. R. Savardekar, D. P. Patra, and A. Nanda, "Tuberculous spondylolisthesis: a reappraisal of the clinicoradiologic spectrum and surgical treatment paradigm," *World Neurosurgery*, vol. 114, pp. 361–367, 2018.

[14] N. Meddeb, N. Rammeh, M. Chahed, H. Sahli, M. Elleuch, E. Cheour et al., "Aspects actuels du mal de Pott en Tunisie. A propos d'une série de 29 cas," *Bull Soc Pathol Exot*, vol. 95, pp. 269–271, 2002.

[15] V. Barrière, P. Gepner, F. Bricaire, O. Blétry, and E. Caumes, "Aspects actuels de la tuberculose vert⊖brale α propos de 16 observations," *Ann Med Interna*, vol. 150, no. 5, pp. 363–369, 1999.

[16] E. Eti, J. C. Daboiko, K. F. Brou, B. Ouali, B. Ouattara, K. D. Koffi et al., "Tuberculose vertébrale Notre expérience à partir d'une étude de 147 cas dans le service de rhumatologie du CHU de Cocody (Abidjan, Côte d'Ivoire)," *Méd Afr Noir*, vol. 57, pp. 287–292, 2010.

[17] F. Z. Bensalah and C. Dziri, "Place de la médecine physique et de réadaptation fonctionnelle dans le traitement des spondy-

lodiscites," *Journal de Réadaptation Médicale : Pratique et Formation en Médecine Physique et de Réadaptation*, vol. 25, no. 3, pp. 119–121, 2005.

[18] A. Zaoui, S. Kanoun, H. Boughamoura et al., "Patients with complicated Pott's disease: Management in a rehabilitation department and functional prognosis," *Annals of Physical and Rehabilitation Medicine*, vol. 55, no. 3, pp. 190–200, 2012.

[19] R. Jain, S. Sawhney, and M. Berry, "Computer tomography of vertebral tuberculosis: Patterns of bone destruction," *Clinical Radiology*, vol. 47, no. 3, pp. 196–199, 1993.

[20] H. S. Sharif and J. L. Morgan, "Role of CT and MR imaging in the management of tuberculous spondylitis," *Radiol Clin North Am*, vol. 33, pp. 787–804, 1995.

[21] A. Cotten, R. M. Flipo, M. H. Drouot, F. Maury, P. Chastanet, B. Duquesnoy et al., "La tuberculose vertébrale: étude des aspects cliniques et radiologiques à partir d'une série de 82 cas," *J Radiol*, vol. 77, pp. 419–426, 1996.

[22] N. Cherif Idrissi El Ganouni, M. Khalil, M. Hiroual et al., "Apport de l'IRM dans les compressions médullaires lentes d'origine tumorale et infectieuse," *Feuillets de Radiologie*, vol. 49, no. 4, pp. 251–262, 2009.

[23] R. K. Garg and D. S. Somvanshi, "Spinal tuberculosis: a review," *The Journal of Spinal Cord Medicine*, vol. 34, no. 5, pp. 440–454, 2011.

[24] M. Gbané-Koné, B. Ouali, A. K. Coulibaly, M. Diomandé, J. C. Yao, E. Eti et al., "Cervical spine in Pott's disease: Epidemiological, clinical and radiological aspects concerning 26 cases," *Mali Méd*, vol. 30, no. 2, pp. 15–18, 2015.

[25] E. S. Nussbaum, G. L. Rockswold, T. A. Bergman, D. L. Erickson, and E. L. Seljeskog, "Spinal tuberculosis: A diagnostic and management challenge," *Journal of Neurosurgery*, vol. 83, no. 2, pp. 243–247, 1995.

[26] B. Eljebbouri, H. Baallal, O. Naama, M. Gazzaz, and M. Boucetta, "Spondylodiscite tuberculeuse multifocale non contiguë," *Rev Mar Rhum*, vol. 20, pp. 42–44, 2012.

[27] A. Ousehal, A. Gharbi, W. Zamiati, A. Saidi, and R. Kadiri, "Imaging findings in 122 cases of Pott's disease," *Neurochirurgie*, vol. 48, no. 5, pp. 409–418, 2002.

[28] J. Yilboudo, S. C. Da, S. I. Nacoulma, and E. Bandre, "Tuberculous spondylodiscitis with neurologic problems: results of surgical treatment," *Med Trop*, vol. 62, pp. 39–46, 2002.

[29] T. Degen and T. Bregenzer, "The treatment of tuberculosis," *Praxis*, vol. 105, no. 8, pp. 457–461, 2016.

[30] F. Tritar, H. Daghfous, S. Ben Saad, and L. Slim-Saidi, "Management of multidrug-resistant tuberculosis," *Revue de Pneumologie Clinique*, vol. 71, no. 2-3, pp. 130–139, 2015.

10

Health Insurance Ownership and Quality of Computed Tomography Requests: Experience from a Peripheral Referral Hospital in Cameroon

Joshua Tambe,[1,2] Yannick Onana,[3] Sylviane Dongmo,[1] Georges Nguefack-Tsague,[4] and Pierre Ongolo-Zogo[2,5]

[1]*Division of Radiology, Department of Internal Medicine and Pediatrics, University of Buea, Buea, Cameroon*
[2]*Department of Public Health, Centre for Research and Training in Graduate Studies in Life, Health and Environmental Sciences, The University of Yaoundé I, Yaoundé, Cameroon*
[3]*Department of Clinical Sciences, University of Ngaoundéré, Ngaoundéré, Cameroon*
[4]*Biostatistics Unit, Department of Public Health, The University of Yaoundé I, Yaoundé, Cameroon*
[5]*Department of Radiology and Radiation Oncology, The University of Yaoundé I, Yaoundé, Cameroon*

Correspondence should be addressed to Joshua Tambe; joshua.tambe@ubuea.cm

Academic Editor: Lorenzo Faggioni

Background. Health insurance ownership facilitates access and minimizes financial hardship after utilization of healthcare services such as computed tomography (CT). Understanding the rational utilization of CT by people with health insurance can help optimize the scheme and provide baseline information for a national universal health coverage program. *Objective.* To assess the relationship between health insurance ownership and the appropriateness of requests for CT in a peripheral referral hospital in Cameroon. *Methods.* A survey of CT users was conducted during which information on health insurance ownership was collected and the request forms for CT assessed for appropriateness using the American College of Radiologists (ACR) Appropriateness Criteria®. *Results.* We consecutively enrolled 372 participants of which 167 (45%) were females. The median age (range) was 52 (18–92) years. Thirty-eight out of 370 participants reported having health insurance (10.3%; 95% confidence interval (CI): 7.2%–13.4%). Twenty-nine out of 352 CT scan requests (8.2%; 95% CI: 5.3–11.0) were judged to be "inappropriate." The proportion of inappropriate scan requests was higher amongst people with health insurance compared to those without health insurance (18.4% vs. 7.0%; $\chi^2 = 5.8$; $p = 0.02$). In the logistic regression analysis, health insurance ownership was associated to the appropriateness of CT requests in the univariate analysis only (OR = 0.33; 95% CI: 0.13–0.84; $p = 0.020$). *Conclusions.* Inappropriate requests for CT were low but nevertheless associated to health insurance ownership. The continuous sensitization and training of physicians would help minimize potential wasteful utilization of resources.

1. Introduction

The continuous development of advanced healthcare technology such as computed tomography (CT) has led to an increase in the cost of healthcare [1]. The utilization of multislice and extreme detector CT equipment with a very broad range of clinical applications has especially led to the price hike of CT procedures [1]. A high cost for healthcare services has the potential to limit access to care as people in need of the services may not be able to afford for them [2, 3]. Affordability of multislice CT technology is therefore perceived to be a barrier to its utilization, especially in settings without any financial protection for health. However, the affordability barrier to CT utilization can be minimized by the implementation of financial protection schemes [3]. Health insurance ownership is therefore expected to protect CT users from impoverishment and financial hardship that could arise from its utilization [3].

In Cameroon, CT scans have been installed in recent years in some peripheral referral hospitals around the country so as to improve upon the geographical accessibility of CT technology. The improved geographical accessibility is expected to reduce the time to obtain CT and also minimize inconveniences linked to long-distance travel to other towns. These peripheral health facilities which have been focusing on primary and secondary care now have to incorporate CT utilization during routine clinical practice with the potential for better health outcomes for patients. Nevertheless, CT, being a referral technology with a high radiation exposure, requires rational cost-effective utilization [1, 4–6]. According to a national survey, 96 to 98% of the general population do not have health insurance [7]. Whilst awaiting the implementation of a national universal health coverage program, available financial protection schemes for health include private insurance policies and community-based mutual and employer-provided insurance schemes.

Given the improved access to healthcare services conferred by health insurance ownership [8, 9], it is important to explore the rational utilization of services such as CT by people who have subscribed to health insurance policies. The information generated can help restructure available private health insurance policies and also shape the planned implementation of a public national universal health coverage scheme. There is paucity of information on the utilization of CT by people with health insurance. A pilot study reported an association between inappropriate CT requests and health insurance ownership in an urban sub-Saharan context [10]. Further studies to ascertain this relationship from different socioeconomic and geographical contexts are important so as to provide empirical evidence. In this study, we explore this relationship in a peripheral intermediate-level referral hospital in Cameroon.

2. Materials and Methods

A cross-sectional survey of CT users was conducted. This study was approved by the institutional ethics committee of the University of Yaoundé 1 (108/UY1/FMSB/VDRC/CSD). Administrative authorization for the study was also obtained from the South-West Regional Delegation for Public Health (R11/MINSANTE/SWR/RDPH/82/786). The study was conducted at the Medical Imaging Centre of Regional Hospital Limbe. Regional Hospital Limbe is an intermediate-level referral hospital in the Southwest Region of Cameroon with the capacity of 200 beds. Designated as a Category 3 referral health facility in the health system pyramid of Cameroon where the categories range from 1 (tertiary care) to 7 (primary care), its main role is to provide secondary care. The geographic location of this health facility is peripheral with respect to the country's political capital Yaoundé. In recent years, Regional Hospital Limbe has benefitted from the installation of a 16-slice CT scanner in an effort by the government to improve on access to health technology.

2.1. Participants. CT users aged 18 years and above who consented to participate in the study were consecutively enrolled between March 2018 and February 2019. Informed consent was written and was obtained either from the patient or the caregiver.

Sample size estimation was done using Cochran's method for surveys with the appropriateness of requests for CT (expressed as a categorical binary variable) being the primary outcome [11]. Given an alpha level of 0.05, a 5% error margin, and a population variance of 0.25, the calculated sample size was 385 participants. Informed by a pilot survey [10], we expected data collection to last for 12 months, period during which an expected 1614 CT scans would be performed as anticipated from the hospital records. The estimated sample size of 385 exceeded 5% of this population, and the Cochran correction formula was applied [11] to give a minimum return sample size of 310 participants. Anticipating a nonresponse rate of 20% [10], a total of 388 potential participants were invited to participate in the study, and enrolment ended when a sufficient sample size was attained. Figure 1 summarizes participant selection.

2.2. Data Collection. Data were collected from March 2018 to February 2019 using standardized forms. There was content validation of the included items on the data forms and pretesting through a pilot survey [10]. Data were collected on age, sex, educational achievement, marital status, occupation, socioeconomic status, health insurance ownership, and type of health insurance. Further information was gathered on the clinical indications for CT, anatomic region, and qualification of the referring healthcare provider. The appropriateness of CT requests was ascertained using the American College of Radiologists (ACR) Appropriateness Criteria® [12], which are guidelines that have been developed in collaboration with specialists from various domains with an aim to help referring healthcare providers to request for the best available imaging modality for specific clinical scenarios. During this study, the request forms for CT were used to determine appropriateness, and the final categorization was consensual between two radiologists (JT and POZ). CT request forms without any clinical indication were excluded from the study, whilst those with insufficient information were ignored from the appropriateness analysis. A research assistant collected all the data under the supervision of the principal investigator (JT).

2.3. Data Analysis. The data forms were transcribed onto a Microsoft Excel® spreadsheet and analyzed using Stata® 12 (StataCorp, Texas, USA). Continuous variables were summarized using the mean and standard deviation or median and range as appropriate. Categorical variables were summarized using frequencies, percentages, and 95% confidence intervals (CIs). Chi-squared tests were performed to compare proportions of inappropriate CT requests among categories of health insurance ownership. Univariate and multivariable logistic regression techniques were used to determine if any factors were associated with the appropriateness of requests for CT. For the multivariable modelling, covariates were entered as a block and included age, sex, educational achievement, socioeconomic status, health insurance ownership, and the qualification of the referring healthcare provider. Statistical tests were two tailed, and p

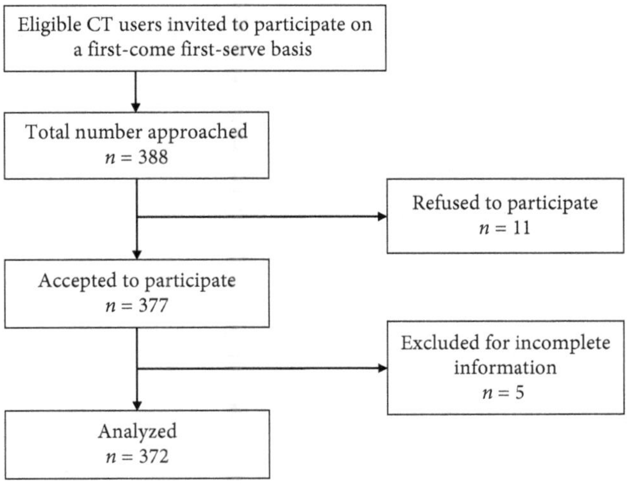

FIGURE 1: Participant selection flowchart.

values less than 0.05 were considered statistically significant. Model fit was assessed using the R^2 statistic. The data were presented using tables.

3. Results

3.1. Participant Characteristics. Three hundred and seventy-two participants were surveyed of which 167 (45%) were females. The median age (range) was 52 (18–92) years. The demographic and socioprofessional characteristics of the participants are presented in Table 1. Thirty-eight out of 370 participants reported having health insurance (10.3%; 95% confidence interval (CI): 7.2%–13.4%). The reported health insurance types are presented in Table 2.

3.2. Appropriateness of CT Requests. Three hundred and fifty-two CT requests could be categorized for appropriateness. Of these, 29 (8.2%; 95% CI = 5.3–11.0) were judged to be "inappropriate." Table 3 shows the categorization of CT appropriateness based on health insurance ownership.

The proportion of inappropriate scan requests was higher amongst people with health insurance compared to those without health insurance (18.4% vs. 7.0%; $\chi^2 = 5.8$; $p = 0.02$). Table 4 summarizes the relationship between health insurance ownership and CT request appropriateness.

In the logistic regression modelling, health insurance ownership was associated with the appropriateness of CT requests in the univariate analysis only (OR = 0.33; 95% CI: 0.13–0.84; $p = 0.020$). However, educational achievement beyond ordinary level was associated with the appropriateness of CT requests both in the univariate (OR = 0.42; 95% CI: 0.18–0.97; $p = 0.043$) and multivariable analysis (aOR = 0.35; 95% CI: 0.13–0.91; $p = 0.032$). The results of the logistic regression analysis are presented in Table 5.

4. Discussion

From the findings of this study, an estimated 10% of the respondents reportedly had health insurance ownership. This is higher than the 2–4% health insurance ownership of the general population following a national survey [7]. This difference could be explained by the fact that this survey focused on a subset of the population utilizing a particular health service and so not representative of the general population. The purchase of healthcare in Cameroon is essentially through direct out-of-pocket (OOP) payments. OOP payments lead to unequal access to care, whilst health insurance ownership minimizes access inequities [13–17]. Many governments around the world seek to improve access to care for its population through the implementation of a universal

TABLE 1: Demographic and socioprofessional characteristics of study participants.

Variables	Frequency (%)
Age group (years; $N = 344$)	
18–24	21 (5.7)
25–34	51 (13.7)
35–44	55 (14.8)
45–54	76 (20.4)
55–64	55 (14.8)
>65	114 (30.6)
Sex ($N = 372$)	
Female	167 (44.9)
Male	205 (55.1)
Marital status ($N = 372$)	
Married	232 (62.7)
Single	83 (22.3)
Widow (er)	42 (11.3)
Divorced	11 (3.0)
Living in union	4 (1.1)
Educational achievement ($N = 347$)	
<O level	158 (45.5)
O level or equivalent	61 (17.6)
A level or equivalent	64 (18.4)
Degree or equivalent	45 (13.0)
Master and above	19 (5.5)
Employment status ($N = 294$)	
Employed, with contract	82 (27.9)
Employed, with no contract	2 (0.7)
Self-employed	115 (39.1)
Unemployed	12 (4.1)
Retired	83 (28.2)
Socioeconomic status quintiles ($N = 370$) from the lowest (1) to the highest (5)	
SES quintile 1	74 (20.0)
SES quintile 2	75 (20.3)
SES quintile 3	75 (20.3)
SES quintile 4	79 (21.4)
SES quintile 5	67 (18.1)
Health insurance ownership ($N = 370$)	
Yes	38 (10.3)
No	332 (89.7)

TABLE 2: Health insurance types.

Insurance type	Frequency (%)
Assistance by a church	2 (5.26)
Private insurance company	5 (13.16)
Insurance provided by the employer	26 (68.42)
Local mutual health insurance scheme	5 (13.16)
Total	38 (100)

Table 3: Health insurance ownership and CT appropriateness.

	CT appropriateness, n (%; 95% CI)			Total, n (%)
	Category A*	Category B	Category C	
No health insurance ownership	218 (69.4; 64.3 – 74.5)	74 (23.6; 18.9 – 28.3)	22 (7.0; 4.2 – 9.8)	314 (100)
Health insurance ownership	25 (65.8; 50.7 – 80.9)	6 (15.8; 4.2 – 27.4)	7 (18.4; 6.1 – 30.7)	38 (100)
Total	243 (69; 64.2 – 73.9)	80 (22.7; 18.3 – 27.1)	29 (8.2; 5.4 – 11.1)	352 (100)

*According to the American College of Radiologists Appropriateness Criteria®, Category A indicates the requested imaging modality (CT in this case) is the most appropriate; Category B indicates the requested study could be appropriate, especially in the absence of any other reasonable alternative; Category C implies the requested imaging study is not appropriate for the clinical indication.

Table 4: Summary analysis of the relationship between CT request appropriateness and health insurance ownership.

	CT appropriateness, n (%; 95% CI)		Total, n (%)
	Category C*	Categories A and B merged	
No health insurance ownership	22 (7.01; 4.2 – 9.8)	292 (92.99; 90.2 – 95.8)	314 (100)
Health insurance ownership	7 (18.42; 6.1 – 30.7)	31 (81.58; 69.3 – 93.9)	38 (100)
Total	29 (8.24; 5.4 – 11.1)	323 (91.76; 88.9 – 94.6)	352 (100)

$\chi^2 = 5.84$; $p = 0.016$. *Category C corresponds to inappropriate CT requests.

Table 5: Regression analysis of the appropriateness of CT requests.

Variables	Univariate analysis		Multivariate analysis	
	Crude OR (95% CI)	p value	Adjusted OR (95% CI)	p value
Age (years, N – 354)	1.00 (098 – 1.02)	0.827	0.98 (0.96 – 1.01)	0.222
Gender (N – 354)				
Female	1		1	
Male	0.53 (0.23 – 1.20)	0.129	0.72 (0.30 – 1.72)	0.461
Education (N – 288)				
Completed ordinary level or less	1		1	
Beyond ordinary level	0.42 (0.18 – 0.97)	0.043	0.35 (0.13 – 0.91)	0.032
Socioeconomic status (N – 352)	1.27 (0.67 – 2.38)	0.462	1.77 (0.92 – 3.43)	0.088
Health insurance (N – 352)				
Yes	0.33 (0.13 – 0.84)	0.020	0.37 (0.14 – 1.01)	0.053
No	1		1	
Healthcare provider (N – 344)				
Specialist doctors	0.79 (0.36 – 1.78)	0.578	0.77 (0.33 – 1.78)	0.540
General physicians	1		1	

Model p value – 0.062; R^2 – 0.062; OR: odds ratio; CI: confidence interval.

health coverage (UHC) scheme [3]. The benefits of UHC cannot be overemphasized, which is the reason why the government of Cameroon has embarked upon the creation of such a scheme in the near future. The anticipation of a UHC scheme motivated the assessment of the rational utilization of CT by people with existing insurance schemes.

The findings of this study support the fact that health insurance ownership confers better access to CT and also potentiates the likelihood of inappropriately using CT as health insurance ownership was independently associated to inappropriate requests for CT. It is likely that people with insurance may have some compulsion to access some health services even when these are not indicated just because they have subscribed to and contribute for such schemes. This may put pressure on healthcare providers to request for CT as they may also fear any potential litigation should they fail to request, and a serious condition is later detected.

Educational achievement beyond ordinary levels was also associated with inappropriate CT requests. Most of the insured participants had an insurance premium provided by the employer, and it is likely that a minimum level of education is required to get employed with a formal contract of employment. Furthermore, people with higher educational qualifications may be more demanding when accessing healthcare services with more pressure to obtain some services even when these might not be needed.

Inappropriate utilization of a health technology such as CT for whatever reason has to be given a serious consideration given that CT is associated to high exposure to ionizing radiation with the potential of radiation-induced cancers [4, 5, 18–21]. The cost of CT is also considerable irrespective of whether payments are made OOP or through insurance [1], and wasteful utilization will strain the pooled resources that have been made available for the scheme [3]. If CT utilization by a smaller population with health insurance shows inappropriate utilization patterns, then it is likely that this effect might be multiplied with the extension of health insurance to a wider population.

Geographic accessibility is fundamental to accessing healthcare services [22, 23]. The installation of CT in peripheral health facilities in cities distant from the capital cities ensures the decentralization of health technology. Patients no longer commute for considerable distances to access some health technologies as was the case, and utilization has all the chances of being timely too. Enhanced geographic access to health technology therefore has the potential to improve the quality of care and health outcomes. Following the introduction of health technology such as CT to peripheral health facilities, health practitioners have to incorporate its use during routine clinical practice. This may be simple for some clear-cut clinical indications and trivial for others. Healthcare practitioners therefore have to step up knowledge usually through refresher courses, continuous medical education seminars, and personal studies to be abreast with the clinical use of health technology.

Strategies to curb inappropriate utilization must therefore be envisaged while the government plans to implement a universal health coverage scheme. Firstly, given the absence of regulations as to who is qualified to request for imaging studies in the study setting, we suggest that CT requests should be approved only when prescribed by duly trained healthcare professionals. Also, consultations with radiologists should be encouraged if uncertain about the role of CT as more cost-effective imaging alternatives might be readily available [24]. Furthermore, continuous training and sensitization, the use of guidelines, and imaging decision support by referring physicians should be encouraged [25, 26]. Finally, a tracking system for all requested CT studies with regular reviews to assess prescription trends and relevance will provide useful feedback on utilization.

CT utilization and health insurance ownership have not been given much attention in the medical literature. Bellolio et al. reported an increase in CT utilization among commercially insured patients but did not assess the appropriateness of CT utilization [27]. Becker et al. also reported inappropriate utilization of both CT and magnetic resonance imaging without any assessment with respect to health insurance ownership [28]. This paper focused on the specific relationship between the health insurance ownership and the appropriateness of CT utilization, providing opportunities for scaling up the use of CT by people with health insurance in resource-poor settings.

4.1. Limitations. As limitations to this study, some CT scan requests could not be categorized for appropriateness due to insufficient clinical information on the forms. Also, reporting bias could have influenced the findings of this study.

5. Conclusions

The findings of this study support the fact that health insurance ownership, despite the proven benefits in minimizing access inequities, can be associated with inappropriate requests for CT in the study setting. This is perceived as an unintended consequence that can be checked by the continuous sensitization and training of physicians, providing them with other cost-effective alternatives to CT as appropriate and encouraging the use of guidelines when uncertain. These measures, in our opinion, could help enhance the rational utilization of CT and reduce unnecessary exposure to ionizing radiation.

Acknowledgments

The authors thank Mrs. Arabella Tambe for manuscript proofreading, language editing, and logistics assistance.

References

[1] W. R. Hendee, G. J. Becker, J. P. Borgstede et al., "Addressing overutilization in medical imaging," *Radiology*, vol. 257, no. 1, pp. 240–245, 2010.

[2] The World Health Report, *Health Systems Financing: The Path to Universal Coverage. 2010*, World Health Organization, Geneva, Switzerland, 2010.

[3] The World Health Report, *The World Health Report 2013: Research for Universal Health Coverage*, World Health Organization, Geneva, Switzerland, 2013.

[4] D. J. Brenner and E. J. Hall, "Cancer risks from CT scans: now we have data, what next?" *Radiology*, vol. 265, no. 2, pp. 330-331, 2012.

[5] D. J. Brenner and E. J. Hall, "Computed tomography—an increasing source of radiation exposure," *New England Journal of Medicine*, vol. 357, no. 22, pp. 2277–2284, 2007.

[6] P. E. Litkowski, G. W. Smetana, M. L. Zeidel, and M. S. Blanchard, "Curbing the urge to image," *The American Journal of Medicine*, vol. 129, no. 10, pp. 1131–1135, 2016.

[7] Institut National de la Statistique (INS), *Enquête Démographique et de Santé à Indicateurs Multiples du Cameroun 2011*, ICF International, Calverton, MD, USA, 2012.

[8] A. Sisira Kumara and R. Samaratunge, "Health insurance ownership and its impact on healthcare utilization," *International Journal of Social Economics*, vol. 47, no. 2, pp. 244–267, 2019.

[9] M. Anderson, C. Dobkin, and T. Gross, "The effect of health insurance coverage on the use of medical services," *American Economic Journal: Economic Policy*, vol. 4, no. 1, pp. 1–27, 2012.

[10] J. Tambe, L. Mbuagbaw, G. Nguefack-Tsague, J. Foyet, and P. Ongolo-Zogo, "Multidetector computed tomography utilization in an urban sub-Saharan Africa setting: user characteristics, indications and appropriateness," *Pan African Medical Journal*, vol. 37, 2020.

[11] J. E. Bartlett II, J. W. Kotrlik, and C. C. Higgins, "Organizational research: determining appropriate sample size in survey research," *Information Technology, Learning, and Performance Journal*, vol. 19, no. 1, pp. 43–50, 2001.

[12] ACR, *ACR Appropriateness Criteria*, https://www.acr.org/Clinical-Resources/ACR-Appropriateness-Criteria, 2019.

[13] C. Zhang, C. Fu, Y. Song, R. Feng, X. Wu, and Y. Li, "Utilization of public health care by people with private health insurance: a systematic review and meta-analysis," *BMC Public Health*, vol. 20, no. 1, p. 1153, 2020.

[14] S. Yaya, F. Da, R. Wang, S. Tang, and B. Ghose, "Maternal healthcare insurance ownership and service utilisation in Ghana: analysis of Ghana Demographic and Health Survey," *PLoS One*, vol. 14, no. 4, Article ID e0214841, 2019.

[15] J. Pan, X. Lei, and G. G. Liu, "Health insurance and health status: exploring the causal effect from a policy intervention," *Health Economics*, vol. 25, no. 11, pp. 1389–1402, 2016.

[16] W. Mao, Y. Zhang, L. Xu, Z. Miao, D. Dong, and S. Tang, "Does health insurance impact health service utilization among older adults in urban China? A nationwide cross-sectional study," *BMC Health Services Research*, vol. 20, no. 1, p. 630, 2020.

[17] C. M. Farrell and A. Gottlieb, "The effect of health insurance on health care utilization in the justice-involved population: United States, 2014–2016," *American Journal of Public Health*, vol. 110, no. S1, pp. S78–S84, 2020.

[18] J. D. Boice, "Radiation epidemiology: a perspective on Fukushima," *Journal of Radiological Protection*, vol. 32, no. 1, pp. N33–N40, 2012.

[19] J. D. Mathews, A. V. Forsythe, Z Brady et al., "Cancer risk in 680,000 people exposed to computed tomography scans in childhood or adolescence: data linkage study of 11 million Australians," *British Medical Journal (Clinical Research edition)*, vol. 346, p. f2360, 2013.

[20] S. P. Power, F. Moloney, M. Twomey, K. James, O. J. O'Connor, and M. M. Maher, "Computed tomography and patient risk: facts, perceptions and uncertainties," *World Journal of Radiology*, vol. 8, no. 12, p. 902, 2016.

[21] R. Smith-Bindman, "Radiation dose associated with common computed tomography examinations and the associated lifetime attributable risk of cancer," *Archives of Internal Medicine*, vol. 169, no. 22, Article ID 2078, 2009.

[22] D. B. Evans, J. Hsu, and T. Boerma, "Universal health coverage and universal access," *Bulletin of the World Health Organization*, vol. 91, no. 8, pp. 546–546A, 2013.

[23] M. Gulliford, J. Figueroa-Munoz, M. Morgan et al., "What does 'access to health care' mean?" *Journal of Health Services Research and Policy*, vol. 7, no. 3, pp. 186–188, 2002.

[24] P. M. Knechtges and R. C. Carlos, "The evolving role of radiologists within the health care system," *Journal of the American College of Radiology*, vol. 4, no. 9, pp. 626–635, 2007.

[25] B. Moifo, A. L. Edzimbi, H. Tebere, J. Tambe, R. N. Samba, and J. G. Fotsin, "Referring physicians' knowledge on justification of medical exposure in diagnostic imaging in a sub-saharan african country, Cameroon," *Open Journal of Radiology*, vol. 04, no. 01, pp. 60–68, 2014.

[26] B. Moifo, U. Tene, J. R. Moulion Tapouh et al., "Knowledge on irradiation, medical imaging prescriptions, and clinical imaging referral guidelines among physicians in a sub-saharan african country (Cameroon)," *Radiology Research and Practice*, vol. 2017, pp. 1–7, 2017.

[27] M. F. Bellolio, S. D. Bellew, L. R. Sangaralingham et al., "Effect on examination ordering by physician attitude, common knowledge, and practice behavior regarding CT radiation exposure," *Radiology*, vol. 129, no. 6, pp. 577–581, 2011.

[28] J. Becker, L. S. Jenkins, M. De Swardt, R. Sayed, and M. Viljoen, "Appropriateness of computed tomography and magnetic resonance imaging scans in the Eden and Central Karoo districts of the Western Cape Province, South Africa," *South African Medical Journal*, vol. 104, no. 11, p. 762, 2014.

11

Real-Life Diagnostic Accuracy of MRI in Prenatal Diagnosis

Manuel Recio Rodríguez,[1] Cristina Andreu-Vázquez,[2] Israel J. Thuissard-Vasallo,[2] Raquel Cano Alonso,[1] Carmina Bermejo López,[3] Ines Tamarit Degenhardt,[4] and Pilar Martínez Ten[3]

[1]*Departamento de Diagnóstico por Imagen, Hospital Universitario Quironsalud Madrid, Madrid, Spain*
[2]*Departamento de Medicina, Facultad de Ciencias Biomédicas, Universidad Europea de Madrid, Madrid, Spain*
[3]*Delta Ecografía, Madrid, Spain*
[4]*Departamento de Obstetricia y Ginecología, Hospital Universitario Quironsalud Madrid, Madrid, Spain*

Correspondence should be addressed to Manuel Recio Rodríguez; mrmrecio@gmail.com

Academic Editor: André Luiz Ferreira Costa

There is some controversy about the value of fetal MRI in prenatal diagnosis, and most of the studies examine its accuracy in central nervous system (CNS) pathology. The objective of this retrospective study was to assess the diagnostic accuracy and usefulness of fetal MRI in the prenatal diagnosis of central nervous system (CNS) pathology and non-CNS pathology. Patients referred to the Radiology Department between 2007 and 2018 for a fetal MRI after detection of an anomaly in the fetal ultrasound, a high-risk pregnancy, or an inconclusive fetal ultrasound ($n = 623$) were included in the study. Postnatal diagnosis was used to assess the diagnostic accuracy of MRI. Fetal MRI was considered to provide additional information over fetal ultrasound when findings of the fetal MRI were not detected in the fetal ultrasound or when established a pathological condition that was not detected in the fetal ultrasound. Fetal MRI provided useful information for the perinatal management and prognosis over fetal ultrasound when findings of the fetal MRI changed the postnatal prognosis, leaded to the decision to legally terminate the pregnancy, changed prenatal or postnatal follow-up, or helped in the planning of prenatal or postnatal treatment. Fetal MRI offered an accurate diagnosis in 97% of cases (compared to 90.4% of fetal ultrasound; $p < 0.001$). Concordance between fetal ultrasound and fetal MRI was 92.1%. Fetal MRI provided additional information over fetal ultrasound in 23.1% of cases. In 11.6% of cases, the information was useful for the perinatal management and prognosis. In 45 cases (7.2%), fetal MRI was the only accurate diagnosis. In conclusion, fetal MRI has a superior diagnostic accuracy, especially in CNS pathology, and provides additional useful information in CNS, thoracic, and abdominal pathology.

1. Introduction

Fetal ultrasound has been described as the first-line diagnostic examination to identify prenatal congenital abnormalities [1], and the majority of fetal ultrasound examinations are diagnostic. However, the technique has technical limitations even in experienced hands. Accordingly, in cases where the pathology is complex, an additional approach is needed to confirm or complement the ultrasound findings. Fetal magnetic resonance (MRI) is a complementary diagnostic technique to fetal ultrasound that does not present the same limitations as the latter in cases of advanced gestational age, oligohydramnios, inadequate fetal position, and maternal obesity. Moreover, fetal MRI visualization of the brain is not affected by interposition of the cranial vault [2].

Although MRI does not use ionizing radiation and is assumed to be safe, not enough research has been carried out to prove long-term safety [3]. Therefore, MRI should be performed when the benefit outweighs the potential side effects [3]. All fetuses should have a screening ultrasonogram for the detection of fetal anomalies and pregnancy complications before performing a fetal MRI [4]. Limitations of fetal MRI include the lack of availability of equipment and radiology expertise, higher cost, and longer time to perform an examination [4] and lower spatial resolution than ultrasound at early gestational age because of the small size of the fetus [5]. Additionally, fetal movement may cause the appearance of artifacts [5]. To avoid this, measures are taken such as fasting the mother in the hours before the exam or ensuring that the she is comfortable during the procedure, especially at advanced gestational age. In addition, current MRI software and hardware allow MRI exams to be performed with high-quality images obtained in less than 1 second, allowing fetal imaging without maternal or fetal sedation [4].

As for all patients, there are absolute contraindications to MRI in pregnant women (e.g., a ferromagnetic cerebral aneurysm clip, cardiac pacemaker), and some patients are too claustrophobic to undergo the examination. In addition, the use of intravenous contrast is not accepted because gadolinium contrast freely passes through the placenta. The transferred gadolinium then passes into the fetal circulation where it is excreted into the urinary tract and subsequently into the amniotic fluid. Some of the gadolinium in the amniotic fluid will be reabsorbed by the maternal circulation, while some will be swallowed and reabsorbed through the fetal GI tract [6]. Furthermore, the half-life of gadolinium in the fetus is unknown. Some authors have recently reported the potential nephrotoxicity risk of gadolinium (nephrogenic systemic fibrosis) [7].

Since the first reports of fetal MRI in 1983 [8], the modality has been increasingly used as an adjunct to ultrasound [9], mainly on cerebral pathology. There are fewer publications describing fetal MRI use in chest and abdominal pathology [10], or other less common anatomical locations such as musculoskeletal pathology [11].

While the diagnostic accuracy of fetal ultrasound (compared with postnatal diagnosis or autopsy) has been widely presented, few studies have assessed the accuracy of fetal MRI in the prenatal diagnosis of different anomalies, and most of these examined central nervous system (CNS) pathology. In a meta-analysis of 34 studies [12], including 959 cases of cerebral fetal MRI confirmed by postnatal surgery or autopsy, the diagnostic accuracy of fetal MRI was approximately 91%, 16 percentage higher than that of fetal ultrasound. Likewise, Gonçalves et al. [13] reported that the sensitivity of fetal MRI in non-CNS-related pathology was 80%, as compared with 77.8% for fetal ultrasound.

There is also some controversy about the value of fetal MRI in prenatal diagnosis and its ability to provide additional information over fetal ultrasound and the extent to which the additional information is useful for perinatal management and prognosis, with published studies providing conflicting findings. In a systematic review of prenatal diagnosis of CNS pathology, it was concluded that fetal MRI provided additional information in approximately 22.1% of cases and resulted in a change in clinical management in some 30% [14]. By contrast, Paladini et al. [15] reported that fetal MRI provided clinically relevant additional information in only 7.9% of cases.

Given the disparity in results from different studies, the objective of the present work was to assess the prenatal diagnostic accuracy and usefulness of fetal MRI in CNS and non-CNS pathology in patients with previous fetal ultrasound examinations referred to the Radiology Department.

2. Materials and Methods

The study protocol was approved by the Medication Research Ethics Board of the Jimenez Diaz Foundation (code EO006-19_HUQM). All patients signed the written informed consent, which includes permission for the use of their clinical data for research purposes, before the fetal MRI was performed.

2.1. Patients. A cohort of pregnant women referred to the diagnostic imaging service of our hospital between January 2007 and December 2018 were studied. In a previous transabdominal fetal ultrasound study (performed and interpreted by qualified gynecologists from 27 different centers), the subjects presented a prenatal anomaly or an indication for fetal MRI for high-risk pregnancy or inconclusive fetal ultrasound.

2.2. Interventions. The diagnosis by fetal MRI was made in the 7 days following fetal ultrasound, without sedation after 4 hours fasting. All fetal MRI studies were performed at the same hospital and interpreted by the same radiologist, with more than 15 years of experience.

2.3. Fetal MRI Procedure. Fetal MRI was carried out using a Signa HDxt 1.5T MRI Scanner (from 2007 to 2010) and an Optima MR450w 1.5T MRI Scanner (from 2010 to 2018) (General Electric, Milwaukee, WI). An 8-channel torso-array coil was used in the Signa HDxt 1.5T MRI Scanner and a 32-channel cardiac or body coil in the Optima MR450w 1.5T MRI Scanner. In all the studies, single-shot Fast Spin Echo T2 (SSFSE T2) sequences, FIESTA (fast imaging employing steady-state acquisition) balanced sequences, T1 weighted sequences (LAVA—liver acquisition with volume acquisition), T2 gradient echo, and diffusion-weighted imaging were generated. Occasionally, recovery-inversion sequences or a cerebral tractography using diffusion tensor imaging were used. Sequence parameters used are shown in Table 1.

2.4. Study Variables and Definitions. Nonpersonal socio-demographic and clinical data were recorded for all patients. Prenatal dates and diagnoses by fetal ultrasound and fetal MRI, gestational age at the time of fetal MRI, and postnatal diagnosis by imaging tests or diagnosis by autopsy were registered. Postnatal diagnosis was made by fetal autopsy in cases of legal termination of pregnancy. In newborns with CNS pathology, postnatal diagnosis was made by ultrasound and MRI. In the cases of thoracic pathology, the postnatal diagnosis was established by chest radiography and/or thoracic computed tomography and, occasionally, thoracic MR. In cases of abdomino-pelvic pathology, ultrasound and, occasionally, MRI were used. In those cases where postnatal surgery was required, the postnatal diagnosis was established during surgery and with the anatomopathological diagnosis of the surgical specimens. Patients with an unknown postnatal diagnosis were excluded from the study.

Table 1: Sequence parameters.

	SSFSE T2 sequences	FIESTA balanced sequences	T1-weighted images (3D LAVA)	Diffusion-weighted imaging	Gradient echo T2	Recovery-inversion sequences SSFSE T2	Diffusion tensor
Repetition time (ms)	1583	5.1	6.2	7706	1125	1955	4278
Echo time (ms)	148	Minimum (1.9)	13.1	72.6	21.8	35.7	104.6
Matrix	320 × 320	192 × 256	192 × 192	128 × 128	128 × 192	160 × 160	64 × 64
Field of view (cm)	32	38	38	40	40	40	20
Bandwidth (kHz)	41.7	83.3	83.3	250	250	41.7	167
Number if excitations	0.5	0.71	0.71	8	4	1	2
Slice thickness (mm)	3 (spacing 0.3 mm)	3	3	3 (spacing 0.3 mm)	3 (spacing 0.3 mm)	3 (spacing 0.3 mm)	3 (spacing 0 mm)
Angle (°)		85°	12°				
Inversion time (ms)				180		1500	
B (s/mm²)				1000			800
Phase-encoding directions							16

FIESTA: fast imaging employing steady-state acquisition, LAVA: liver acquisition with volume acquisition, SSFSE: single-shot fast spin echo.

The following terms were defined. Accurate fetal ultrasound/MRI diagnosis: the prenatal diagnosis by fetal ultrasound/MRI coincides with the postnatal diagnosis or autopsy. Concordant fetal ultrasound and fetal MRI diagnosis: the prenatal diagnosis by fetal ultrasound coincides with the prenatal diagnosis by fetal MRI. Fetal MRI provides additional information over fetal ultrasound: the fetal MRI diagnosis coincides with the fetal ultrasound diagnosis, and findings of the fetal MRI were not detected in the fetal ultrasound, or the fetal MRI established a pathological condition that was not detected in the fetal ultrasound. Fetal MRI provides useful information for perinatal management and prognosis over fetal ultrasound: fetal MRI diagnosis is concordant with fetal ultrasound diagnosis, and the findings of the fetal MRI [1] change the postnatal prognosis, [2] lead to the decision to legally terminate the pregnancy, [3] result in a change in prenatal or postnatal follow-up, or [4] help in the planning of prenatal or postnatal treatment. The fetal MRI is the only accurate diagnosis: fetal MRI diagnosis is accurate and nonconcordant with that of fetal ultrasound (i.e., MRI diagnosis accurate and fetal ultrasound diagnosis inaccurate).

2.5. Statistical Analysis. For the descriptive analysis, absolute (n) and relative frequencies (%) were used to express the qualitative variables. The parametric behavior of the quantitative variables was verified and variables were described using the mean ± standard deviation (SD) if they followed a normal distribution or using the median (interquartile range (IQR)) if they did not.

To study the statistical significance between the diagnostic accuracy of fetal ultrasound and fetal MRI, and the concordance between both diagnostic techniques in the different indications, Chi-squared tests or Fischer's exact tests were performed. Similarly, the proportion of cases in which fetal MRI provided additional information and useful information for perinatal management and prognosis over fetal ultrasound are described and compared among the different indications. Data were analyzed using the SPSS statistical package, v21.0 (IBM Corp., Armonk, NY). A significance level <5% was used.

3. Results

A total of 694 pregnant women were attended in our hospital for a fetal MRI complementary to fetal ultrasound between January 2007 and December 2018. Diagnostic confirmation was not possible in 71 women because of a lack of postnatal follow-up, and so 623 women were included in the final study (Figure 1).

The median age in the study population on the day of MRI was 35.1 (5.1) years. Median gestational age was 29.4 (8.2) weeks, and in 147 cases (23.6%), gestational age was ≤24 weeks. Forty of the 623 gestations (6.4%) were twins.

Table 2 shows the indications for the 623 cases included in the study. Most of them (429 cases; 68.9%) corresponded to CNS pathology, 37 cases (5.9%) to thoracic pathology, 61 cases (9.8%) to abdominal pathology, and 96 cases (15.4%) to other indications.

3.1. Diagnostic Accuracy and Fetal MRI and Fetal Ultrasound Concordance. The diagnostic accuracy of the fetal ultrasound and the fetal MRI and the concordance between the two tests are shown in Table 3. The diagnostic accuracy of the fetal MRI was higher than that of fetal ultrasound in all cases and all indications. The differences in diagnostic accuracy between fetal ultrasound and fetal MRI were significant for all cases (90.4% vs 97%; $p < 0.001$) and for CNS pathology (89.7% vs 98.1%; $p < 0.001$).

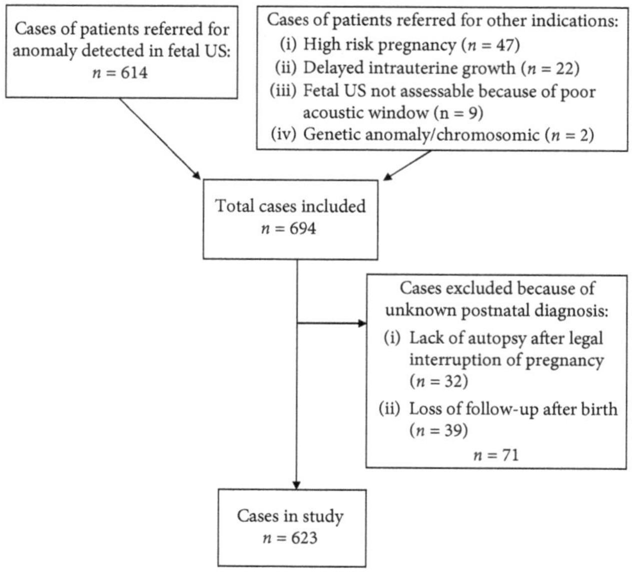

Figure 1: Flow diagram. Cases of patients referred for prenatal diagnosis by magnetic resonance imaging between January 2007 and December 2018.

Table 2: Indications of the 623 cases with a previous ultrasound study referred for fetal MRI between January 2007 and December 2018.

	Indication	*n* (%)
CNS pathology		**429 (68.9)**
	Ventriculomegaly	148 (34.5)
	Posterior fossa malformations	71 (16.6)
	Abnormalities of the corpus callosum	58 (13.5)
	Other midline anomalies	38 (8.9)
	Infectious pathology	30 (7.0)
	Ischemic/hemorrhagic pathology	25 (5.8)
	Tumoral pathology and lesions of the cranial vault, neck or orbits	24 (5.6)
	Spinal column pathology	12 (2.8)
	Tuberous sclerosis	13 (3.0)
	Malformations of cortical development	10 (2.3)
Thoracic pathology		**37 (5.9)**
	Parenchymatous lesions	22 (59.5)
	Congenital diaphragmatic hernia	12 (32.4)
	Mediastenic or pleural pathology	3 (8.1)
Abdominal pathology		**61 (9.8)**
	Digestive pathology	28 (45.9)
	Urogenital pathology	12 (19.7)
	Abdominal masses	13 (21.3)
	Abdominal wall defects	4 (6.6)
	Vascular pathology	4 (6.6)
Other indications		**96 (15.4)**
	Normal ultrasound in high-risk pregnancy	47 (49.0)
	Intrauterine growth retardation	22 (22.9)
	Ultrasound not valid due to poor acoustic window	9 (9.4)
	Placental pathology	9 (9.4)
	Musculoskeletal pathology	7 (7.3)
	Genetic or chromosomal abnormality	2 (2.1)

Fetal ultrasound and fetal MRI were concordant in 574 of the 623 cases (92.1%). The greatest concordance between diagnoses was recorded in the group of other indications (97.9%), and concordance was less in CNS pathology (90.2%).

The diagnostic accuracy of fetal MRI was not significantly different between cases with gestational age ≤24 weeks and cases with gestational age >24 weeks (97.3% and 96.9%, $p = 1.000$). Differences in the diagnostic accuracy of fetal

Table 3: Diagnostic accuracy of fetal ultrasound and fetal magnetic resonance relative to the postnatal diagnosis or autopsy and concordance ($n = 623$).

Indication	Diagnostic accuracy relative to postnatal diagnosis					Concordance between fetal ultrasounsd and MRI n (%)	
	Of fetal ultrasound n (%)		Of fetal MRI n (%)		p-value		
Total	593	(90.4)	604	(97.0)	<0.001	574	(92.1)
CNS pathology ($n = 429$)	385	(89.7)	421	(98.1)	<0.001	387	(90.2)*
Thoracic pathology ($n = 37$)	33	(89.2)	34	(91.9)	1.000	36	(97.3)
Abdominal pathology ($n = 61$)	52	(85.2)	54	(88.5)	0.592	57	(93.4)
Other indications ($n = 96$)	93	(96.9)	95	(99.0)	0.621	94	(97.9)*

p-value of the Chi-squared test for the differences in diagnostic accuracy of fetal ultrasound (US) and fetal magnetic resonance imaging (MRI) for all indications and for each indication. The asterisk (*) indicates a statistically significant difference (Chi-squared test or Fischer's exact test, $p < 0.05$) in the concordance between fetal US and fetal MRI for the different indications.

MRI between cases of gestational age less or greater than 24 weeks were not observed for the different indications.

The cases where the diagnosis by fetal MRI and fetal ultrasound did not match with the postnatal diagnosis or autopsy (inaccurate diagnosis) are recorded in Table 4. There were 45 cases in which fetal MRI was the only accurate diagnosis, while only four cases had an accurate diagnosis by fetal ultrasound but an inaccurate diagnosis by fetal MRI. Inaccurate diagnosis by fetal MRI and also by fetal ultrasound occurred in 15 cases.

3.2. Additional Information and Useful Information for Perinatal Management and Prognosis of Fetal MRI Over Fetal Ultrasound. Table 5 shows the proportion of cases in which fetal MRI provides additional information and useful information for perinatal management and prognosis over fetal ultrasound. Fetal MRI provided additional information in 23.1% of cases and useful information for perinatal management and prognosis over fetal ultrasound in 11.6% of cases. Fetal MRI was the only accurate diagnosis in 7.2%. In the CNS pathology indication, fetal MRI was the only accurate diagnosis in 39 of the 429 cases (9.1%) and provided additional information and useful information for perinatal management and prognosis over fetal ultrasound in 96 (22.1%) and 47 cases (11%), respectively (Figures 2–4). The greatest contribution of additional information and useful information for perinatal management and prognosis over fetal ultrasound occurred in cases with thoracic pathology indication (56.8% and 35.1%, respectively), while fetal MRI was the only accurate diagnosis in 2.7% of cases (Figure 5). The abdominal pathology was the second indication in which fetal MRI provided more additional information and useful information for perinatal management and prognosis over fetal ultrasound (27.9% and 11.5%, respectively), and MRI was the only accurate diagnosis in 4.9% of the cases (Figure 6). Overall, fetal MRI provided less additional information and less useful information over fetal ultrasound in cases referred with other indications (10.4% and 5.2%, respectively), and MRI was the only accurate diagnosis in 2.1% of the cases.

3.3. Accuracy, Concordance, and Usefulness of Fetal MRI in Cases Referred from Reference and Nonreference Ultrasound Centers. Of the 623 cases, 362 (58.1%) were referred from centers considered to be ultrasound reference centers and 261 (41.9%) from centers considered not to be reference centers. The accuracy of fetal ultrasound was not significantly different between centers (90.1% vs 89.7%; $p = 0.608$), but the MRI provided additional information and useful information for perinatal management and prognosis over fetal ultrasound to a greater extent when cases were referred from ultrasound reference centers than from nonreference centers (Table 6).

4. Discussion

The present study, based on 623 cases treated during the last 11 years in the Radiology Department, confirms the usefulness of fetal MRI as an adjunct to fetal ultrasound, especially in those cases referred with CNS pathology. In fact, CNS pathology was the most frequent indication in our study, corresponding to 68.9% of cases. The diagnostic accuracy of fetal MRI and fetal ultrasound in the detection of CNS pathology was 98.1% and 89.7%, respectively. These values are slightly higher for fetal MRI and lower for fetal ultrasound than reported by Paladini et al. [15] (94.4% and 91.3%, respectively) and are higher for both techniques than those reported in the meta-analysis of Jarvis et al. [12] (91% and 75%, respectively). In the multicenter MERIDIAN study [16], the values of diagnostic accuracy were 95% for fetal MRI and 82% for fetal ultrasound. The concordance between the fetal MRI and fetal ultrasound diagnosis in the 429 cases described in the present study with indication of CNS pathology was 90.2%, which is slightly higher than that reported by Paladini et al. [15] based on 126 cases (86.5%). In the present study, no significant differences were found in

Table 4: Cases with inaccurate diagnosis by fetal ultrasound and/or fetal magnetic resonance imaging (MRI).

Inaccurate diagnosis by fetal ultrasound	Accurate diagnosis by fetal MRI	Postnatal diagnosis	Cases (*n*)
Total			45
CNS pathology			39
Hypoplasia of corpus callosum	Normal	Normal	7
Partial agenesis of the corpus callosum	Normal	Normal	4
Agenesis of the SP	Normal	Normal	5
Poor visualization of CSP	Polymicrogyria and heterotopias that deform the CSP	Polymicrogyria and heterotopias that deform the CSP	1
Small-sized CSP	Complete agenesis of the corpus callosum and the SP	Complete agenesis of the corpus callosum and the SP	1
Hydranencephaly	Alobar holoprosencephaly	Alobar holoprosencephaly	1
Severe ventriculomegaly and interhemispheric cyst	Semilobar holoprosencephaly	Semilobar holoprosencephaly	1
Ventriculomegaly	Ventriculomegaly and venous infarction.	Ventriculomegaly and venous infarction.	1
Ventriculomegaly	Normal	Normal	4
Lissencephaly	Normal	Normal	1
Closed lip schizencephaly	Normal	Normal	1
Posterior fossa arachnoid cyst	Mega cisterna magna	Mega cisterna magna	2
Dandy walker complex	Mega cisterna magna	Mega cisterna magna	1
Dandy walker complex	PHACE syndrome	PHACE syndrome	1
Inferior vermis hypoplasia	Normal	Normal	1
Posterior fossa mass lesion	Dural sinus malformation and thrombosis	Dural sinus malformation and thrombosis	1
Dandy walker complex	Mega cisterna magna	Mega cisterna magna	1
Microcephaly	Normal	Normal	1
Tethered spinal cord	Normal	Normal	1
Blakes pouch cyst	Mild vermian hypoplasia	Mild vermian hypoplasia	1
Cleft lip	Normal	Normal	2
Thoracic pathology			**1**
CPAM	Congenital diaphragmatic hernia	Congenital diaphragmatic hernia	1
Abdominal pathology			**3**
Renal cyst	Congenital adrenal cyst	Congenital adrenal cyst	1
Ileal atresia	Normal	Normal	1
Bilateral adrenal hyperplasia	Normal	Normal	1
Other indications			**2**
IUGR	Normal	Normal	2
Inaccurate diagnosis by fetal ultrasound	Inaccurate diagnosis by MRI	Postnatal diagnosis	Cases (*n*)
Total			**15**
CNS pathology			5
Occipital soft-tissue hemangioma	Occipital soft-tissue hemangioma	Fibrosarcoma	1
Hydrocephalus	Hydrocephalus and ischemic sequelae	Hydrocephalus and cerebral toxoplasmosis with intraparenchymal lesion	1
Mild ventriculomegaly	Mild ventriculomegaly	Mild ventriculomegaly and malformation of the outer ear	1
Epidural hematoma	Bone lesion: Sarcoma or fibrous dysplasia	Intraosseous hemangioma	1
Mega cisterna magna and frontal polymicrogyria	Mega cisterna magna frontal polymicrogyria	Mega cisterna magna	1
Thoracical pathology			**3**
CPAM type 3	CPAM type 3	Normal (vanishing lesion of the lung)	1
Pulmonary hybrid lesion	Pulmonary hybrid lesión	Type 1 CPAM	1
Left atrial myxoma	Left atrial myxoma	Left atrial hemangioma	1
Abdominal pathology			**6**
Perirenal hematoma	Perirenal lymphangioma	Perirenal urinoma without hydronephrosis	1
Mild dilation of ileal loops	Hypoplastic colon syndrome without ileal dilatation	Ileal atresia	1
Esophageal atresia	Esophageal atresia	Esophageal duplication cyst	1
Left adrenal neuroblastoma	Left adrenal neuroblastoma	Infradiaphragmatic bronchopulmonary sequestration	1

Table 4: Continued.

Inaccurate diagnosis by fetal ultrasound	Accurate diagnosis by fetal MRI	Postnatal diagnosis	Cases (*n*)
Renal cyst	Pyeloureteral junction stenosis	Pyeloureteral junction stenosis and mesoblastic nephroma in calyceal wall	1
Other indications			**1**
Placenta increta	Placenta increta	Normal placenta	1
Accurate diagnosis by fetal ultrasound	**Inaccurate diagnosis by fetal MRI**	**Postnatal diagnosis**	**Cases (*n*)**
Total			**4**
CNS pathology			**3**
Scoliosis and dorsal hemivertebrae	Dorsal scoliosis	Scoliosis and dorsal hemivertebrae	3
Abdominal pathology			**1**
Hepatic calcifications	Normal liver	Hepatic calcifications	1

CNS: central nervous system, SP: septum pellucidum, CSP: cavum septum pelludidum, IUGR: intrauterine growth restriction, CPAM: congenital pulmonary airway malformation.

the diagnostic accuracy of fetal MRI between those cases with a gestational age of 24 weeks or less and those with a gestational age above 24 weeks. This contrasts with the study by Paladini et al. [15], who described a diagnostic accuracy of fetal MRI lower than that of fetal ultrasound when the former was carried out before week 24 of gestation (90.4% vs 93.1% for fetal MRI and fetal ultrasound, respectively). Nevertheless, caution should be exercised when interpreting fetal MRI performed before week 24-25 of gestation (10), as several CNS pathologies cannot be accurately diagnosed until the gestational age is greater than 24 weeks, such as the delay in the rotation of the vermis [17], or in the resolution of Blake's pouch cyst [18], which may be mistaken for vermian hypoplasia. When performed before week 24, MRI also has a low sensitivity in the diagnosis of heterotopias [19]. In this regard, the discrepancy between our results and those of Paladini et al. [15] is likely due to the lower number of cases with these pathologies in our study.

Assessing the usefulness of fetal MRI is more controversial, and different studies report highly variable values. Despite the fact that, like fetal ultrasound, fetal MRI is commonly considered a non-operator-dependent technique, both the equipment used to perform the test and the radiologist's experience in interpreting the results in complex pathologies can affect assessment of the usefulness of fetal MRI. Likewise, there is no consensus on the definition of useful information for perinatal management and prognosis over fetal ultrasound, and this also contributes to the variability of the results across the different studies. In our study, fetal MRI contributed 22.4% of additional information over fetal ultrasound, and 11% of useful information for perinatal management and prognosis over fetal ultrasound in cases with CNS pathology, which supports the usefulness of fetal MRI even when the concordance between the diagnoses exceeds 90%. Fetal MRI provided useful information for perinatal management and prognosis over fetal ultrasound in a large number of cases with ischemic-hemorrhagic pathology and tuberous sclerosis, although it was less useful in conditions affecting the corpus callosum, other midline defects, ventriculomegaly, and malformations of the posterior fossa. Similar to our study, Paladini et al. [15] reported that fetal MRI provided clinically relevant information in 7.9% of cases. By contrast, the MERIDIAN study [16] reported that fetal MRI provided additional information over fetal ultrasound in 49% of cases and modified the prognostic information in 20%. The aforementioned study has received some criticism, especially from Paladini et al. in a letter to the Lancet [20], which emphasized the importance of using transvaginal ultrasound with high-resolution transducers in neurosonography studies (not used in the MERIDIAN study) that, presumably, would have reduced the prognostic information provided by fetal MRI.

Thoracic pathology was evident in 5.9% of cases in our study, with pulmonary parenchymatous lesions being the commonest indication. From a clinical perspective, however, the main value of fetal MRI in this clinical scenario is to study congenital diaphragmatic hernia [21], in spite of its low incidence [22]. Fetal MRI provided additional information in 56.8% of the cases and useful information for perinatal management and prognosis over fetal ultrasound in 35.1%. This high figure is mainly due to the 12 cases of congenital diaphragmatic hernia, where fetal MRI could accurately detect the presence of the hernia and the compromised abdominal internal organs, measure the pulmonary volume and its signal, determine the degree of hypoplasia, and quantify the percentage of hepatic herniation, permitting a neonatal prognosis to be established [23–25]. In the study of pulmonary pathology by Levine et al. [26], fetal MRI provided additional information over fetal ultrasound in 38% of cases and resulted in a change in treatment in 8%.

Abdominal pathology corresponded to 9.8% of the cases in our study, in which fetal MRI and fetal ultrasound showed similar accuracies. The fetal MRI provided additional information and useful information for perinatal management and prognosis over fetal ultrasound in 27.9% and 11.5% of the cases. The most frequent cases referred were those with gastrointestinal pathology (28 cases), with fetal MRI providing additional information and useful information for perinatal management and prognosis in 5 and 4, and producing the only accurate diagnosis in one case. The values of

Table 5: Usefulness of fetal magnetic resonance as a complementary procedure to fetal ultrasound in the 623 cases referred between January 2007 and December 2018.

Indication	MRI concordant with fetal ultrasound *n* (%)	MRI provides additional information *n* (%)	MRI provides useful information *n* (%)	MRI is the only accurate diagnosis *n* (%)
Total (n = 623)	**574 (92.1)**	**144 (23.1)**	**72 (11.6)**	**45 (7.2)**
CNS pathology (n = 429)	**387 (90.2)**	**96 (22.4)**	**47 (11.0)**	**39 (9.1)**
Ventriculomegaly	142 (95.9)	22 (14.9)	10 (6.8)	6 (4.1)
Posterior fossa malformations	65 (91.5)	9 (12.7)	4 (5.6)	6 (8.5)
Abnormalities of the corpus callosum	45 (77.6)	17 (29.3)	8 (13.8)	13 (22.4)
Other midline abnormalities	32 (84.2)	10 (26.3)	4 (10.5)	6 (15.8)
Infectious pathology	30 (100.0)	9 (30.0)	3 (10.0)	0 (0.0)
Ischemic/hemorrhagic pathology	23 (92.0)	14 (56.0)	9 (36.0)	2 (8.0)
Tumoral pathology and lesions of the cranial vault, neck, or orbits	21 (87.5)	7 (29.2)	4 (16.7)	3 (12.5)
Spinal column pathology	8 (66.7)	1 (8.3)	1 (8.3)	1 (8.3)
Tuberous sclerosis	13 (100.0)	6 (46.2)	4 (30.8)	0 (0.0)
Malformations of cortical development	8 (80.0)	1 (10.0)	0 (0.0)	2 (20.0)
Thoracic pathology (n = 37)	**36 (97.3)**	**21 (56.8)**	**13 (35.1)**	**1 (2.7)**
Parenchymatous lesions	21 (95.5)	9 (40.9)	1 (4.5)	1 (4.5)
Congenital diaphragmatic hernia	12 (100.0)	12 (100.0)	12 (100.0)	0 (0.0)
Mediastenic or pleural pathology	3 (100.0)	0 (0.0)	0 (0.0)	0 (0.0)
Abdominal pathology (n = 61)	**57 (93.4)**	**17 (27.9)**	**7 (11.5)**	**3 (4.9)**
Digestive pathology	26 (92.9)	5 (17.9)	4 (14.3)	1 (3.6)
Urogenital pathology	11 (91.7)	2 (16.7)	0 (0.0)	1 (8.3)
Abdominal masses	12 (92.3)	4 (30.8)	1 (7.7)	1 (7.7)
Abdominal wall defects	4 (100.0)	2 (50.0)	0 (0.0)	0 (0.0)
Vascular pathology	4 (100.0)	4 (100.0)	2 (50.0)	0 (0.0)
Other indications (n = 96)	**94 (97.9)**	**10 (10.4)**	**5 (5.2)**	**2 (2.1)**
Normal ultrasound in high-risk pregnancy	47 (100.0)	2 (4.3)	1 (2.1)	0 (0.0)
IUGR	20 (90.9)	2 (9.1)	3 (13.6)	2 (9.1)
Ultrasound not assessable (poor acoustic window)	9 (100.0)	3 (33.3)	0 (0.0)	0 (0.0)
Placental pathology.	9 (100.0)	1 (11.1)	0 (0.0)	0 (0.0)
Musculoskeletal pathology	7 (100.0)	2 (28.6)	1 (14.3)	0 (0.0)
Genetic or chromosomal abnormality	2 (100.0)	0 (0.0)	0 (0.0)	0 (0.0)

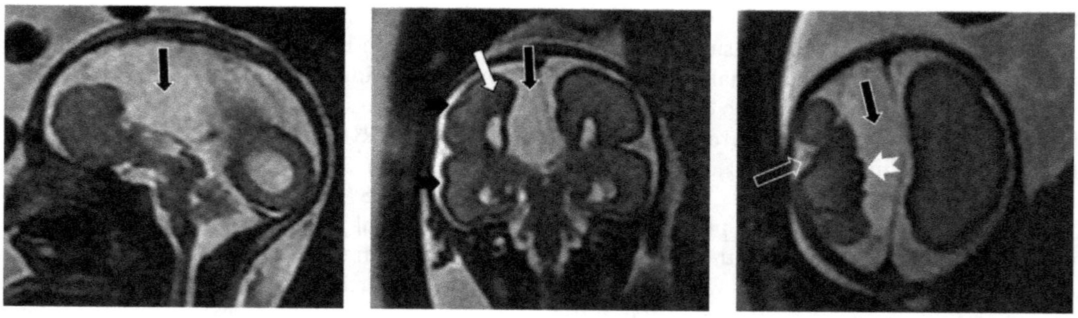

(a) (b) (c)

Figure 2: Complete agenesis of corpus callosum. Gestational age: 27 weeks. (a) Sagittal SSFSE T2. (b) Coronal SSFSE T2. (c) Axial SSFSE T2. Complete agenesis of corpus callosum with right interhemispherical cyst with mass effect (solid black arrow) is shown. The right cerebral hemisphere is smaller in size, and malformation of cortical development is evident, with multiple anomalous sulci, bumpy cortical surface (solid black arrowhead), and cortical invaginations (empty white arrow). Regions of associated polymicrogyria (solid white arrowhead) and heterotopias bulging on the ventricle wall are depicted (solid white arrow). Fetal MRI provides useful information for perinatal management and prognosis over fetal ultrasound by detecting anomalies of the cerebral cortex and heterotopies not visible in the fetal ultrasound.

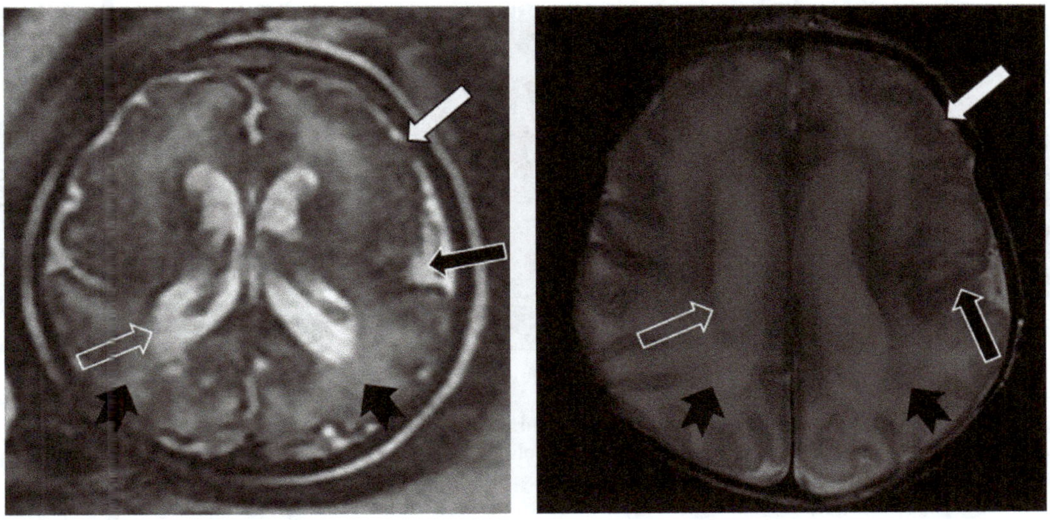

(a) (b)

Figure 3: CMV infection. Gestational age: 35 weeks. (a) Fetal Axial SSFSE T2. (b) Postnatal cerebral MRI at 8 days of life, axial FSE T2. The presence of diffuse affectation of the white matter of parietal predominance (solid black arrowhead) with mild ventriculomegaly (empty white arrow) is shown. Fetal MRI provided useful information for perinatal management and prognosis over fetal ultrasound by detecting left frontal (solid white arrow) and left Sylvian fissure (solid black arrow) polymicrogyria not visible in the fetal ultrasound.

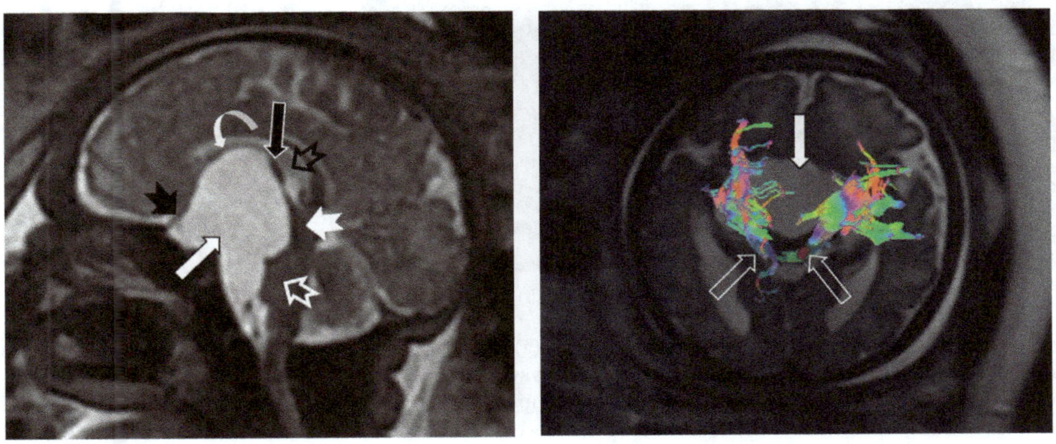

(a) (b)

Figure 4: Arachnoid cyst associated with persistence of Liliequist membrane. Gestational age: 36 weeks and 2 days. (a) Sagittal SSFSE T2. Large-sized arachnoid cyst (solid white arrow) anterior to the mesencephalon extending into the prepontine cistern and suprasellar region is shown. The cyst produces a slight mass effect of the protuberance (empty white arrowhead) and an important mass effect on the mesencephalon (solid white arrowhead), hypothalamic region (empty black arrowhead), mammillary bodies (solid black arrow), the floor of the third ventricle (curved white arrow), and optic chiasm (solid black arrowhead). (b) Diffusion tensor with axial tractography image. The cyst (solid white arrow) extends towards the interpeduncular cistern of the mesencephalon and displaces the corticospinal tracts in a posterolateral direction (empty white arrows). Fetal MRI provides additional information because the real extent of the lesion is better evaluated than with ultrasound.

additional information and useful information for perinatal management and prognosis over fetal ultrasound are lower than those reported by Manganaro et al. [27] in a prospective study of 38 cases, wherein fetal MRI provided additional information in more than 60% of cases, ruled out the presence of anomalies diagnosed in the fetal ultrasound in 5.2% of cases, and changed the fetal ultrasound diagnosis in 5.2% of cases. Once again, the lack of consensus in the definitions of additional and useful information could explain the discrepancies between the results.

Regarding those cases with indication for urogenital pathology, fetal MRI provided additional over fetal ultrasound in 16.7% of cases. Nonetheless, it is noteworthy that these results are only based on 12 cases. In a study of 46 fetuses with urogenital anomalies, Kajbafzadeh et al. [28] reported that MRI provided additional information in 37% of cases.

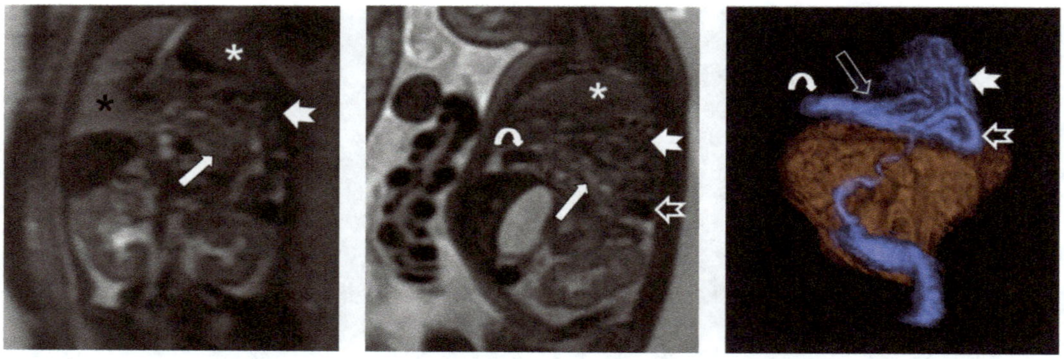

(a) (b) (c)

Figure 5: Left diaphragmatic hernia. Gestational age: 27 weeks and 6 days. (a) Coronal SSFSE T2. (b) Sagittal SSFSE T2. (c) Volume rendering coronal reconstruction. Complete herniation of jejunal (solid white arrow) and ileal (solid white arrowhead) loops is observed. Herniation of the hepatic angle of the colon (curved white arrow), ascending colon and cecum (empty white arrow) is also observed, and they are located above the splenic angle of the colon (empty white arrowhead). The left lung is hypoplastic and is collapsed in the left upper hemithorax (white asterisk). The cardiomediastenic displacement towards the right hemithorax and normal right lung (black asterisk) is shown. No hepatic or gastric herniation is observed. Relative pulmonary volume is 72.64%; the intensity ratio of the pulmonary parenchyma relative to the hepatic parenchyma is >1 and the intensity ratio of the pulmonary parenchyma in relation to the CSF is 0.78, implying a good prognosis. Fetal MRI provided useful information for perinatal management and prognosis over the fetal ultrasound.

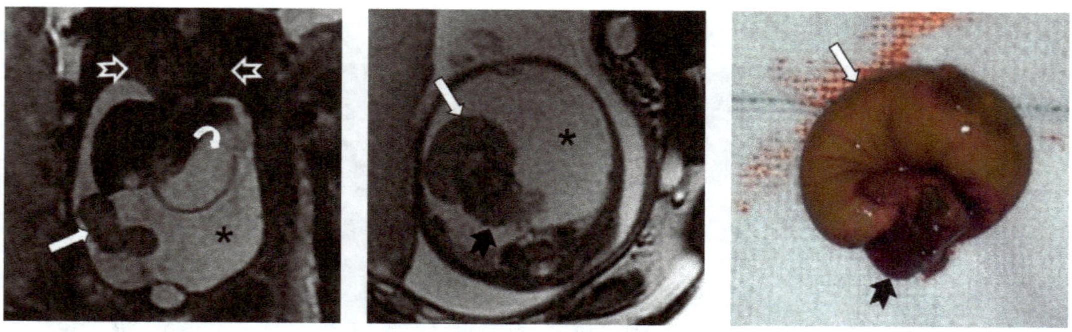

(a) (b) (c)

Figure 6: Intestinal volvulus. Gestational age 28 weeks and 2 days. (a) Coronal SSFSE T2. (b) Axial SSFSE T2. (c) Photograph of surgical specimen. Bichorial biamniotic gestation. One of the twins presents with an intestinal volvulus, along with meconial ileus and meconial peritonitis. The presence of massive ascites (black asterisk) that compress both lungs (empty white arrowhead) is shown. The stomach is dilated (curved white arrowhead). Dilated and volvulated ileal loops (solid white arrow) with distal necrosed clustered loops (solid black arrowhead) are shown. Fetal MRI diagnosed intestinal volvulus not described in fetal ultrasound providing useful information for perinatal management and prognosis over fetal ultrasound.

Table 6: Diagnostic accuracy of the fetal ultrasound relative to postnatal diagnosis, concordance, and usefulness of fetal MRI of the 623 cases referred from reference and non-reference ultrasound centers.

	Fetal ultrasound studies performed in centers of reference ($n = 362$)	Fetal ultrasound studies not performed in centers of reference ($n = 261$)	p-value
Diagnostic accuracy of fetal ultrasound	329 (90.9%)	234 (89.7%)	0.608
Concordance between fetal ultrasound and MRI	338 (93.4%)	236 (90.4%)	0.177
MRI provides additional information over fetal ultrasound	96 (26.5%)	48 (18.4%)	0.018
MRI provides additional information useful for perinatal management and prognosis over fetal ultrasound	53 (14.6%)	19 (7.3%)	0.004
MRI is the only accurate diagnosis	22 (6.1%)	23 (8.8%)	0.193

p-value of the chi-squared tests for the differences in diagnostic accuracy of fetal ultrasound, concordance, and usefulness of MRI between cases referred from ultrasound reference and nonreference centers.

Overall, fetal MRI provided additional information in 23.1% of the 623 cases, which corresponded to useful information for perinatal management and prognosis in 11.6%. Fetal MRI was the only accurate diagnostic method in 45 cases (7.2%). To our knowledge, our study represents the largest number of cases describing the value of fetal MRI both in CNS-related and non-related pathologies.

5. Conclusions

Fetal MRI has a superior diagnostic accuracy, especially in CNS pathology, and provides additional useful information in CNS, thoracic, and abdominal pathology. The combination of fetal MRI with high-quality ultrasound facilitates additional diagnostic information, which widens the possibilities for detecting early perinatal development disorders.

References

[1] F. V. Coakley, O. A. Glenn, A. Qayyum, A. J. Barkovich, R. Goldstein, and R. A. Filly, "Fetal MRI:A developing technique for the developing patient," *American Journal of Roentgenology*, vol. 182, no. 1, pp. 243–252, 2004.

[2] D. Levine, "Ultrasound versus magnetic resonance imaging in fetal evaluation," *Topics in Magnetic Resonance Imaging*, vol. 12, no. 1, pp. 1225–1238, 2001.

[3] N. R. Valevičienė, G. Varytė, J. Zakarevičienė, E. Kontrimavičiūtė, D. Ramašauskaitė, and D. Rutkauskaitė-Valančienė, "Use of magnetic resonance imaging in evaluating fetal brain and abdomen malformations during pregnancy," *Medicina (Kaunas)*, vol. 55, no. 2, p. 55, 2019.

[4] U. M. Reddy, R. A. Filly, and J. A. Copel, "Prenatal imaging," *Obstetrics & Gynecology*, vol. 112, no. 1, pp. 145–157, 2008.

[5] O. A. Glenn and A. J. Barkovich, "Magnetic resonance imaging of the fetal brain and spine: an increasingly important tool in prenatal diagnosis, part 1," *AJNR. American Journal of Neuroradiology*, vol. 27, no. 8, pp. 1604–1611, 2006.

[6] L. J. Salomon, N. Siauve, D. Balvay et al., "Radiology imaging with contrast agents in a mouse model 1," *Radiology*, vol. 5, pp. 73–80, 2005.

[7] T. Grobner and F. C. Prischl, "Gadolinium and nephrogenic systemic fibrosis," *Kidney International*, vol. 72, no. 3, pp. 260–264, 2007.

[8] F. Smith, A. H. Adam, and W. D. Phillips, "NMR imaging in pregnancy," *The Lancet*, vol. 321, no. 8314-8315, pp. 61-62, 1983.

[9] S. Yagel, S. M. Cohen, S. Porat et al., "Detailed transabdominal fetal anatomic scanning in the late first trimester versus the early second trimester of pregnancy," *Journal of Ultrasound in Medicine*, vol. 34, no. 1, pp. 143–149, 2015.

[10] L. Manganaro, A. Antonelli, S. Bernardo et al., "Highlights on MRI of the fetal body," *La Radiologia Medica*, vol. 123, no. 4, pp. 271–285, 2018.

[11] R. d. A. Nogueira, H. Werner Júnior, P. Daltro, G. M. Lima, A. D. Barbosa, and E. Araujo Júnior, "The role of a novel magnetic resonance imaging sequence in the evaluation of the fetal skeleton: a pilot study," *Radiologia Brasileira*, vol. 51, no. 5, pp. 303–307, 2018.

[12] D. Jarvis, C. Mooney, J. Cohen et al., "A systematic review and meta-analysis to determine the contribution of mr imaging to the diagnosis of foetal brain abnormalities in Utero," *European Radiology*, vol. 27, no. 6, pp. 2367–2380, 2017.

[13] L. F. Gonçalves, W. Lee, S. Mody, A. Shetty, H. Sangi-Haghpeykar, and R. Romero, "Diagnostic accuracy of ultrasonography and magnetic resonance imaging for the detection of fetal anomalies: a blinded case-control study," *Ultrasound in Obstetrics & Gynecology*, vol. 48, no. 2, pp. 185–192, 2016.

[14] A. C. Rossi and F. Prefumo, "Additional value of fetal magnetic resonance imaging in the prenatal diagnosis of central nervous system anomalies: a systematic review of the literature," *Ultrasound in Obstetrics & Gynecology*, vol. 44, no. 4, pp. 388–393, 2014.

[15] D. Paladini, M. Quarantelli, G. Sglavo et al., "Accuracy of neurosonography and MRI in clinical management of fetuses referred with central nervous system abnormalities," *Ultrasound in Obstetrics & Gynecology*, vol. 44, no. 2, pp. 188–196, 2014.

[16] P. D. Griffiths, M. Bradburn, M. J. Campbell et al., "Use of MRI in the diagnosis of fetal brain abnormalities in utero (MERIDIAN): a multicentre, prospective cohort study," *The Lancet*, vol. 389, no. 10068, pp. 538–546, 2017.

[17] J. Pinto, D. Paladini, M. Severino et al., "Delayed rotation of the cerebellar vermis: a pitfall in early second-trimester fetal magnetic resonance imaging," *Ultrasound in Obstetrics & Gynecology*, vol. 48, no. 1, pp. 121–124, 2016.

[18] A. J. Robinson, "Inferior vermian hypoplasia—preconception, misconception," *Ultrasound in Obstetrics & Gynecology*, vol. 43, no. 2, pp. 123–136, 2014.

[19] O. A. Glenn, A. A. Cuneo, A. J. Barkovich, Z. Hashemi, A. I. Bartha, and D. Xu, "Malformations of cortical development: diagnostic accuracy of fetal MR imaging," *Radiology*, vol. 263, no. 3, pp. 843–855, 2012.

[20] D. Paladini, G. Malinger, G. Pilu, I. Timor-Trisch, and P. Volpe, "The MERIDIAN trial: caution is needed," *The Lancet*, vol. 389, no. 10084, p. 2103, 2017.

[21] A. M. Johnson and A. M. Hubbard, "Congenital anomalies of the fetal/neonatal chest," *Seminars in Roentgenology*, vol. 39, no. 2, pp. 197–214, 2004.

[22] N. Butler and A. E. Claireaux, "Congenital diaphragmatic hernia as a cause of perinatal mortality," *The Lancet*, vol. 279, no. 7231, pp. 659–663, 1962.

[23] M. Yamoto, T. Iwazaki, K. Takeuchi et al., "The fetal lung-to-liver signal intensity ratio on magnetic resonance imaging as a predictor of outcomes from isolated congenital diaphragmatic hernia," *Pediatric Surgery International*, vol. 34, no. 2, pp. 161–168, 2018.

[24] R. Ruano, D. A. Lazar, D. L. Cass et al., "Fetal lung volume and quantification of liver herniation by magnetic resonance imaging in isolated congenital diaphragmatic hernia," *Ultrasound in Obstetrics & Gynecology*, vol. 43, no. 6, pp. 662–669, 2014.

[25] M. Weis, S. Hoffmann, C. Henzler et al., "Isolated impact of liver herniation on outcome in fetuses with congenital diaphragmatic hernia—a matched-pair analysis based on fetal MRI relative lung volume," *European Journal of Radiology*, vol. 105, pp. 148–152, 2018.

[26] D. Levine, C. E. Barnewolt, T. S. Mehta, I. Trop, J. Estroff, and G. Wong, "Fetal thoracic abnormalities: MR imaging," *Radiology*, vol. 228, no. 2, pp. 379–388, 2003.

[27] L. Manganaro, M. Saldari, S. Bernardo et al., "Role of magnetic resonance imaging in the prenatal diagnosis of gastrointestinal fetal anomalies," *La Radiologia Medica*, vol. 120, no. 4, pp. 393–403, 2015.

[28] A.-M. Kajbafzadeh, S. Payabvash, Z. Sadeghi et al., "Comparison of magnetic resonance urography with ultrasound studies in detection of fetal urogenital anomalies," *Journal of Pediatric Urology*, vol. 4, no. 1, pp. 32–39, 2008.

12

Comparative Study of Multiple High-Signal-Intensity Spots on 3D and 2D Magnetic Resonance Sialography for Patients with Sjögren's Syndrome

Yusuke Shimada, Ikuho Kojima, and Masahiro Iikubo

Department of Dental Informatics and Radiology, Tohoku University Graduate School of Dentistry, 4-1 Seiryo-machi, Aoba-ku, Sendai 980-8575, Japan

Correspondence should be addressed to Ikuho Kojima; ikuhokojima@tohoku.ac.jp

Academic Editor: André Luiz Ferreira Costa

We investigated the sensitivities of 2-dimensional (2D) magnetic resonance sialography (MR-S) and unilateral sagittal and axial 3-dimensional (3D) MR-S using a surface coil and their combination in diagnosing patients with Sjögren's syndrome (SS). We retrospectively analyzed the 3D and 2D MR-S results of 78 patients with SS. We evaluated the sensitivities of multiple high-signal-intensity spots and staging on MR sialograms and analyzed the efficient imaging methods and cross section for diagnosing patients with SS. The sensitivities of MR-S for detecting abnormal findings (i.e., MR-S stage 1 or higher) were as follows: 65 cases (83.3% [95% confidence interval (CI): 73.2–90.8]) for unilateral sagittal 3D MR-S; 62 cases (79.4% [95% CI: 68.8–87.8]) for axial 3D MR-S; 66 cases (84.6% [95% CI: 74.7–91.8]) for combined unilateral sagittal and axial 3D MR-S; and 32 cases (41.0% [95% CI: 30.0–52.7]) for bilateral sagittal 2D MR-S. The ratio of the abnormal finding of MR-S was tested using the two-tailed Fisher's exact test. Unilateral sagittal, axial, and combined unilateral sagittal and axial 3D MR-S showed significantly higher sensitivity than bilateral sagittal 2D MR-S, respectively ($P < 0.001$). Most cases upstaged by 3D MR-S were those positive (stage 1 or higher) among the stage 0 cases detected by 2D MR-S. Axial 3D MR-S, compared with 2D MR-S, understaged four cases, which was due to the imaging range of the axial 3D MR-S. We concluded that a single unilateral sagittal 3D MR-S was sufficient and axial 3D MR-S was unnecessary for SS staging. T1- and T2-weighted images are essential for investigating the salivary glands in patients with SS. Therefore, we also concluded that bilateral sagittal 3D MR-S of the parotid glands in addition to T1- and T2-weighted imaging is necessary, sufficient, and most efficient for precise MR imaging examination of the salivary glands, including diagnosing SS.

1. Introduction

Magnetic resonance (MR) imaging has become widely used for assessing salivary gland diseases and is useful for the diagnosis of Sjögren's syndrome (SS). X-ray sialography, whose apple tree appearance has been adopted for some SS criteria [1, 2], cannot simultaneously and bilaterally examine the three pairs of major salivary glands (i.e., parotid, submandibular, and sublingual glands) and is invasive and requires the use of contrast medium. Conversely, MR imaging, including MR sialography (MR-S), can bilaterally evaluate all major salivary glands simultaneously without contrast medium. MR imaging of patients with SS shows characteristic findings of the parotid gland, including a heterogeneous signal-intensity distribution (HD) on T1- and T2-weighted images (salt and pepper appearance) [3, 4], multiple high-signal-intensity spots (MHS) on MR-S (apple tree appearance) [5, 6], and swelling or atrophy of the parotid gland [4, 7]. Moreover, MR-S has a higher sensitivity (>82%) for the diagnosis of SS than conventional MRI, salivary gland scintigraphy, or ultrasonography [8–12]. Diffusion-weighted MRI also possessed only additional utility to MR-S in the diagnosis of SS [13]. Thus, MR-S is expected to be an alternative to conventional X-ray sialography for the diagnosis of SS.

Three-dimensional (3D) MR-S techniques facilitate the reliable prediction of ductal dilatation, stenosis, and damage better than the two-dimensional (2D) techniques [14–16]. Moreover, high-resolution MR-S using a small surface coil has been reported [17, 18]. MR-S using a combination of the constructive interference in steady-state sequence and the half-fourier acquisition single-shot turbo spin-echo sequence have been reported to be useful for patients with inflammatory salivary gland disorder [15]. However, these studies were mainly aimed at depicting detailed salivary gland ducts, and none of them mentioned the diagnostic accuracy of SS. Moreover, there is no study comparing the diagnostic accuracy of SS between 3D and 2D MR-S. The longer duration of acquisition (more than a few minutes per cross section imaging) and narrow range of acquisition (less than approximately 30 mm width) are major disadvantages of 3D MR-S for routine clinical use relative to 2D MR-S (imaging time less than approximately 20 s). Additionally, sagittal 3D MR-S of the bilateral parotid glands and axial 3D MR-S are time-consuming. The use of special coils, which are not used for other MR imaging techniques, such as high-resolution small surface coils, is also time-consuming and difficult. Furthermore, the contribution of 3D MR-S in combination with 2D MR-S to the sensitivity of the diagnosis of SS in individual patients has not been established. Therefore, we investigated the sensitivities of 2D MR-S and sagittal/axial 3D MR-S using a regular surface coil and their combination in diagnosing SS.

2. Materials and Methods

The procedures in this study adhered to the Helsinki Declaration of 1975, as revised in 1983. This retrospective study was approved by our institutional review board (no. 2012-24-1). Informed patient consent was obtained via an opt-out system on our institutional website displaying information about the study objectives and procedures.

2.1. Patients. We retrospectively reviewed the MR images of 78 patients (76 women and 2 men; age, 19–79 years; mean age, 55 years) clinically diagnosed with SS based on the chief complaint of xerostomia, positive histopathological findings of labial gland biopsy, and positive serologic evidence of anti-SS-A/Ro and/or anti-SS-B/La antibodies. Autoimmune disease specialists diagnosed all the patients with SS; the patients were negative for human immunodeficiency virus and sarcoidosis. We adopted labial gland biopsy as a criterion for all patients and graded the histopathological findings using focal scores according to previously established criteria [19]. We determined the histopathological findings based on the focal scores with focal aggregates of 50 lymphocytes per 4 mm^2 of salivary gland tissue. Therefore, positive histopathological findings, the chief complaint of oral dryness, and anti-SS-A/Ro and/or anti-SS-B/La antibodies formed the basis of a definitive diagnosis of SS according to the criteria proposed by the American-European Consensus Group [1], American College of Rheumatology [20], and revised Japanese criteria [2].

2.2. MR Imaging Technique. We performed MR imaging with a 1.5- or 3.0-Tesla MR unit (Achieva 1.5 T or Achieva 3.0 T; Royal Philips Electronics, Eindhoven, the Netherlands) using the surface coils with a loop diameter of 11 cm. Transverse T1-weighted images (TR/TE, 477–619/7–12 ms) and fat-suppressed T2-weighted images (TR/TE, 4000–5711/54–90 ms) were obtained using the spin-echo and fast-spin-echo techniques, respectively. The section thickness of the transverse T1- and T2-weighted images was 5 mm with an intersection gap of 1 mm, acquisition matrix of 512 × 358, and field of view (FOV) of 210 mm. MR-S was performed using a high-resolution technique and a heavily T2-weighted 3D fast-spin-echo sequence (TR/TE/number of signal-intensity acquisitions, 5000/602–675 ms/2) according to a previous report that a heavily T2-weighted 3D fast-spin-echo sequence is the most suitable for the evaluation of thin salivary gland ducts (section thickness: 1 mm, gapless image, number of slices: 20, pixel size: 0.45–0.55 mm × 0.55–0.79 mm, FOV: 200 mm; scan time: 185 s) [21]. The 2D MR-S was performed using a single-shot 2D sequence (TR/TE, 8000–9000/800–914, the slice thickness: 30 mm, pixel size: 0.88 mm × 1.08 mm, FOV: 200 mm, scan time: 18–25 sec.). The MRI protocol for routine clinical practice was as follows: first, we performed T1- and T2-weighted imaging of the salivary glands, followed by the bilateral sagittal 2D MR-S of the parotid glands. Second, we performed axial 3D MR-S, which involved the bilateral parotid gland ducts. Finally, unilateral sagittal 3D MR-S was performed for the parotid gland. The laterality of the sagittal 3D MR-S was decided by the oral and maxillofacial radiologists based on the following: we selected the side that clearly showed the MHS on 2D MR-S. If MHS was not observed bilaterally, we assessed the T1- and T2-weighted images and proceeded with the side with strong HD findings.

2.3. Imaging Analysis and Sensitivity for Sjögren's Syndrome. Two oral and maxillofacial radiologists with 11 and 19 years of experience, respectively, evaluated the coded and randomly presented unilateral sagittal 3D MR-S, axial 3D MR-S, and bilateral sagittal 2D MR-S for the presence or absence of MHS based on a previous report [6]. Both radiologists were blinded to the histopathological grading and T1- and T2-weighted imaging findings. The radiologists used digital imaging and communications in medicine viewer and processing software (nv-1000; Hitachi Medical Corporation, Tokyo, Japan) and were free to use the available image-enhancement options (density, contrast, and magnification) to perform visual assessments on the same 29.7-inch display (2560 × 1600 screen resolution, RadiForce RX440; EIZO Corporation, Ishikawa, Japan). Using the X-ray sialography criteria established in previous reports, we staged the MHS measured the size of the maximum diameter of the high-signal-intensity spots, which represented saliva leaked from peripheral ducts [10] by the viewer software on display (Figure 1). MHS was classified as stages 0 (no cavities found), 1 (cavities ≤1 mm in diameter), 2 (cavities 1-2 mm in

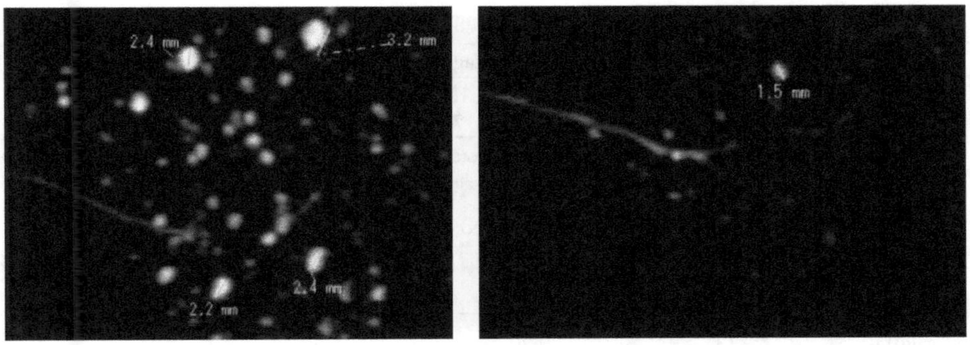

(a) (b)

FIGURE 1: Analysis and measurement of MHS on MR-S. We staged the presence or absence of MHS and measured the size of the maximum diameter of the high-signal-intensity spots by the viewer software on display. A case of stage 3 with the maximum cavity >2 mm (a) and another case of stage 2 with the maximum cavity of 1-2 mm (b). MHS: multiple high-signal-intensity spots; MR-S: magnetic resonance sialography.

diameter), 3 (cavities >2 mm in diameter), or 4 (severe irregular dilatation of the main duct with bizarrely patterned cavities). After an independent evaluation, the reviewers compared and discussed their staging. Any differences in interpretation were discussed, and a consensus was reached.

2.4. Statistical Analysis. Categorical variables are presented as counts and percentages. We determined the sensitivity of the MHS (according to previous reports [10], stage 0 is normal and stage 1 or higher is abnormal), and the sensitivity (ability to detect abnormalities) were compared between 3D MR-S and 2D MR-S for each sagittal image of 98 sides, and between the unilateral sagittal 3D MR-S, axial 3D MR-S, combined unilateral sagittal + axial 3D MR-S, and bilateral sagittal 2D MR-S patientwise in 78 patients, which were tested using the two-tailed Fisher's exact test. In case of significant association for categorical variables with a multiple comparison (patientwise comparison), pairwise comparison using adjustment methods of the Bonferroni correction was implemented. All P values were two-sided, and statistical significance was set at $P < 0.05$. Interobserver agreement between the two reviewers in the imaging analysis was evaluated using the kappa coefficient (κ). The strength of agreement was classified as slight (0.01 to 0.20), fair (0.21 to 0.40), moderate (0.41 to 0.60), substantial (0.61 to 0.80), or excellent (0.81 to 1.00). The sample size calculation for this study was based on Fisher's exact test for a power of 80% with reference to the accuracy of MR-S in a previous report [8]. A total of 92 samples would be required to test the association at 5% levels using a two-tailed test. EZR software (Saitama Medical Center, Jichi Medical University, Saitama, Japan), providing a graphical interface for *R* (v3.2.2; The *R* Foundation for Statistical Computing, Vienna, Austria), was used for statistical analyses.

3. Results

In the imaging analysis for the staging of MR-S, which indicates the detection of the MHS and measurement of the diameter of the MHS, the kappa values for the interobserver agreement of the sagittal 3D MR-S, axial 3D MR-S, and sagittal 2D MR-S were 0.92 (95% confidence interval [CI], 0.808–1.02), 0.96 (95% CI, 0.881–1.04), and 0.85 (95% CI, 0.744–0.957), respectively. All the values showed high agreement (excellent).

The MR-S staging on 98 sides of 78 patients with SS is shown in Table 1. The sagittal 3D MR-S identified MHS in 21 stage 0 cases, 40 stage 1 cases, 24 stage 2 cases, 12 stage 3 cases, and 1 stage 4 case. The sagittal 2D MR-S showed MHS for 58 stage 0 cases, 10 stage 1 cases, 22 stage 2 cases, 7 stage 3 cases, and 1 stage 4 case. Focusing on the frequencies of cases of stages 0–4, the 3D MR-S can detect more cases of stage 1 or higher than stage 0 than 2D MR-S. MR-S showed a statistically significant difference between the sensitivity for detecting abnormal findings of MHS between the two imaging methods: 78.6% (95% CI, 69.1–86.2%) on the 77 sides for 3D MR-S and 40.8% (95% CI, 31–51.2%) on the 40 sides for 2D MR-S ($P = 0.000000106$).

The patientwise MR-S staging for SS based on imaging findings and cross section is shown in Table 2. MR-S showed abnormal findings of MHS (i.e., stage 1 or higher): 65 cases (83.3%; 95% CI, 73.2–90.8%) for unilateral sagittal 3D MR-S; 62 cases (79.4%; 95% CI, 68.8–87.8%) for axial 3D MR-S; 66 cases (84.6%; 95% CI, 74.7–91.8%) for unilateral sagittal + axial 3D MR-S; and 32 cases (41.0%; 95% CI, 30–52.7%) for bilateral sagittal 2D MR-S. Unilateral sagittal, axial, and combined unilateral sagittal + axial 3D MR-S had significantly higher sensitivity than bilateral sagittal 2D MR-S ($P = 0.00000043$, $P = 0.00000889$, and $P = 0.00000014$, respectively). We checked the T1- and T2-weighted images and assessed the side with strong HD findings or tendencies if MHS was not observed bilaterally on bilateral 2D MR-S (Figure 2). As a result, the unilateral sagittal 3D MR-S images using this criterion had higher sensitivity than the axial 3D MR-S, including the bilateral parotid ducts.

Most cases designated as stage 2 or higher based on 3D MR-S could also be designated as stage 1 or higher by 2D MR-S (Figure 3). Most cases upstaged by 3D MR-S could be detected as positive (stage 1 or higher) from stage 0 by 2D MR-S (Figure 4). The unilateral sagittal, axial, and combined unilateral sagittal + axial 3D MR-S detected (upstaging) 33, 30, and 33

Table 1: MR-S staging by sagittal images of 98 sides.

	Stage 0	Stage 1	Stage 2	Stage 3	Stage 4	Sensitivity (%) [95% CI]	
3D MR-S (sagittal)	21	40	24	12	1	78.6 [69.1–86.2]	***
2D MR-S (sagittal)	58	10	22	7	1	40.8 [31.0–51.2]	$P < 0.001$[a]

***, $P < 0.001$, comparison of sensitivities of 3D and 2D MR-S by [a]Fisher's exact test. MR-S: magnetic resonance sialography; CI: confidence interval.

Table 2: Patientwise MR-S staging stratified by imaging method and cross section.

	Stage 0	Stage 1	Stage 2	Stage 3	Stage 4	Sensitivity (%) [95% CI]	
3D MR-S (unilateral sagittal)	13	35	20	9	1	83.3 [73.2–90.8]	*** $P < 0.001$[a] (vs. 2D MR-S)
3D MR-S (axial)	16	31	24	6	1	79.4 [68.8–87.8]	*** $P < 0.001$[a] (vs. 2D MR-S)
3D MR-S (unilateral sagittal + axial)	12	33	22	10	1	84.6 [74.7–91.8]	*** $P < 0.001$[a] (vs. 2D MR-S)
2D MR-S (bilateral sagittal)	46	6	20	5	1	41.0 [30.0–52.7]	

***, $P < 0.001$, multiple comparisons of sensitivities by [a]Fisher's exact test and pairwise comparisons with the Bonferroni correction. MR-S: magnetic resonance sialography; CI: confidence interval.

positive cases of stage 1 or higher, respectively, from stage 0 cases of 2D MR-S. The unilateral sagittal and axial 3D MR-S understaged 1 and 4 cases, respectively, compared to the staging of 2D MR-S. Some cases of understaging by axial 3D MR-S were due to the imaging range of MR-S (Figure 5). The one case of understaging by unilateral sagittal 3D MR-S was due to MHS on the opposite side.

4. Discussion

A comparison of the 3D and 2D techniques for sagittal MR-S (78 patients, 98 sides: Table 1) showed that 3D sagittal MR-S had significantly higher sensitivity than 2D MR-S. Similarly, unilateral sagittal, axial, and combined sagittal + axial 3D MR-S had significantly higher sensitivity for detecting SS-related findings than bilateral 2D MR-S by patientwise MR-S staging (Table 2). Three-dimensional MR-S enables the precise assessment of salivary gland ductal systems and detects early stages of SS with 91–100% accuracy [5]. Takagi et al. [18] demonstrated high diagnostic performance with MRI using a 47 mm microscopic coil, with an area under the curve of 0.91 in the receiver operating characteristics curve analysis for MR-S lesion counts. The ability of 3D MR-S to detect ductal structures is better than that of 2D MR-S, and the sensitivity is much better than the results of this study. The present findings indicated that 3D MR-S without the high-resolution coil and using a normal surface coil had a relatively high sensitivity for SS diagnosis, which was significantly superior to 2D MR-S. Although a simple comparative study between 2D and 3D methods would not be useful, this study examined the combination of 2D and 3D MR-S for efficient imaging by considering the imaging duration and cross section and the number of images.

Our results indicate that unilateral sagittal 3D MR-S is comparable to or better than axial 3D MR-S in diagnosing SS (Table 2). The axial 3D MR-S was unable to detect MHS at the upper and lower ends of the parotid gland for several cases because the imaging range was limited to 30 mm. In one case, unilateral sagittal 3D MR-S was unable to detect MHS because of presence on the opposite side. Moreover, bilateral sagittal MRI is not only recommended for MR-S-based staging but also for the diagnosis of the bilateral parotid duct because it covers both sides of the parotid gland within the imaging range. Kojima et al. [8] analyzed the diagnostic performance of MR imaging and MR-S of the three major salivary glands for SS and demonstrated low sensitivity and high specificity for the submandibular glands and low diagnostic performance for the sublingual gland. For detecting SS, MR-S of other salivary glands is not necessary. 3D MR-S of the parotid gland is sufficient. Several cases undergoing MR-S with 3D and high-resolution imaging using special coils have been reported [14–18]. However, no study has examined the combination of imaging methods that are efficient in terms of imaging duration, imaging cross section, and the number of images for each case. We concluded that a single unilateral sagittal 3D MR-S was sufficient and axial 3D MR-S was not necessary for SS staging.

In the abovementioned study that examined the diagnostic accuracy of SS [8], the MHS findings on MR-S and HD findings on T1- and T2-weighted images were compared. The results demonstrated that the MHS of MR-S of the parotid gland was the most sensitive at 82%, followed by the HD findings on T1- and T2-weighted images of the parotid gland, and then the HD findings of the submandibular gland, at 67% and 58%, respectively. Furthermore, the HD findings on T1- and T2-weighted images have been reported to be more greatly associated with the salivary secretion in patients with SS than MHS findings on MR-S [9]. In the present study, we checked the T1- and T2-weighted images and assessed the side with strong HD findings or tendencies if MHS was not observed bilaterally on bilateral 2D MR-S. The unilateral sagittal 3D MR-S images using this criterion had higher sensitivity than the axial 3D MR-S, including the bilateral parotid ducts. Therefore, considering the usefulness of the diagnostic value by previous reports and HD findings by the present study, T1- and T2-weighted images are essential for investigating the salivary glands in patients with SS.

Several stages of SS by 3D MR-S (unilateral sagittal, axial, and unilateral sagittal + axial) were upstaged from 2D MR-S.

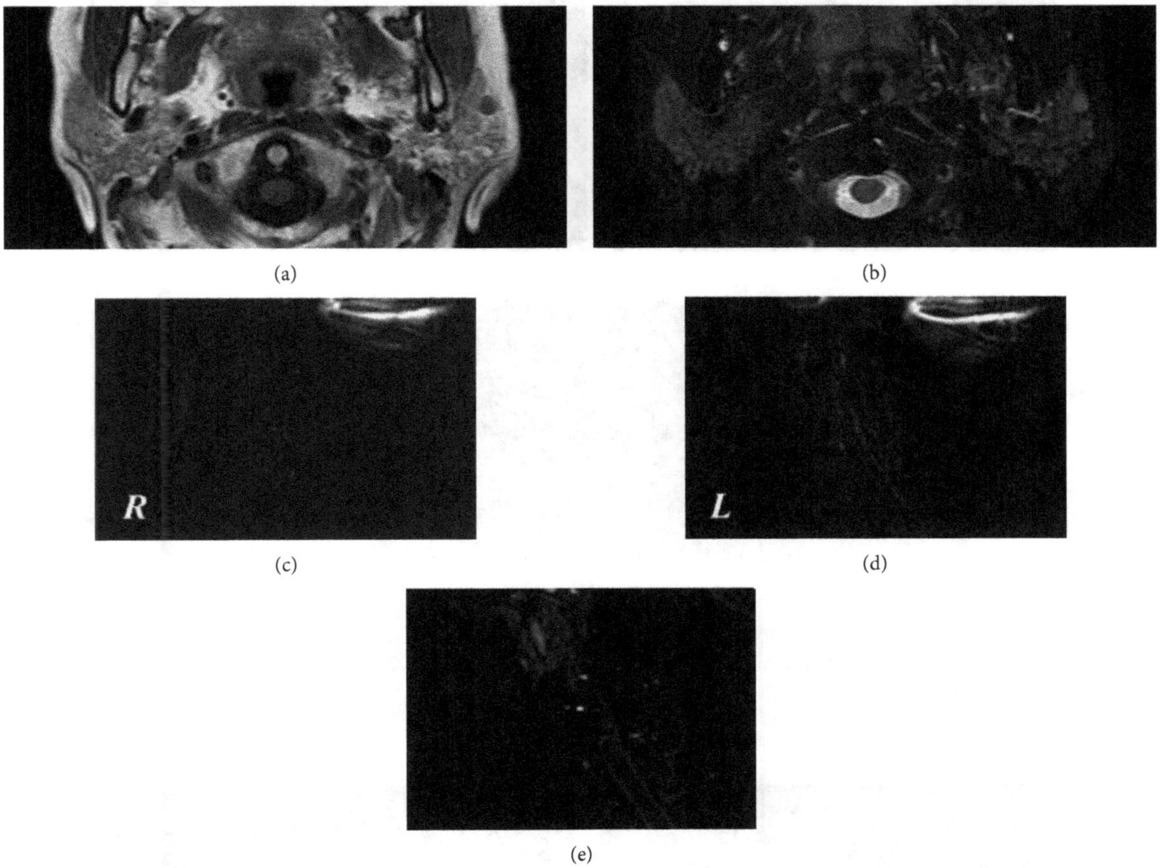

FIGURE 2: A case of the usefulness in determining the imaging side for unilateral sagittal 3D MR-S with T1- and T2-weighted images. T1-weighted image (a) and fat-suppressed T2-weighted image (b) showed HD of the parotid gland with left predominance. This case had no MHS in bilateral 2D MR-S (c, d). We determined the imaging side (right or left) for unilateral sagittal 3D MR-S by evaluating the HD on T1- and T2-weighted images (b, c). Unilateral left 3D MR-S (e) clearly depicted MHS. MR-S: magnetic resonance sialography; HD: heterogeneous distribution; MHS: multiple high-signal-intensity spots.

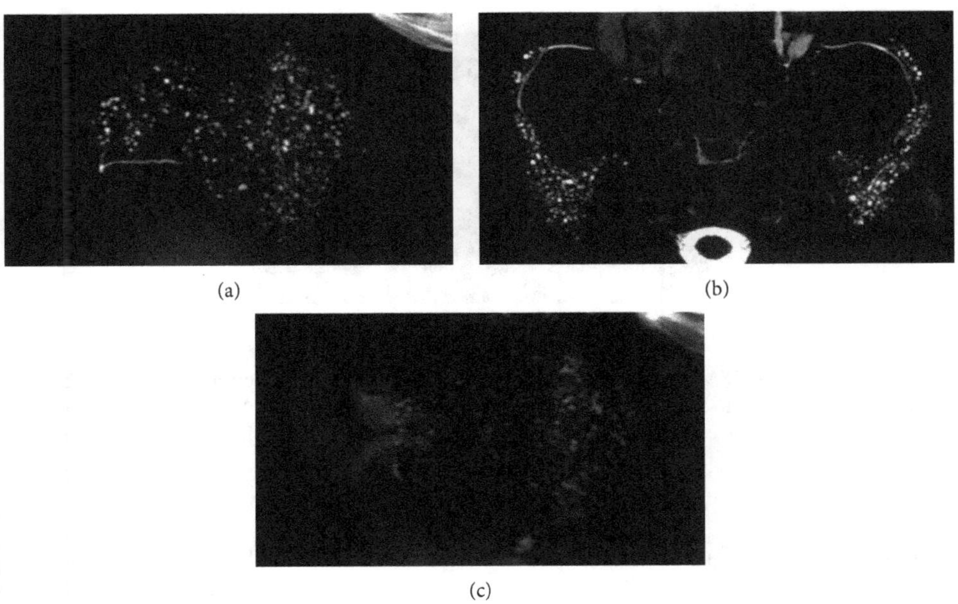

FIGURE 3: A case of detectable MHS on 3D and 2D MR-S. The sagittal 3D MR-S (a), axial 3D MR-S (b), and sagittal 2D MR-S (c) detected MHS and graded it as stage 2. MHS: multiple high-signal-intensity spots; MR-S: magnetic resonance sialography.

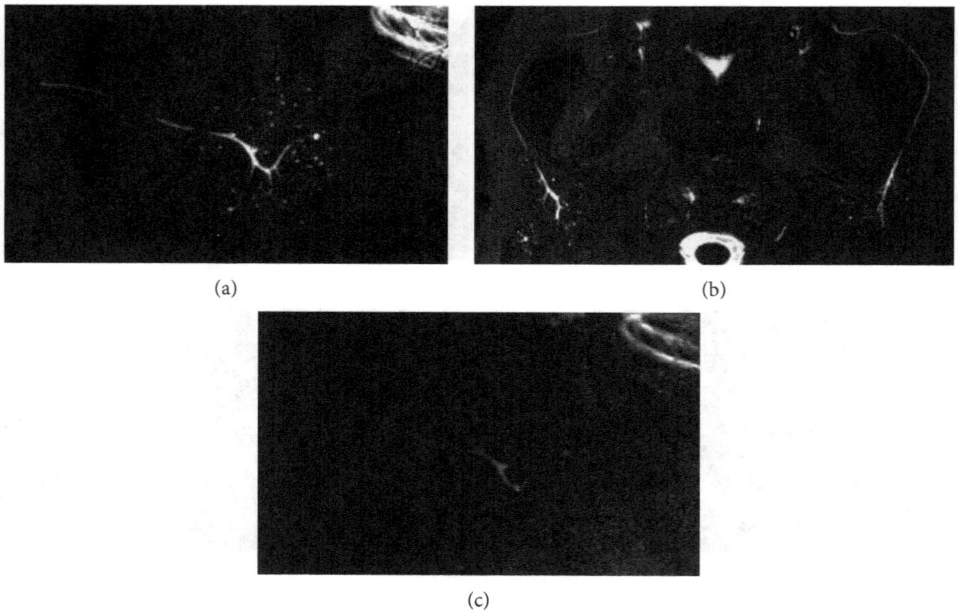

Figure 4: A case of detectable MHS only by 3D MR-S. The sagittal 3D MR-S (a) and axial 3D MR-S (b) were able to detect MHS and graded it as stage 1. The sagittal 2D MR-S (c) was not able to detect MHS and graded it as stage 0. MHS: multiple high-signal-intensity spots; MR-S: magnetic resonance sialography.

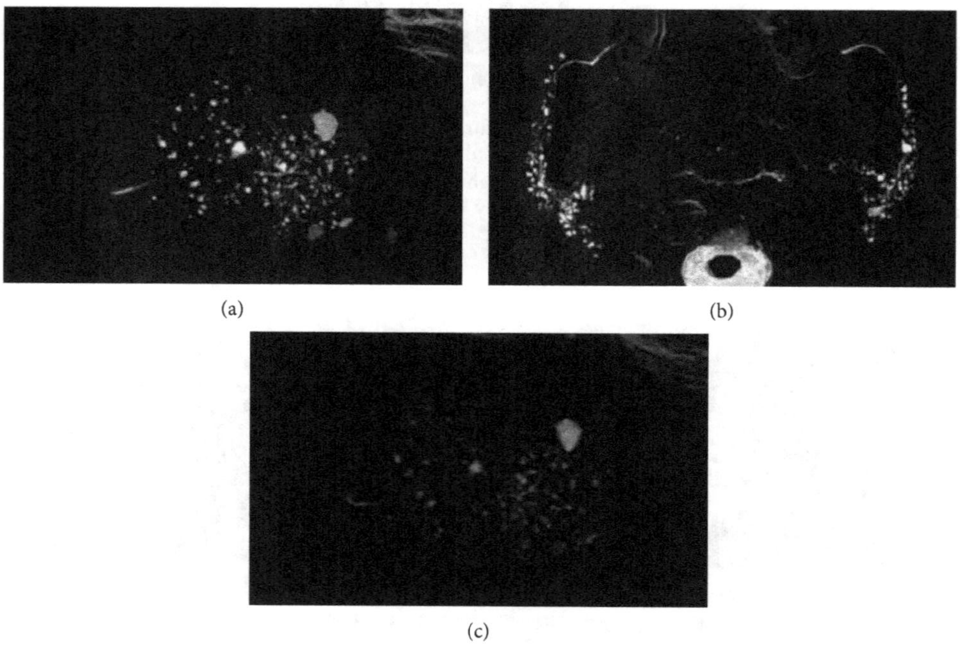

Figure 5: A case of understaging by axial 3D MR-S compared with the staging by 2D MR-S. Sagittal 3D (a), axial 3D (b), and sagittal 2D MR-S can all detect MHS. While the axial 3D MR-S (b) result was stage 2, sagittal 3D (a) and 2D (c) MR-S results indicated stage 3. The axial 3D MR-S (b) was not able to detect a larger size of MHS due to being out of imaging range. MR-S: magnetic resonance sialography; MHS: multiple high-signal-intensity spots.

Most of them converted to stage 1 or more from stage 0 designated by 2D MR-S: unilateral sagittal 3D MR-S, 33 cases; axial 3D MR-S, 30 cases; and unilateral sagittal + axial 3D MR-S, 33 cases, respectively. In other words, because 2D MR-S often provides false-negative results, additional 3D MR-S imaging is necessary. A few 3D MR-S cases were understaged from the stage for SS on 2D MR-S: 3 cases by axial 3D MR-S and one case by unilateral sagittal 3D MR-S.

The axial 3D MR-S results for some of these cases were due to the imaging range of MR-S, as described above. In the one unilateral sagittal 3D MR-S case, MHS could not be detected on the opposite side, which was due to the imaging range of MR-S. In addition, in the longitudinal parotid gland, the MHS can be easily distinguished from the thin parotid duct on sagittal 3D MR-S. Conversely, in axial 3D MR-S, the MHS and relatively thick parotid ducts are densely packed and overlap, making it difficult to distinguish between them, which is considered to result in understaging. Some cases of understaging by unilateral sagittal and axial MR-S may be misled as upstaging on 2D MR-S because of the partial volume effect on 2D MR-S with poor spatial resolution.

A limitation of this study was that we could not compare the sensitivities for detecting abnormal findings of the MHS for unilateral and bilateral 3D MR-S. Since we did not perform bilateral sagittal 3D MR-S and axial 3D MR-S at our hospital because of the limited imaging duration, the imaging side for sagittal 3D MR-S was decided during the examination by the oral and maxillofacial radiologists.

Another limitation of this study is the further improvement of the MR-S imaging technique, which should be considered in future studies. The development of imaging methods using phantoms of a wide range of imaging thickness and shorter duration of the imaging acquisition while maintaining the MR-S image quality and evaluating the diagnostic accuracy of these improved MR-S techniques is warranted.

5. Conclusions

We concluded that a single unilateral sagittal 3D MR-S was sufficient and axial 3D MR-S was not necessary for SS staging. T1- and T2-weighted images are essential for investigating the salivary glands in patients with SS. Therefore, we also concluded that bilateral sagittal 3D MR-S of the parotid glands in addition to T1- and T2-weighted imaging is necessary, sufficient, and most efficient for precise MRI examination of diagnosing SS.

Acknowledgments

This work was supported by the Japan Society for the Promotion of Science (JSPS) Grants-in-Aid for Scientific Research (Grant nos. 18K09804 and 19K18983). The authors would like to thank Editage (http://www.editage.com) for English language editing.

References

[1] C. Vitali, S. Bombardieri, R. Jonsson, H. M. Moutsopoulos, E. L. Alexander, and S. E. Carsons, "Classification criteria for Sjögren's syndrome: a revised version of the European criteria proposed by the American-European Consensus Group," *Annals of the Rheumatic Diseases*, vol. 61, no. 6, pp. 554–5588, 2002.

[2] T. Fujibayashi, S. Sugai, N. Miyasaka, Y. Hayashi, and K. Tsubota, "Revised Japanese criteria for Sjögren's syndrome (1999): availability and validity," *Modern Rheumatology/the Japan Rheumatism Association*, vol. 14, no. 6, pp. 425–434, 2004.

[3] M. Izumi, K. Eguchi, and M. Ohki, "MR imaging of the parotid gland in Sjögren's syndrome: a proposal for new diagnostic criteria," *AJR American journal of roentgenology*, vol. 166, no. 6, pp. 1483–1487, 1996.

[4] T. J. Vogl, S. H. Dresel, and G. Grevers, "Sjögren's syndrome: MR imaging of the parotid gland," *European Radiology*, vol. 6, no. 1, pp. 46–51, 1996.

[5] N. Ohbayashi, I. Yamada, N. Yoshino, and T. Sasaki, "Sjögren's syndrome: comparison of assessments with MR sialography and conventional sialography," *Radiology*, vol. 209, no. 3, pp. 683–688, 1998.

[6] H. Tonami, Y. Ogawa, and M. Matoba, "MR sialography in patients with Sjögren's syndrome," *AJNR American journal of neuroradiology*, vol. 19, no. 7, pp. 1199–1203, 1998.

[7] Y. Kimura, Y. Hotokezaka, and M. Sasaki, "Magnetic resonance imaging-based differentiation between juvenile recurrent parotitis and juvenile Sjögren's syndrome," *Oral Radiology*, vol. 27, no. 1, pp. 73–77, 2011.

[8] I. Kojima, M. Sakamoto, and M. Iikubo, "Diagnostic performance of MR imaging of three major salivary glands for Sjögren's syndrome," *Oral Diseases*, vol. 23, no. 1, pp. 84–90, 2017.

[9] I. Kojima, M. Sakamoto, M. Iikubo, Y. Shimada, T. Nishioka, and T. Sasano, "Relationship of MR imaging of submandibular glands to hyposalivation in Sjögren's syndrome," *Oral Diseases*, vol. 25, no. 1, pp. 117–125, 2019.

[10] R. K. Niemela, E. Paakko, I. Suramo, R. Takalo, and M. Hakala, "Magnetic resonance imaging and magnetic resonance sialography of parotid glands in primary Sjögren's syndrome," *Arthritis & Rheumatism*, vol. 45, no. 6, pp. 512–518, 2001.

[11] R. K. Niemela, R. Takalo, and E. Paakko, "Ultrasonography of salivary glands in primary Sjögren's syndrome. A comparison with magnetic resonance imaging and magnetic resonance sialography of parotid glands," *Rheumatology*, vol. 43, no. 7, pp. 875–879, 2004.

[12] H. Tonami, K. Higashi, M. Matoba, H. Yokota, I. Yamamoto, and S. Sugai, "A comparative study between MR sialography and salivary gland scintigraphy in the diagnosis of Sjögren's syndrome," *Journal of Computer Assisted Tomography*, vol. 25, no. 2, pp. 262–268, 2001.

[13] M. Regier, T. Ries, and C. Arndt, "Sjögren's syndrome of the parotid gland: value of diffusion-weighted echo-planar MRI for diagnosis at an early stage based on MR sialography grading in comparison with healthy volunteers," *Röfo*, vol. 181, no. 3, pp. 242–248, 2009.

[14] M. Becker, F. Marchal, and C. D. Becker, "Sialolithiasis and salivary ductal stenosis: diagnostic accuracy of MR sialography with a three-dimensional extended-phase conjugate-symmetry rapid spin-echo sequence," *Radiology*, vol. 217, no. 2, pp. 347–358, 2000.

[15] A. Gadodia, A. Seith, R. Sharma, A. Thakar, and R. Parshad, "Magnetic resonance sialography using CISS and HASTE sequences in inflammatory salivary gland diseases: comparison with digital sialography," *Acta Radiologica*, vol. 51, no. 2, pp. 156–163, 2010.

[16] Y. Morimoto, T. Tanaka, S. Kito, K. Tominaga, I. Yoshioka, and Y. Yamashita, "Utility of three dimension fast asymmetric spin-echo (3D-FASE) sequences in MR sialographic sequences: model and volunteer studies," *Oral Diseases*, vol. 11, no. 1, pp. 35–43, 2005.

[17] Y. Takagi, M. Sumi, M. Van Cauteren, and T. Nakamura, "Fast and high-resolution MR sialography using a small surface coil," *Journal of Magnetic Resonance Imaging: JMRI*, vol. 22, no. 1, pp. 29–37, 2005.

[18] Y. Takagi, M. Sumi, T. Sumi, Y. Ichikawa, and T. Nakamura, "MR microscopy of the parotid glands in patients with Sjögren's syndrome: quantitative MR diagnostic criteria," *AJNR American journal of neuroradiology*, vol. 26, no. 5, pp. 1207–1214, 2005.

[19] J. S. Greenspan, T. E. Daniels, N. Talal, and R. A. Sylvester, "The histopathology of Sjögren's syndrome in labial salivary gland biopsies," *Oral Surgery, Oral Medicine, Oral Pathology*, vol. 37, no. 2, pp. 217–229, 1974.

[20] S. C. Shiboski, C. H. Shiboski, L. Criswell, A. Baer, S. Challacombe, and H. Lanfranchi, "American College of Rheumatology classification criteria for Sjögren's syndrome: a data-driven, expert consensus approach in the Sjogren's International Collaborative Clinical Alliance cohort," *Arthritis Care & Research*, vol. 64, no. 4, pp. 475–487, 2012.

[21] M. Sakamoto, T. Sasano, and S. Higano, "Evaluation of pulse sequences used for magnetic resonance sialography," *Dentomaxillofacial Radiology*, vol. 30, no. 5, pp. 276–284, 2001.

13

What Radiologist Should Know about MRI Translational Forces and Hazard: An Ex-Vivo Simulation of Retained Metallic Shrapnel

Ali Kanj,[1] **Ibrahim Ghosn**,[2] **Assaad Mohanna**,[3] **and Georges Rouhana**[3]

[1]*Radiology Department, Hammoud Hospital University Medical Center, Saida, Lebanon*
[2]*Fellow of Radiology, Radiology Department, Faculty of Medical Sciences, Lebanese University, Hadath, Lebanon*
[3]*Radiology Department, Faculty of Medical Sciences, Lebanese University, Hadath, Lebanon*

Correspondence should be addressed to Ali Kanj; kanj.ali1974@gmail.com

Academic Editor: Lorenzo Faggioni

Background. In a country immersed in endless rounds of wars, retained metallic foreign bodies remain a significant dilemma in the daily practice of every Lebanese radiologist. When a shrapnel's hazard is of concern, the decision between performing or refusing a justified MRI exam is not always straightforward. In this small trial, we aimed to better understand the shrapnel's MRI safety by mimicking our daily practice. *Methods.* Five shrapnel with an incremental increase in their long axis were put in an animal flesh and then introduced into a 3 T magnetic field. The behavior of each shrapnel was concretely assessed by performing before and after magnetic field exposure CT acquisitions. *Results.* Translation along the z-axis ranged from 0.9 mm to 2.8 mm. Torque angle ranged between 2.8 and 54 degrees with an average of 15.62 degrees. *Conclusions.* Shrapnel's movements in the magnetic field are not negligible during the acute phase of injury where there is no reinforcing fibroblastic reaction and invite us to reconsider the MRI safety of these metallic foreign bodies. Standard radiographs may be sufficient, but a targeted CT scan may be of better value for a confident decision for assessment of shrapnel position near viscera and major vessels.

1. Background

Lebanon, a more than 6 million population country [1], witnessed multiple consecutive wars and conflicts, generating hundreds of thousands of deaths and a higher number of injuries. After the recovery of material losses, war-related injuries and retained metallic foreign bodies are still buried in a considerable number of Lebanese people's organs. It could be secondary to explosive weapon-related fragments, Cluster Munitions, and the Anti-Personnel mine called shrapnel or gunshot-bonded bullets and pellets [2].

Surgical removal of the retained fragment from the human body is not always feasible or indicated. Surgeons usually decide by weighing benefits versus operation risk [3]. Therefore, the fate of these patients was to carry within their bodies these metallic fragments without problems until an MRI is judged necessary.

Almost on a daily basis, the Lebanese radiologists find themselves in a hard dilemma between the risk of hazardous incidence and the justified indication of MRI. Solving this dilemma is essential due to its medico-legal aspect and more importantly to insure patients' safety and optimal care [4]. With the advancement in MRI technology and the introduction of high field MRI systems as well as the increase of MRI implication in patient's management, the MRI safety issue should be re-evaluated or at least should be better understood.

To understand the factors influencing the MRI induced hazards, we present in this article a small ex-vivo trial of 5 different metallic shrapnel retained within an animal flesh simulating human extremity to assess the eventual torque and displacement in a 3 T MRI magnet.

2. Methods

Multiple studies are available in the literature concerning foreign bodies and MRI especially those performed to assess the MRI safety of metallic implants and orthopedic materials [5]. These studies were conducted under strict measures detailed by the American Society for Testing and Materials (ASTM). In this article we tried to simulate these methods with a simplified approach mimicking our daily practice.

2.1. Model. Knowing that the relative risk of injury is determined by the characteristics of the foreign body in question (ferromagnetic properties, geometry and dimensions) as well as by the strength of the static magnetic field, we tried to simulate a daily scenario when an MRI is ordered for a patient with a history of blast injury.

(i) Steel shrapnel was cut into 5 smaller pieces of almost the same thickness but with a 3 mm incremental increase in the long axis (Figure 1).

The size, volume, and weight of obtained shrapnel are shown in Table 1.

(ii) An animal flesh was used as the container to simulate the consistency and the histology of the muscular compartment of a human extremity.

One shrapnel was introduced at a time during each trial.

2.2. Simulation. 3 steps were performed consecutively:

(i) A baseline CT acquisition was performed using a GE 64-MDCT scan to assess the initial position and orientation of the fragment within the flesh.

(ii) The model was put on the table of a 3T GE Discovery 750 W MRI and then slid through the magnet portal and toward the isocenter of MRI gantry. The model was then left for 5 min in the isocenter of the magnetic field and then slid back to the initial position through the magnet portal.

(iii) A second CT acquisition was performed using the same CT machine and centering parameters to assess the new position and orientation of the shrapnel.

2.3. Measurements. All measurements were done on Advantage Window Workstation AW4.6 from GE.

(i) Pre- and postmagnetic field exposure CT images were fused, and a qualitative visual assessment of their rotation around their centers was done

(ii) Shrapnel translation was measured relatively to the meat's plate

(iii) Rotational angle (RA) was calculated on the fused images between the initial and new position of the long axis of each shrapnel along the z-axis of the magnet and the xy plane orthogonal to the z-axis

3. Results

The translation and the rotation of studied shrapnel are shown in Table 2.

3.1. Translation. The five shrapnel of incremental size difference experienced a subtle translation along the z-axis. Their translation ranged from 0.9 mm to 2.8 mm. The minimal translation was noted with the smallest shrapnel size (shrapnel A), whereas the maximum translation was seen with the shrapnel D. Only 0.5 mm difference is noted when comparing the translation of the shrapnel D to the largest shrapnel (shrapnel E).

3.2. Torque. All the five shrapnel experienced rotation along the B_0 axis and in the xy plane.

We calculated the alignment within the z-axis by measuring, on the sagittal plane, the angle between the greater axis of the shrapnel and the greatest axis of the flesh (parallel to the z-axis). It ranged between 2.8 and 54 degrees with an average of 15.62 degrees (Figure 2).

The average rotation angle for the 5 shrapnel in the coronal plane was 72.18 degrees.

The average rotation angle of the five shrapnel in the xy plane was 54.26 degrees.

4. Discussion

Shrapnel is a major foreign body issue encountered in our daily practice especially in a country immersed in endless rounds of wars. It got its name from General Henry Shrapnel [6] of the British Army's Royal Artillery who invented during the Peninsular War an exploding shell that broke apart and shattered when it was detonated.

Because of their ferromagnetic potential, they are considered to be a relative contraindication to MRI exams [7]. However the word "relative" is somewhat confusing and absurd and carries a lot of interpretations.

We tried to better understand their behavior by simplifying the physics of interactions between the retained objects and the magnetic field and by mimicking our daily practice with this trial using readily available materials.

4.1. Magnetic Field Interaction with Retained Metallic Shrapnel. When a metallic object is placed in a magnetic field, it will be subject to a magnetic force. This force is due to different factors related to the magnetic field itself (strength and spatial gradient strength) and other factors related to the metallic object put in the field (volume, surface shape, and composition determining its ferromagnetic characteristics) [8].

The magnetic field strength used in our daily practice varies between 0.3 T and 3 T and corresponds to B_0. The spatial gradient of the magnetic field B_0 is a major parameter in determining the interaction force exerted over a ferromagnetic object. It is defined as the change in the strength of the magnetic field proportional to distance and is measured in Tesla per meter (T/m) or in Gauss per centimeter (G/cm), where (1 T/m = 100 G/cm). This magnetic force can be further divided into two kinetic forces: the translational force and the torque force. The former is responsible for the displacement of an object within a magnetic field

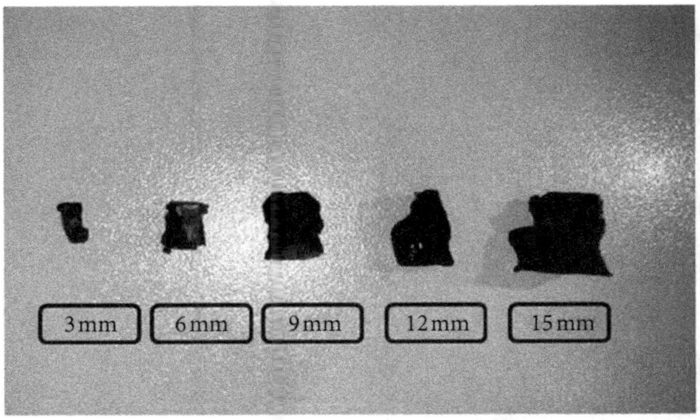

FIGURE 1: Shrapnel (dimensions of each long axis are shown).

TABLE 1: Shrapnel characteristics.

	A	B	C	D	E
Shrapnel size (mm)	1 × 3	5 × 6	8 × 9	8 × 12	11 × 15
Shrapnel weight (g)	0.29	1.11	1.99	3.06	6.9
Shrapnel volume (mm^3)	80	200	450	500	900

TABLE 2: Shrapnel translation and rotation.

Shrapnel	A	B	C	D	E
Translation (mm)	0.9	1.4	2.2	2.8	2.3
Rotation angle in coronal plane (degree)	88.3	49.2	73.2	85.4	64.8
Rotation angle in axial plane (degree)	90	88.7	10.9	53.6	28.1
Alignment along B_0 (after exposure)	5	54	15.4	2.8	0.9

(translation and diversion), and the latter is responsible for the object's rotation movement [9].

4.1.1. Translational Force or Displacement (F). The translational force (F) exerted on a ferromagnetic shrapnel of a certain volume V with magnetic susceptibility X is proportional to the product of the static field (B) and the spatial gradient [8]:

$$F \propto X \cdot VB \cdot \frac{dB}{dz}. \quad (1)$$

According to this equation; the maximal amplitude of (F) is as close to the opening of the magnet bore.

In MRI magnet, the direction of the magnetic field vector (B_0) is horizontal; in 3 T MRI systems, the highest gradient occurs at a position range from 10 to 30 cm from laser point locator.

In contrast to torque force (T), translational force or displacement is minimal at the isocenter of the magnetic field.

When evaluating an implant deflection (translation), this can be easy extrapolated to any ferromagnetic foreign body. The ASTM considers a deflection of less than 45° insignificant, because the magnetically induced deflection force is less than the force on the implant due to gravity (the weight of the implant). Therefore, we can consider that any risk induced by a similar ferromagnetic force is no greater than any risk imposed by normal daily activity in the Earth's gravitational field.

In this trial, all shrapnel presented a minimal degree of translation ranging from 0.9 to 2.8 mm.

4.1.2. Rotational Force or Torque (T). The rotational force on a shrapnel dipole (μm) in a magnetic field B is equal to the vector product of μm and B:

$$T = \mu m \cdot B. \quad (2)$$

This explains why the torque force (T) is maximum where the strength of B_0 itself is maximum [9] independent of the spatial gradient amplitude. Therefore, the maximum torque occurs within the magnet bore in the isocenter, and it is proportional to the field strength, B_0, which is constant (3 T) in our study. Its amplitude decreases as the shrapnel moves out of the isocenter.

If shrapnel has longitudinal shape, it will be exposed to the twisting magnetic force or torque (T). This force tends to align the shrapnel to the field and this force magnitude will be related to the angle between the shrapnel's long axis and the field direction.

For this reason and for irregular shaped ferromagnetic shrapnel retained in the body, the torque force (T) may be the essential safety issue as compared to translational force (F) especially when present in the proximity of a major vessel or nerve.

4.2. MRI Safety and Shrapnel. Shrapnel lodged in human bodies are considered relative contraindication for MRI and therefore leaving the final decision for radiologists. In front of a similar scenario, we are obliged to perform a full survey starting with shrapnel localization, dating the exposure, weighing the risk versus the benefit of the MRI, and also considering the availability of other alternative exams.

At least two significant MRI hazardous morbidity and mortality were reported in the literature; one with metallic clip with secondary rupture and bleeding after exposure to the magnetic field [10] and the second one for ocular injury related to missed intraorbital foreign body [11].

Other than shrapnel in/near the ocular globe that constitute the clearest contraindication, the shrapnel position near viscera and major vessels should be a concern while accepting to perform an MRI exam. Standard radiographies may be sufficient, but a targeted CT scan may be of better value for a confident decision.

In this small ex-vivo trial, we aimed to realize a simulation of circumstances that we encounter in our daily practice by using animal flesh composed of muscles, fat, and fascia's and thereby histologically similar to human extremity.

Our primary limitation was the lack of surrounding scar tissue and fibrosis, a factor that could fix and retain the metallic shrapnel reducing the degree of translation and

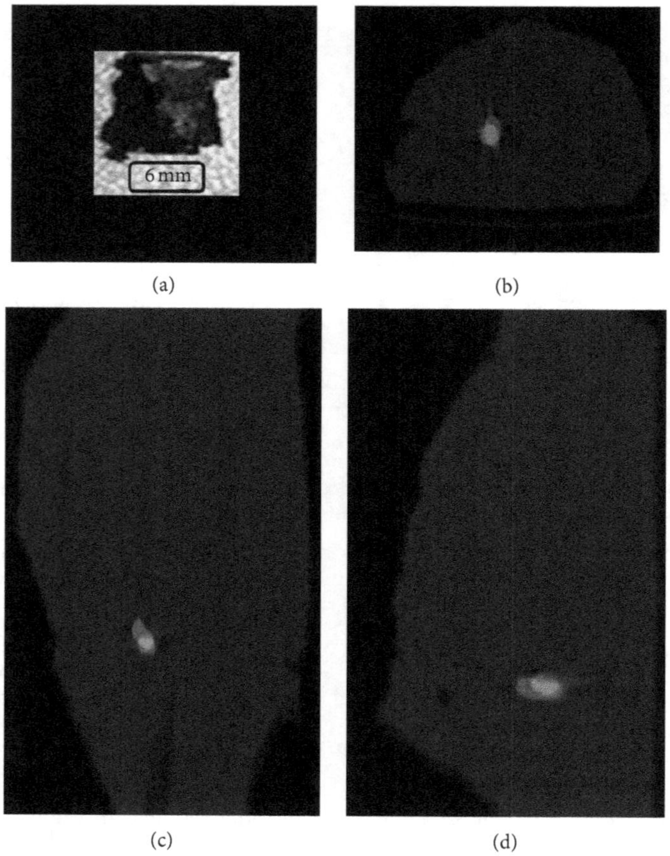

FIGURE 2: Shrapnel *B* (a). Fused images before and after MRI exposure in axial (b), coronal (c), and sagittal (d) plans.

torque. And this factor could explain the paucity of reported hazards in our practice with patients reporting shrapnel exposure.

The second limitation is the small number of studied shrapnel. The aim of this study is to understand the physics of MRI/foreign bodies' interactions rather than extracting formulas and statistical analysis and to encourage a better investment in this contradictory yet important issue.

5. Conclusions

Shrapnel-related MRI safety will remain a daily issue in our practice; better understanding of its behavior in MRI is mandatory for optimal patients' safety. This article proved that shrapnel's movements in the magnetic field is not negligible at least during acute phase of injury where there is no reinforcing fibrotic matrix and invites us to reconsider the MRI safety of these metallic foreign bodies and to look to this issue with mistrust in our future decision making. This article also shed some light on the usefulness of CT scan as a readily available tool to assess the position of the shrapnel and its relation to the surrounding noble structures helping the radiologist to take a more straightforward decision.

Abbreviations

MRI: Magnetic resonance imaging
CT: Computed tomography
T: Torque force
F: Translation force
ASTM: American Society for Testing and Materials.

Acknowledgments

The authors would like to thank the Radiology Department at Hammoud Hospital UMC for their contributions and effort to accomplish this work.

References

[1] The World Bank, *Population, Total—Lebanon*, 2020, https://data.worldbank.org/indicator/SP.POP.TOTL?locations=LB.

[2] Geneva International Centre for Humanitarian Demining, "Explosive weapon effects," 2017, https://www.gichd.org/en/resources/publications/detail/publication/explosive-weapon-effects/.

[3] A. Guermazi, D. Hayashi, S. E. Smith, W. Palmer, and J. N. Katz, "Imaging of blast injuries to the lower extremities sustained in the Boston marathon bombing," *Arthritis Care & Research*, vol. 65, no. 12, pp. 1893–1898, 2013.

[4] MRI Safety, "Pellets, Bullets, and Shrapnel," 2020, http://www.mrisafety.com/SafetyInformation_view.php?editid1=192Shellock 2019.

[5] C. McComb, D. Allan, and B. Condon, "Evaluation of the translational and rotational forces acting on a highly ferromagnetic orthopedic spinal implant in magnetic resonance imaging," *Journal of Magnetic Resonance Imaging*, vol. 29, no. 2, pp. 449–453, 2009.

[6] H. Shrapnel, *Encyclopædia Britannica*, 2020, https://www.britannica.com/biography/Henry-Shrapnel.

[7] UCSF Radiology, "Relative contraindications," 2020, https://radiology.ucsf.edu/patient-care/patient-safety/mri/relative-contraindications#accordion-sh rapnel.

[8] L. P. Panych and B. Madore, "The physics of MRI safety," *Journal of Magnetic Resonance Imaging*, vol. 47, no. 1, pp. 28–43, 2018.

[9] P. Shokrollahi, J. Drake, and A. Goldenberg, "Quantification of force and torque applied by a high-field magnetic resonance imaging system on an ultrasonic motor for MRI-guided robot-assisted interventions," *Actuators*, vol. 6, no. 4, p. 29, 2017.

[10] D. McRobbie, E. Moore, M. Graves, and M. Prince, *MRI from Picture To Proton*, Cambridge University Press, Cambridge, MA, USA, 2017.

[11] N. Mamas, K. Andreanos, D. Brouzas et al., "Acute ocular pain during magnetic resonance imaging due to retained intraocular metallic foreign body: the role of ultrasonography and ultrasound biomicroscopy in diagnosis and management of this condition," *Journal of Ultrasound*, vol. 21, no. 2, pp. 159–163, 2018.

14

Hearing Thresholds Changes after MRI 1.5T of Head and Neck

Maryam Bahaloo,[1] Mohammad Hossein Davari,[1] Mohammad Sobhan,[2] Seyyed Jalil Mirmohammadi,[1] Mohammad Taghi Jalalian,[3] Mohammad Javad Zare Sakhvidi,[4] Farimah Shamsi,[5] Sam Mirfendereski,[6] Abolfazl Mollasadeghi,[1] and Amir Houshang Mehrparvar[1]

[1]*Industrial Diseases Research Center, Shahid Sadoughi University of Medical Sciences, Yazd 89138-14389, Iran*
[2]*Department of Radiology, Shahid Sadoughi University of Medical Sciences, Yazd 89138-14389, Iran*
[3]*Department of Occupational Medicine, Shahid Sadoughi University of Medical Sciences, Yazd 89138-14389, Iran*
[4]*Department of Occupational Health, Shahid Sadoughi University of Medical Sciences, Yazd 89138-14389, Iran*
[5]*Shahid Sadoughi University of Medical Sciences, Yazd 89138-14389, Iran*
[6]*Department of Radiology, Faculty of Medicine, Shahrekord University of Medical Sciences, Shahrekord 8815713471, Iran*

Correspondence should be addressed to Mohammad Taghi Jalalian; mtg_mtg2002@yahoo.com

Academic Editor: Henrique M. Lederman

Introduction. Exposure to high intensity noise produced by MRI is a cause for concern. This study was conducted to determine the temporary and permanent effects of exposure to noise created by performing MRI on the hearing threshold of the subjects using conventional and extended high frequency audiometry. *Methods.* This semiexperimental study was performed on 35 patients referred to Shahid Rahnemoun Hospital for head and neck MRI due to different clinical conditions. The hearing threshold of patients was measured before, immediately after, and 24 hours after performing 1.5 Tesla MRI using conventional and extended high frequency audiometry. SPSS version 18 was used to compare the mean hearing thresholds before and after MRI using paired T test and repeated measures analysis. *Results.* Comparison of auditory thresholds in conventional and extended high frequencies before and immediately after MRI showed a significant shift at 4 KHz (P = 0.008 and P = 0.08 for right and left ears), 6 KHz (P = 0.03 and P = 0.01 for right and left ears), and 14 KHz (P =0.03 and P = 0.31 for right and left ears). However, there was no significant difference between audiometric thresholds before and 24 hours after MRI. *Conclusion.* Noise due to 1.5 Tesla MRI can only cause transient threshold shift.

1. Introduction

High levels of noise can temporary impair hearing thresholds and cause temporary threshold shift (TTS) which is probably reversed after abstinence from noise exposure. Permanent threshold shift (PTS) occurs after a mechanical injury to hair cells due to exposure to noise [1, 2]. According to Occupational Safety and Health Association (OSHA), permissible exposure limit for noise in an 8-hour work shift is 90 dBA [3].

Magnetic resonance imaging (MRI) is an ever-increasing imaging modality used to detect many lesions in the body. New MRI devices, due to their detailed imaging and three-dimensional measurements, are widely used for central nervous system imaging. MRI device produces noise during imaging which is positively related to the strength of magnetic field (in Tesla) and may affect patient's hearing [4–6]. Studies showed that MRI creates higher levels of noise during last gradient echo pulse sequence [7].

Head and neck MRI especially may affect hearing due to the closeness of the device to the ear. Hearing damage after exposure to MRI noise depends on the frequency and intensity of the noise and duration of the exposure and also the distance between ear and MRI device [8].

Some previous studies have found that MRI may affect hearing by oxidative stress and cochlear hair cells injury [9].

The noise produced by MRI devices is dependent on MRI strength, so that the MRI devices with different powers (0.2

to 3 Tesla) produce varying noise levels from 101 to 131 dBA [10, 11]. The frequency of noise produced by MRI devices is mostly around 4 KHz [4, 11]. According to National Institute for Occupational Safety and Health (NIOSH) guidelines, recommended exposure limit to noise with 120 dBA intensity is 7 s. Radomskij et al. in a study on dogs found that hearing threshold was increased about 2-5 dB after exposure to MRI noise in 50% of dogs [9].

The studies about the effect of MRI noise on hearing thresholds are few and controversial. Some case reports have found MRI as the cause of TTS [5, 12] and PTS [13] in humans. Lim et al. could not find the effect of MRI noise on hearing thresholds in both conventional (500-8000 Hz) and extended high frequencies (10000–14000 Hz). They used 3 Tesla MRI and all patients had used ear plugs during imaging [14]. Jin et al. found that 3 Tesla MRI noise can induce TTS in healthy subjects, even with the use of ear protectors [15]. We could not find a study on 1.5 Tesla MRI which is the most commonly used intensity for head and neck imaging.

This study was performed to define the effect of noise produced by 1.5 Tesla MRI on hearing thresholds in different audiometric frequencies (500-16000 Hz) in patients referred for head and neck MRI.

2. Materials and Methods

This was a before-after study performed in Shahid Rahnemoun Hospital. Participants were selected by consecutive sampling from patients referred to MRI center of Shahid Rahnemoun Hospital to perform head and neck MRI with different indications during January till December 2017. An informed consent was obtained from each participant. Patients older than 50 years were not selected and those with moderate hearing loss (hearing threshold higher than 40 dB at each frequency) and conductive hearing loss were excluded from the study after performing baseline audiometry.

MRI device was a Siemens (Avanto, B19, Germany) with magnetic field intensity of 1.5 Tesla. Five steps were performed for each imaging: localizing (10 s), T1 axial (90 s), T2 axial (120 s), T2 trim (180 s), T2 sagittal (90 s), T2 sagittal (90 s), and T2 coronal (90 s) with 1-2-second interval between each protocol. Totally, imaging lasted about 10 minutes for head and 7 minutes for neck.

Pure-tone audiometry (PTA) was done using a diagnostic audiometer (device: Interacoustic AC40, Denmark, headphone: TDH-39 for conventional and Koss R/80 for extended high frequencies, oscillator B70 for bone conduction) by an expert audiologist for each participant at three occasions: (1) 10 minutes before imaging (baseline); (2) during 1 hour after imaging (to detect TTS); and (3) between 24 and 48 hours after imaging (to detect PTS). Hearing threshold for air conduction (AC) and bone conduction (BC) was measured for each frequency in each ear separately. Hearing frequencies which were tested by PTA included 500, 1000, 2000, 3000, 4000, 6000, 8000, 10000, 12000, 14000, and 16000 Hz.

Data were analyzed by SPSS ver. 19 using paired T test and repeated measures analysis.

3. Results

Initially 62 patients between 14 and 45 years old were selected. After the first audiometry, 29 patients were excluded due to moderate hearing loss or conductive hearing loss, and at last 33 patients continued the study.

Mean (±SD) of age was 31 (±9.7) years (range: 16-45). Threshold shift was observed after MRI and the highest threshold shift one hour after MRI was observed at 4 KHZ and 14 KHz in conventional and extended high frequency audiometry in both ears. Table 1 compares hearing threshold of different frequencies before, 1 hour after, and 24 hour after MRI.

Table 2 shows the P value for the comparison of mean hearing thresholds at different frequencies at three occasions (baseline, 1 hour, and 24 hours after MRI) calculated by repeated measures analysis.

4. Discussion

Hearing damage due to loud noise can be temporary or permanent. Many individuals experience a TTS after exposure to loud noise which disappears some hours after the termination of exposure; but in some individuals the hearing loss may exist even after several hours of abstinence from exposure to noise. In permanent hearing loss, hair cells of the organ of Corti are damaged due to some mechanisms.

MRI is a widely used imaging method in different disciplines of medicine and due to its advantages, its application is being increased. Exposure to high levels of noise is one of the problems which the patients may experience during imaging and this loud noise may cause TTS or PTS. Wagner et al. found that MRI produces a sound pressure level at the patient's ear between 79.5 to 86.5 dBA and sort-term peaks up to 120 dB [16].

In this study, we examined the effect of noise produced by 1.5 Tesla MRI on hearing status of the patients. We assessed both TTS and PTS at conventional and extended high frequencies. The results showed that TTS was observed at 4, 6, 8, and 14 KHz frequencies, but this threshold shift disappeared after 24 hours, so no PTS was observed.

The results of the studies on hearing loss after MRI are controversial. Most studies have assessed TTS at conventional frequencies [5, 12, 13]. A study showed that those who undergone 0.5 Tesla MRI without wearing hearing conservation devices experienced headache, earache, and tinnitus after imaging [17]. Govindaraju et al. found TTS and tinnitus after exposure to 3 Tesla MRI of spine, but the hearing loss was disappeared after 3 days, and tinnitus remained [5]. These results are in accordance with the results of the present study. Mollasadeghi et al. reported a case of permanent hearing loss after exposure to MRI noise [13].

The results of the present study showed that bilateral hearing loss was observed at 4, 6, and 14 KHz which are the most common frequencies affected by continuous noise in occupational settings [18–20]. Hearing loss at 14 and 16 KHz has been also shown after exposure to MRI noise [20–23].

Radomskij et al. found that 1.5 tesla MRI caused 68% more hearing changes measured by OAEs in patients not wearing

TABLE 1: Comparison of mean of hearing thresholds at different frequencies of both ears before MRI (baseline), 1 hour after MRI (TTS), and 24 hours after MRI (PTS).

Frequency (KHz)	Ear	Mean (SD) of Hearing thresholds (dB)			Comparison between baseline and 1 hr after MRI		Comparison between baseline and 24 hr after MRI	
		Baseline	after MRI 1 hr	after MRI 24 hrs	Mean difference	P-value	Mean difference	P-value
0.5	Right	9.39 (2.07)	9.39 (2.07)	9.39 (2.07)	0	1	0	1
	Left	9.54 (1.92)	9.54 (1.92)	9.54 (1.92)	0	0.31	0	1
1	Right	10.90 (4.23)	11.06 (4.09)	11.06 (4.09)	0.97	0.31	0.16	0.31
	Left	10.15 (4.23)	10.30 (4.13)	10.30 (4.13)	0.30	1	0.15	0.31
2	Right	10.15 (4.4)	10.15 (4.1)	10.15 (4.1)	0.45	0.18	0	1
	Left	11.51 (5.51)	11.21 (5.59)	11.21 (5.59)	0.15	0.15	-0.30	0.31
3	Right	11.36 (4.55)	11.51 (4.41)	11.51 (4.41)	0.60	0.1	0.15	0.31
	Left	11.81 (7.37)	11.81 (7.37)	11.81 (7.37)	0.91	0.70	0	1
4	Right	11.36 (6.76)	11.51 (5.37)	11.51 (5.37)	1.06	0.008	0.15	0.73
	Left	13.03 (7.17)	13.18 (7.16)	13.18 (7.16)	1.06	0.08	0.15	0.31
6	Right	16.96 (7.8)	17.27 (7.71)	17.27 (7.71)	0.91	0.03	0.31	0.37
	Left	18.33 (7.14)	18.48 (7.44)	18.48 (7.44)	1.03	0.01	0.15	0.78
8	Right	16.06 (9.16)	16.21 (7.6)	16.21 (7.6)	1.06	0.19	0.15	0.48
	Left	17.12 (9.01)	17.27 (8.93)	17.27 (8.93)	0.75	0.04	0.15	0.31
10	Right	10.45 (12.7)	10.45 (12.7)	10.45 (12.7)	0	1	0	1
	Left	7.87 (13.23)	7.87 (13.23)	7.87 (13.23)	0.31	0.32	0	1
12	Right	15.45 (15.73)	15.30 (15.6)	15.30 (15.6)	0.45	0.18	-0.15	0.55
	Left	14.09(13.31)	14.24 (13.23)	14.24 (13.23)	0.60	0.32	0.13	0.31
14	Right	16.21 (19.72)	16.36 (19.77)	16.36 (19.77)	1.21	0.03	0.15	0.31
	Left	13.78 (18.49)	14.54 (13.23)	14.54 (13.23)	1.22	0.31	0.76	0.1
16	Right	29.09 (22.51)	29.09 (22.51)	29.09 (22.51)	0.30	0.31	0	1
	Left	26.96 (22.6)	27.12 (22.6)	27.12 (22.6)	0.46	0.1	0.16	0.31

TABLE 2: P value of the comparison of mean hearing thresholds at three occasions (baseline, 1 hour, and 24 hours after MRI).

Frequency	Right ear	Left ear
500	0.983	0.876
1000	0.372	0.226
2000	0.167	0.591
3000	0.114	0.047
4000	0.025	0.005
6000	0.028	0.012
8000	0.194	0.465
10000	0.728	0.374
12000	0.239	0.114
14000	0.026	0.015
16000	0.374	0.096

ear plugs compared those wearing ear plugs [9]. They did not assess PTS. Lim et al. and Wagner et al. did not find any changes in hearing status in patients undergoing MRI who used hearing protection devices [14, 16].

In the present study, patients had authority to use hearing protection devices and some of them used them. Jin et al. used ABR for assessing the effect of 3 Tesla MRI noise on hearing and found only TTS in the patients who wore hearing protection devices, which was consistent with the results of the present study [15].

5. Conclusion

This study showed that noise produced by 1.5 Tesla MRI during head and neck MRI probably causes TTS without permanent hearing threshold shift.

Disclosure

This research did not receive any specific grant from funding agencies in the public, commercial, or not-for-profit sectors.

Acknowledgments

The authors are grateful to Sommaye Shirmohammadi for her kind collaboration in this project.

References

[1] D. I. Nelson, R. Y. Nelson, M. Concha-Barrientos, and M. Fingerhut, "The global burden of occupational noise-induced hearing loss," *American Journal of Industrial Medicine*, vol. 48, no. 6, pp. 446–458, 2005.

[2] M. H. Baradarnfar, K. Karamifar, A. H. Mehrparvar et al., "Amplitude changes in otoacoustic emissions after exposure to industrial noise," *Noise & Health*, vol. 14, no. 56, pp. 28–31, 2012.

[3] C. D. Reese and J. V. Eidson, *Handbook of OSHA Construction Safety and Health*, CRC Press, 2006.

[4] A. Moelker, R. A. J. J. Maas, F. Lethimonnier, and P. M. T. Pattynama, "Interventional MR imaging at 1.5 T: Quantification of sound exposure," *Radiology*, vol. 224, no. 3, pp. 889–895, 2002.

[5] R. Govindaraju, R. Omar, R. Rajagopalan, R. Norlisah, and N. Kwan-Hoong, "Hearing loss after noise exposure," *Auris Nasus Larynx*, vol. 38, no. 4, pp. 519–522, 2011.

[6] W. A. Edelstein, R. A. Hedeen, R. P. Mallozzi, S.-A. El-Hamamsy, R. A. Ackermann, and T. J. Havens, "Making MRI quieter," *Magnetic Resonance Imaging*, vol. 20, no. 2, pp. 155–163, 2002.

[7] S. Ahmed and F. G. Shellock, "Magnetic resonance imaging safety: Implications for cardiovascular patients," *Journal of Cardiovascular Magnetic Resonance*, vol. 3, no. 3, pp. 171–182, 2001.

[8] M. McJury and F. G. Shellock, "Auditory noise associated with MR procedures: A review," *Journal of Magnetic Resonance Imaging*, vol. 12, no. 1, pp. 37–45, 2000.

[9] P. Radomskij, M. A. Schmidt, C. W. Heron, and D. Prasher, "Effect of MRI noise on cochlear function," *The Lancet*, vol. 359, no. 9316, pp. 1485-1486, 2002.

[10] D. L. Price, J. P. De Wilde, A. M. Papadaki, J. S. Curran, and R. I. Kitney, "Investigation of acoustic noise on 15 MRI scanners from 0.2 T to 3 T," *Journal of Magnetic Resonance Imaging*, vol. 13, no. 2, pp. 288–293, 2001.

[11] Y. Hattori, H. Fukatsu, and T. Ishigaki, "Measurement and evaluation of the acoustic noise of a 3 Tesla MR scanner," *Nagoya Journal of Medical Science*, vol. 69, no. 1-2, pp. 23–28, 2007.

[12] R. E. Brummett, J. M. Talbot, and P. Charuhas, "Potential hearing loss resulting from MR imaging," *Radiology*, vol. 169, no. 2, pp. 539-540, 1988.

[13] A. Mollasadeghi, A. H. Mehrparvar, S. Atighechi, M. H. Davari, P. Shokouh, M. Mostaghaci et al., "Sensorineural hearing loss after magnetic resonance imaging," *Case Reports in Radiology*, vol. 2013, Article ID 510258, 3 pages, 2013.

[14] E. Y. L. Lim, I. P. Tang, M. Peyman, N. Ramli, P. Narayanan, and R. Rajagopalan, "3 Tesla magnetic resonance imaging noise in standard head and neck sequence does not cause temporary threshold shift in high frequency," *European Archives of Oto-Rhino-Laryngology : Official Journal of the European Federation of Oto-Rhino-Laryngological Societies (EUFOS) : Affiliated with the German Society for Oto-Rhino-Laryngology - Head And Neck Surgery*, vol. 272, no. 11, pp. 3109–3113, 2015.

[15] C. Jin, H. Li, X. Li et al., "Temporary hearing threshold shift in healthy volunteers with hearing protection caused by acoustic noise exposure during 3-T multisequence MR neuroimaging," *Radiology*, vol. 286, no. 2, pp. 602–608, 2018.

[16] W. Wagner, I. Staud, G. Frank, F. Dammann, S. Plontke, and P. K. Plinkert, "Noise in magnetic resonance imaging: No risk for sensorineural function but increased amplitude variability of otoacoustic emissions," *The Laryngoscope*, vol. 113, no. 7, pp. 1216–1223, 2003.

[17] J. P. De Wilde, D. Grainger, D. L. Price, and C. Renaud, "Magnetic resonance imaging safety issues including an analysis of recorded incidents within the UK," *Progress in Nuclear Magnetic Resonance Spectroscopy*, vol. 51, no. 1, pp. 37–48, 2007.

[18] D. E. Dunn and P. M. Rabinowitz, "Noise," *Textbook of Clinical Occupational and Environmental Medicine*, pp. 893–901, 2005.

[19] D. I. McBride and S. Williams, "Audiometric notch as a sign of noise induced hearing loss," *Occupational and Environmental Medicine*, vol. 58, no. 1, pp. 46–51, 2001.

[20] A. H. Mehrparvar, S. J. Mirmohammadi, M. H. Davari et al., "Conventional audiometry, extended high-frequency audiometry, and dpoae for early diagnosis of NIHL," *Iranian Red Crescent Medical Journal*, vol. 16, no. 1, p. e9628, 2014.

[21] A. H. Mehrparvar, S. J. Mirmohammadi, A. Ghoreyshi, A. Mollasadeghi, and Z. Loukzadeh, "High-frequency audiometry: A means for early diagnosis of noise-induced hearing loss," *Noise & Health*, vol. 13, no. 55, pp. 402–406, 2011.

[22] S. Türkkahraman, U. Gök, T. Karlidag, E. Keleş, and A. Oztürk, "Findings of standard and high-frequency audiometry in workers exposed to occupational noise for long durations," *Kulak burun bogaz ihtisas dergisi : KBB = Journal of ear, nose, and throat*, vol. 10, no. 4, pp. 137–142, 2003.

[23] G. Somma, A. Pietroiusti, A. Magrini et al., "Extended high-frequency audiometry and noise induced hearing loss in cement workers," *American Journal of Industrial Medicine*, vol. 51, no. 6, pp. 452–462, 2008.

15

Postcontrast Fluid-Attenuated Inversion Recovery (FLAIR) Sequence MR Imaging in Detecting Intracranial Pathology

Ajit Mahale, Shaloo Choudhary, Sonali Ullal, Merwyn Fernandes, and Sonali Prabhu

Department of Radiodiagnosis, Kasturba Medical College Mangalore, MAHE Dakshina Kannada, Karnataka 575001, India

Correspondence should be addressed to Ajit Mahale; ajitmahale137@gmail.com

Academic Editor: André Luiz Ferreira Costa

Background. Imaging sequences for detection of meningeal and parenchymal lesions are critical in intracranial pathology. Our study analysed FLAIR MRI sequence for evaluating postcontrast enhancement. *Objectives.* FLAIR imaging sequences have been used in evaluation of enhancement in the brain. We conducted a study of FLAIR imaging sequences to better delineate postcontrast enhancement. *Materials and Methods.* In this prospective hospital-based observational study, postcontrast T1 MTC and delayed postcontrast T2 FLAIR and T1 FLAIR images of 66 patients with intracranial pathology were assessed by experienced radiologists from November 2017 to November 2019. *Results.* 28 cases of meningeal enhancement were identified in delayed postcontrast T2 FLAIR images. Low-grade gliomas included in the study showed postcontrast enhancement on postcontrast T1 MTC images. Multiple sclerosis lesions were better seen on postcontrast T1 FLAIR. In extraaxial lesions of 11 cases of meningioma, brighter enhancement was seen on delayed postcontrast T2 FLAIR images. *Conclusion.* We found that delayed postcontrast T2 FLAIR was better in detection of meningeal enhancement in infectious meningitis and in meningitis carcinomatosis than T1 MTC images. In delayed postcontrast T2 FLAIR images, intra-axial parenchyma lesions appeared more conspicuous or similar to T1 MTC images. Delayed postcontrast T1 FLAIR images provided better anatomic delineation of intra-axial lesions.

1. Introduction

The role of imaging sequences for more accurate detection of meningeal and parenchymal lesions is critical in diagnosis [1, 2]. Some studies performed in the last decade show that postcontrast T2 FLAIR is a useful imaging sequence for evaluation enhancement [3]. There are not many studies done to determine the utility of postcontrast T1 FLAIR in intracranial pathologies. The greatest advantage of CE FLAIR seems to be for detecting subtle abnormalities such as leptomeningeal carcinomatosis, where there is no mass effect [4, 5]. We conducted a study to validate utilization of FLAIR sequences in delineating postcontrast enhancement.

2. Methods and Materials

In this prospective hospital-based observational study, postcontrast T1 MTC and delayed postcontrast T2 FLAIR and T1 FLAIR images of 66 patients—32 patients with meningeal enhancement (28 cases of infectious etiology and 4 with tumoral meningeal lesions-metastasis), 23 parenchymal enhancing lesions (7 patients with infection (5 cases tuberculomas and 2 toxoplasmosis), 2 patients with demyelination (multiple sclerosis), 6 patients with primary tumors (4 low-grade gliomas and 2 high-grade gliomas), and 8 patients with metastatic lesions), and 11 patients with extraaxial lesions(meningiomas)—were assessed by experienced radiologists during a study period from November 2017 to November 2019.

The study was approved by the institutional ethics committee. Data were collected from all age groups of patients who were referred to the department of radio diagnosis for MRI brain study with contrast, to rule out meningeal or parenchymal lesions.

Data were collected from the patients referred to the department of radio diagnosis, for MR imaging of the brain, in the teaching hospitals attached to Kasturba Medical College, Mangalore. MR examinations were performed on 1.5 Tesla (Magnetom Siemens Avanto).

Gadolinium dimeglumine (0.5 mmol/ml) was administered.

Sequential order of postcontrast sequences was as follows: T1W postcontrast sequence was run prior to delayed postcontrast FLAIR (fluid attenuation inversion recovery) sequences.

2.1. Scanning Parameters

Imaging parameters for delayed (10 min) postcontrast T2 FLAIR imaging:

TR:9000
TE:92
TI:2500
Slice thickness: 5 mm

Imaging parameters for postcontrast T1W FLAIR:

TR:2000
TI:860
TE:59
Slice thickness: 5 mm

Imaging parameters for postcontrast T1W MTC images:

TR:741
TE:17
Slice thickness: 5 mm

2.2. Inclusion Criteria. Patients referred for gadolinium-enhanced brain imaging.

2.3. Exclusion Criteria

(1) Patients with intracranial aneurysm clips.
(2) Patients with intraorbital metal fragments, any electrically, magnetically, and mechanically activated implants (cardiac pacemakers, biostimulators, neurostimulators, cochlear implants, and hearing aids).
(3) Patients having renal failure or raised creatinine (1.6 mg/dl) levels.

3. Results

Out of the 28 cases with clinical diagnosis of leptomeningitis, in all of the 28 cases, meningeal enhancement was easily identified in delayed postcontrast T2 FLAIR images. In comparison, in postcontrast T1 MTC images, differentiation of meningeal enhancement from vascular enhancement was difficult and could have been missed easily. CSF studies were positive in all 28 cases. On the contrary, delayed postcontrast T1 FLAIR images demonstrated minimal meningeal enhancement in 26 cases out of the 28 cases of leptomeningitis, and the enhancement was inferior to T1 MTC images in all of these 28 cases (Figure 1).

Out of the 23 cases of intra-axial parenchymal lesions included in the study, in 2 cases, postcontrast T1 FLAIR was not done. In rest of 21 cases, delayed postcontrast T1 FLAIR was done, out of which 13 cases showed brighter and thicker enhancement of solid components and peripheral walls of the lesions. It provided better delineation of lesion. These 13 cases included 4 cases of solid cystic parenchymal mass lesions (2 primary and 2 metastatic), 2 cases of peripherally enhancing primary cystic tumors, 2 cases of cystic metastasis, 4 cases of infection (3 tuberculomas and 1 toxoplasmosis), and 1 case of demyelination (multiple sclerosis). In such cases, characteristics of the wall of peripherally enhancing tumors/infectious lesions were better defined by delayed postcontrast T1 FLAIR images as compared to postcontrast T1 MTC.

In three out of four low-grade glioma included in the study, subtle postcontrast enhancement seen on postcontrast T1 MTC images could not be well appreciated on delayed postcontrast T2 FLAIR images due to the intrinsic FLAIR hyperintense nature of the lesions (Figure 2). Subtle enhancement noted in postcontrast T1 MTC images in all 4 low-grade gliomas was better delineated on delayed postcontrast T1 FLAIR images.

Postcontrast enhancement could not be well appreciated on delayed postcontrast T2 FLAIR images in two cases of multiple sclerosis as compared to postcontrast T1 MTC images. In patients with multiple lesions delayed T1 postcontrast FLAIR images picked up almost the same number of lesions as compared to postcontrast T1 MTC images.

Out of the 11 cases of meningioma, brighter enhancement was seen on delayed postcontrast T2 FLAIR images as compared to postcontrast T1 MTC images. Dural tail was easier to identify on delayed postcontrast T2 FLAIR images in 8 out of 11 cases due to brighter enhancement as compared to postcontrast T1 MTC images. In one case of meningioma, dural tail was less well appreciated than in postcontrast T1 MTC images. CSF cleft was better appreciated on postcontrast T2 FLAIR images than on postcontrast T1 MTC images in 8 out of 11 cases (Figure 3).

Dural tail and extraaxial nature of the lesion was better appreciated on postcontrast T2 FLAIR images than postcontrast T1 MTC images.

4. Discussion

Our results are similar to a report published by Kremer et al. [6] which compared unenhanced, enhanced, and delayed enhanced T2 FLAIR images with enhanced T1 MTC images in 10 patients and concluded that delayed enhanced T2 FLAIR MR sequence seems to improve the detection of lesions. The main reason for better detection of meningeal enhancement on postcontrast T2 FLAIR images is lack of vascular enhancement [7] unlike postcontrast T1 MTC images, where it becomes difficult to differentiate between the vascular enhancement of congested slow flowing vessels from meningeal enhancement (Figure 4).

Parmar et al. [8] in an in vitro phantom study showed that FLAIR was more sensitive to gadolinium effects at four times lower concentrations than T1-weighted images.

Studies done by Splendiani et al. and Artzi et al. [9] show similar results with overall sensitivity of enhanced FLAIR sequence to be 100% and 85%, respectively.

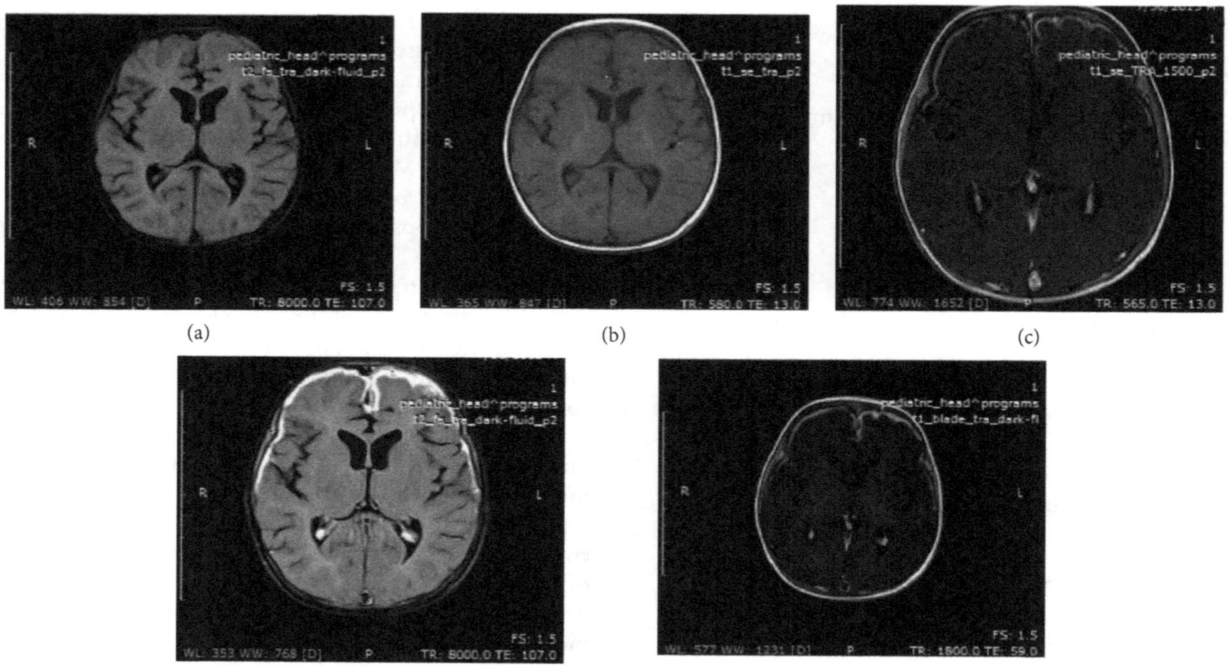

(a) (b) (c) (d) (e)

FIGURE 1: Case of meningitis: (a) unenhanced T2 FLAIR image; (b) unenhanced T1 image; (c) postcontrast T1 MTC image; (d) delayed postcontrast T2 FLAIR image; (e) delayed postcontrast T1 FLAIR image.

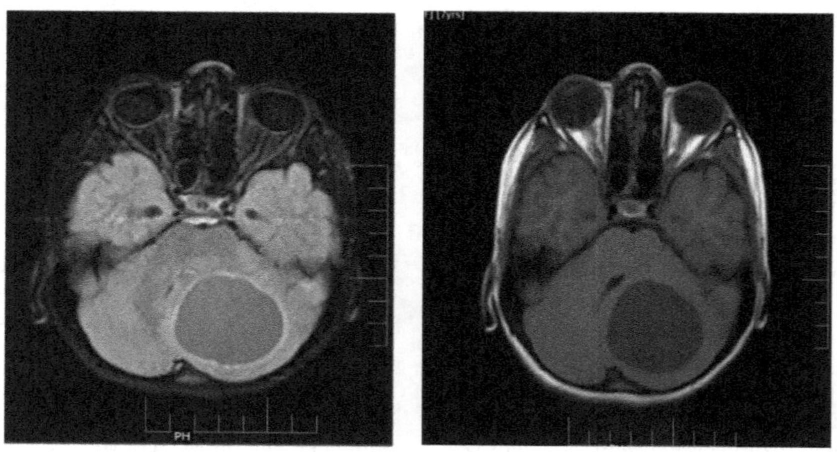

(a) (b)

FIGURE 2: Continued.

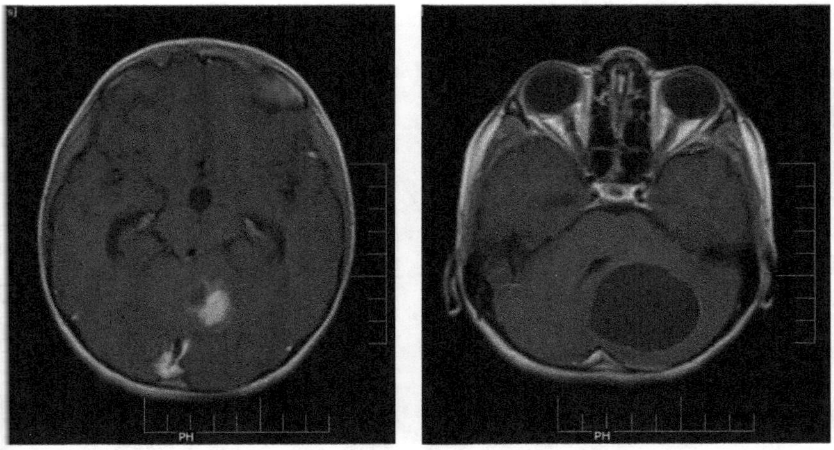

(c) (d)

Figure 2: Pilocytic astrocytoma: (a) unenhanced FLAIR images; (b) unenhanced T1 images; (c, d) postcontrast T1 MTC.

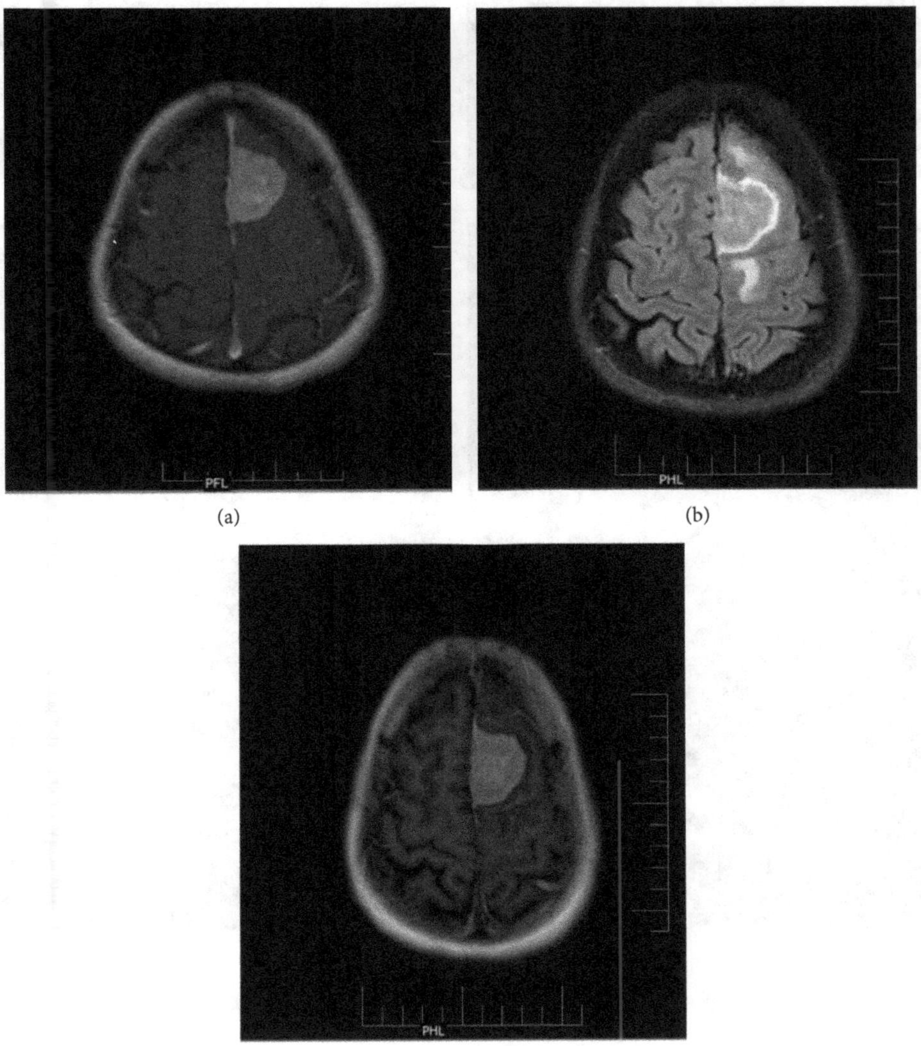

(a) (b) (c)

Figure 3: Case of meningioma: (a) postcontrast T1 MTC image; (b) delayed postcontrast T2 FLAIR image; (c) delayed postcontrast T1 FLAIR image.

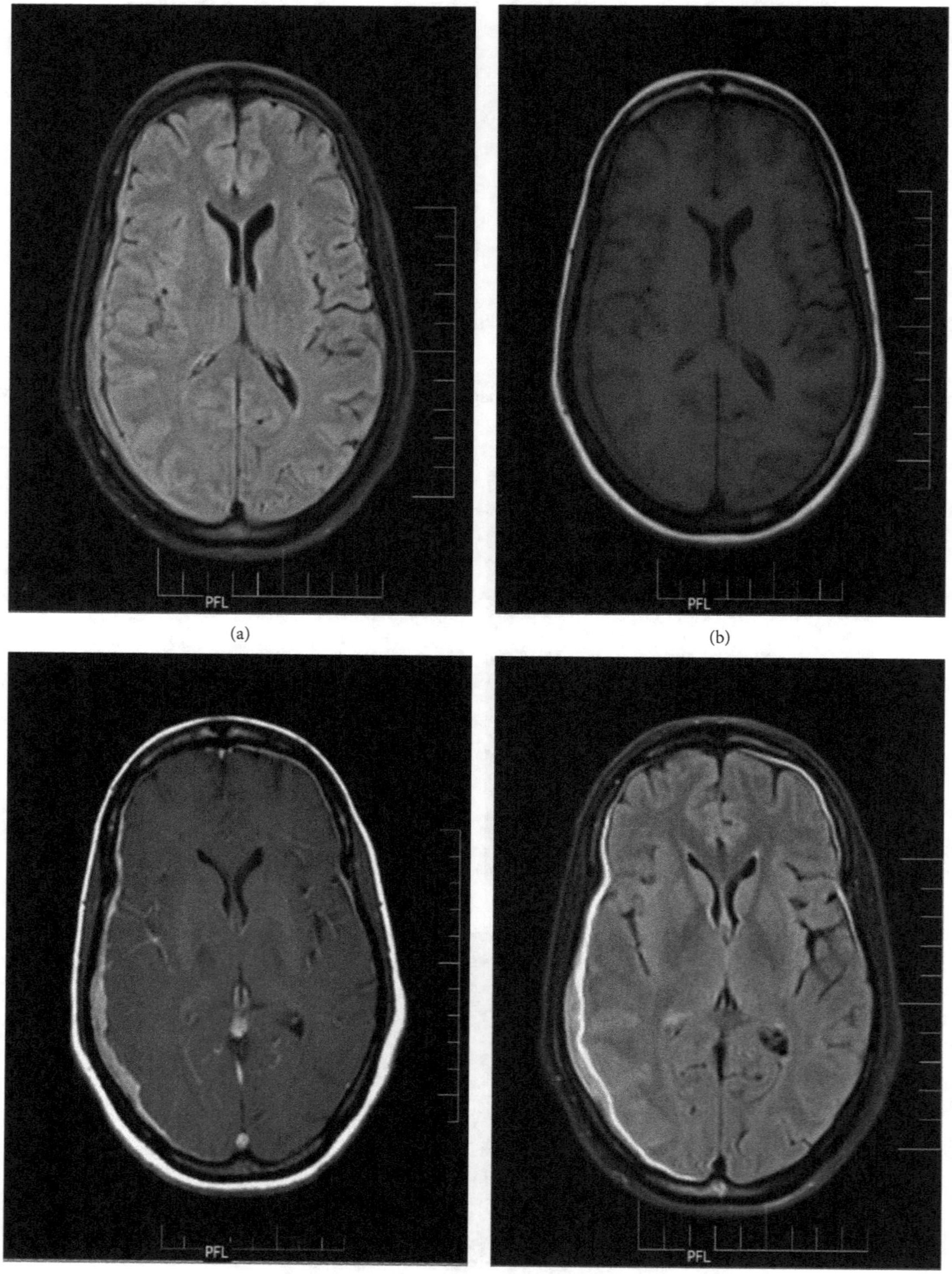

(a) (b)

(c) (d)

FIGURE 4: Continued.

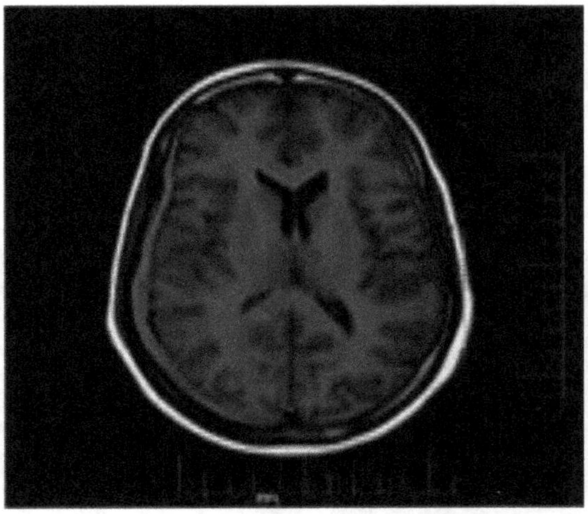

(e)

FIGURE 4: Case of meningeal metastasis: (a) unenhanced FLAIR image; (b) unenhanced T1 image; (c) postcontrast T1 MTC images; (d) delayed postcontrast T2 FLAIR image; (e) delayed postcontrast T1 FLAIR image.

We have found that in delayed postcontrast T1 and T2 FLAIR images, most of the intra-axial parenchyma lesions appeared more conspicuous or similar to T1 MTC images. Flair images show increased signal intensity because the T1 and T2 effects of various tissues supplement each other.

In a study done by Hakyemez et al. [10] in patients with glioblastoma multiforme, nonenhancing FLAIR hyperintense areas surrounding the enhancing lesion represented vasogenic edema, and further evaluation of this nonenhancing FLAIR hyperintense area was done with perfusion and spectroscopy to rule out tumor infiltration.

However, in our study, we found that delayed postcontrast FLAIR images can be helpful in differentiating between metastatic disease and high-grade glioma as a greater degree of perilesional signal change representing edema is more indicative of metastatic disease, as described in another study [11].

In our study, we found that delayed postcontrast T1 FLAIR images were not sensitive for detection of leptomeningeal enhancement. Any leak of gadolinium into the CSF space may shorten the TI of CSF enough so that the longitudinal magnetization recovers before the null point of CSF on T2 FLAIR images; however, this leak of gadolinium is not enough for the recovery of CSF signal intensity on T1 FLAIR images due to the shorter TI time and more T1 weightage of the images as compared to T2 FLAIR images.

Postcontrast T1 FLAIR images provided better anatomic delineation, with a better contrast between the gray and white matter and also between gray matter and the lesion, and T2 FLAIR showed delineation between lesion and CSF due to the darker CSF on T2 FLAIR images.

We found that delayed postcontrast T1 FLAIR images provided better anatomic delineation with intense enhancement of high-grade tumors, large metastatic, and infectious ring-enhancing lesions (Figure 5).

Thickened walls of chronic lesions have increased vascularity which leads to accumulation of gadolinium within the lesions, and high-grade tumors with increased perfusion show increased gadolinium retention in blood pool or within the tumor. Retention of gadolinium results in decrease of TI in CSF so that it is no longer nulled by the inversion pulse and appears bright. The cystic nonenhancing components within the lesion appear even more hypointense (than on T1 MTC) due to the inversion pulse.

Increased contrast between enhancing hyperintense and nonenhancing cystic component of the lesions along with the intrinsic high CNR of lesions on T1 FLAIR images provides excellent delineation of lesions on delayed postcontrast T1 FLAIR images. Our findings were consistent with those of Al-Saeed et al. [12].

The overall image contrast was judged to be superior on T1-weighted FLAIR images compared with T1-weighted FSE images by all neuroradiologists [12] (Figure 6).

Delayed postcontrast T2 and T1 FLAIR images showed better enhancement of meningeal and parenchymal lesions and detected more number of lesions as compared to postcontrast T1 MTC. Delayed postcontrast T2 FLAIR images provided better delineation of extraaxial mass lesions with more conspicuous enhancement and better demarcation of dural tail.

Hence, we concluded that delayed postcost contrast T2 FLAIR images should be included in the routine protocol for contrast MRI brain study.

On the contrary, postcontrast T1 FLAIR had no added advantage over T1 MTC images in detection of meningeal lesions. Although T1 FLAIR images provided better delineation of the extraaxial mass lesions, the degree of enhancement was either inferior or similar to T1 MTC images.

Postcontrast T1 FLAIR provides better enhancement and delineation of intraparenchymal high-grade vascular tumors and large tuberculomas than postcontrast T1 MTC.

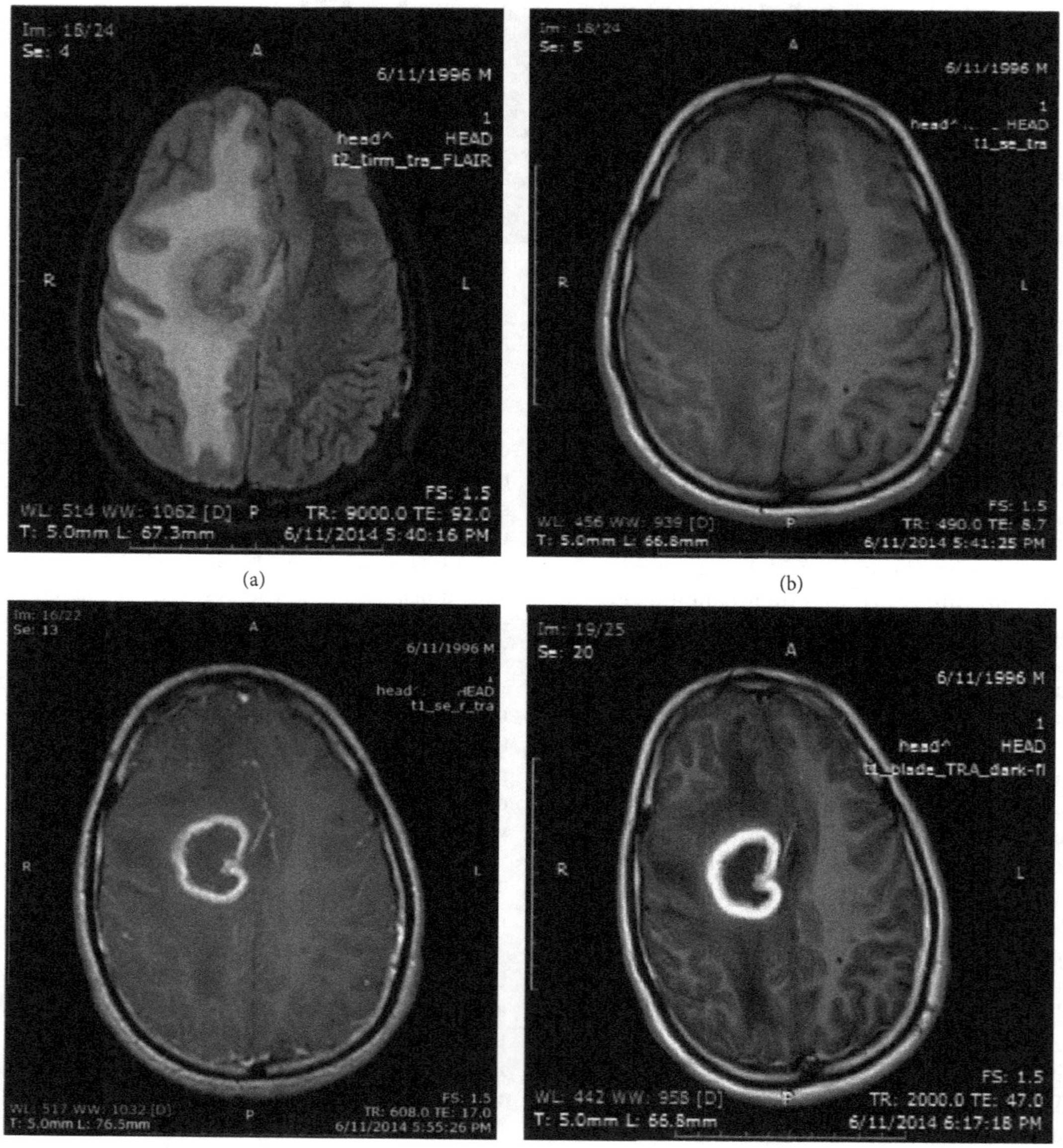

Figure 5: Continued.

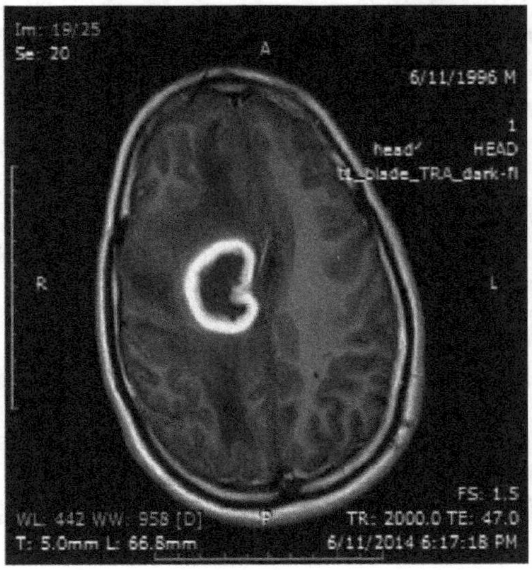

(e)

FIGURE 5: Ring enhancing lesion-tuberculoma: (a) unenhanced FLAIR image; (b) unenhanced T1 image; (c) postcontrast T1 MTC image; (d) delayed postcontrast T1 FLAIR image; (e) delayed postcontrast T1 Flair.

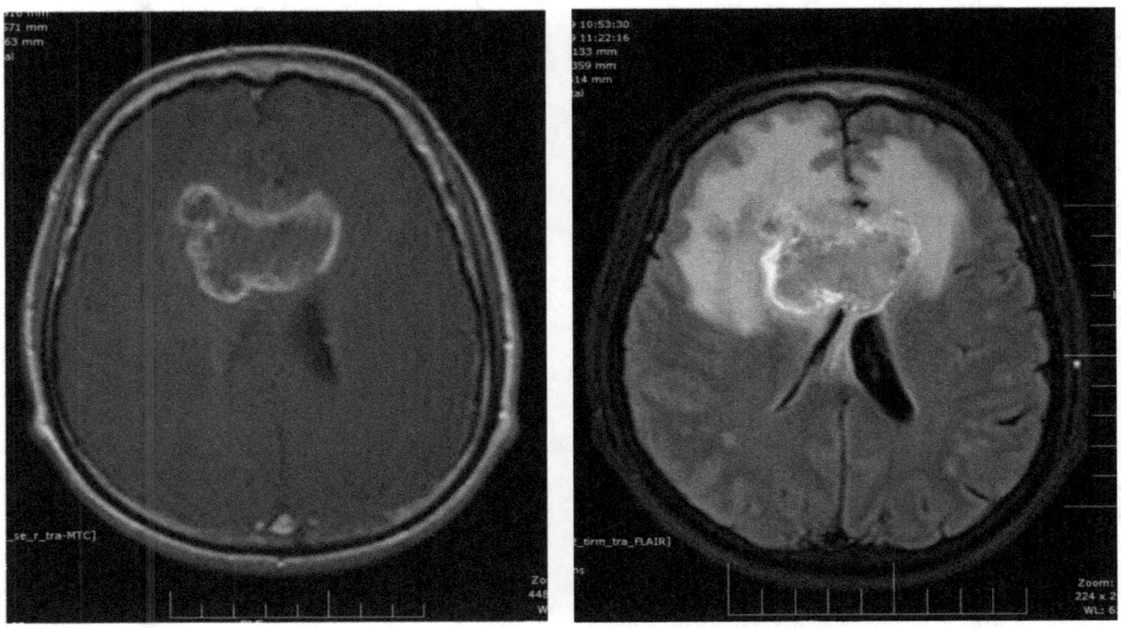

(a) (b)

FIGURE 6: Continued.

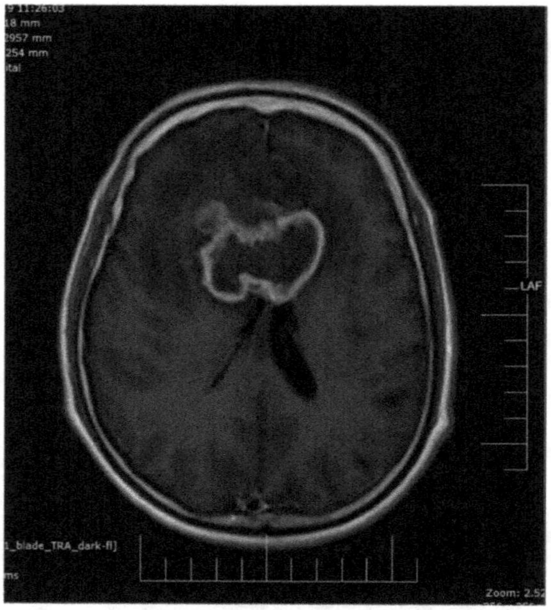

(c)

Figure 6: Butterfly glioma: (a) T1 MTC postcontrast; (b) T2 FLAIR postcontrast; (c) TI FLAIR postcontrast.

References

[1] W. Galassi, W. Phuttharak, J. R. Hesselink, J. F. Healy, R. B. Dietrich, and S. G Imbesi, "Intracranial meningeal disease: comparison of contrast-enhanced MR imaging with fluid-attenuated inversion recovery and fat-suppressed T1-weighted sequences," *AJNR. American Journal of Neuroradiology*, vol. 26, no. 3, pp. 553–559, 2005.

[2] S. K. Singh, N. E. Leeds, and L. E. Ginsberg, "MR imaging of leptomeningeal metastases: comparison of three sequences," *AJNR. American Journal of Neuroradiology*, vol. 23, no. 5, pp. 817–821, 2002.

[3] V. P. Mathews, K. S. Caldemeyer, M. J. Lowe, S. L. Greenspan, D. M. Weber, and J. L. Ulmer, "Brain: gadolinium-enhanced fast fluid-attenuated inversion-recovery MR imaging," *Radiology*, vol. 211, no. 1, pp. 257–263, 1999.

[4] Y.-F. Qian, C.-L. Yu, C. Zhang, and Y.-Q. Yu, "MR T1-eighted inversion recovery imaging in detecting brain metastases: could it replace T1-eighted spincho imaging?" *American Journal of Neuroradiology*, vol. 29, no. 4, pp. 701–704, 2008.

[5] L. Penev, "Diagnostic value of contrast-enhanced fluid-attenuated inversion recovery MR imaging of intracranial metastases," *Rentgenologiya i Radiologiya*, vol. 50, no. 3, pp. 207–212, 2011.

[6] S. Kremer, M. Abu Eid, G. Bierry et al., "Accuracy of delayed post-contrast FLAIR MR imaging for the diagnosis of leptomeningeal infectious or tumoral diseases," *Journal of Neuroradiology*, vol. 33, no. 5, pp. 285–291, 2006.

[7] A. C. Mamourian, P. J. Hoopes, and L. D. Lewis, "Visualization of intravenously administered contrast material in the CSF on fluid-attenuated inversion-recovery MR images: an in vitro and animal- model investigation," *American Journal of Neuroradiology*, vol. 21, no. 1, pp. 105–111, 2000.

[8] H. Parmar, Y.-Y. Sitoh, P. Anand, V. Chua, and F. Hui, "Contrast-enhanced flair imaging in the evaluation of infectious leptomeningeal diseases," *European Journal of Radiology*, vol. 58, no. 1, pp. 89–95, 2006.

[9] M. Artzi, F. Bokstein, D. T. Blumenthal et al., "Differentiation between vasogenic-edema versus tumor-infiltrative area in patients with glioblastoma during bevacizumab therapy: a longitudinal MRI study," *European Journal of Radiology*, vol. 83, no. 7, pp. 1250–1256, 2014.

[10] B. Hakyemez, C. Erdogan, G. Gokalp, a. Dusak, and M. Parlak, "Solitary metastases and high-grade gliomas: radiological differentiation by morphometric analysis and perfusion-weighted MRI," *Clinical Radiology*, vol. 65, no. 1, pp. 15–20, 2010.

[11] O. L Alkan, O. Kizilkiliç, T. Yildirim, and S. Alibek, "Comparison of contrast-enhanced T1-weighted FLAIR with BLADE, and spin-echo T1-weighted sequences in intracranial," *Diagnostic and Interventional Radiology*, vol. 15, no. 2, pp. 75–80, 2009.

[12] O. Al-Saeed, M. Ismail, R. P. Athyal, M. Rudwan, and Khafajee, "T1-weighted fluid-attenuated inversion recovery and T1-weighted fast spin-echo contrast-enhanced imaging: a comparison in 20 patients with brain lesions," *Journal of Medical Imaging and Radiation Oncology*, vol. 53, no. 4, pp. 366–372, Aug 2009.

16

Comparison of MRI and CT in the Evaluation of Unilateral Maxillary Sinus Opacification

Elise Chua ,[1] Annakan V. Navaratnam ,[2] Dominic St Leger,[1,3] Vincent Lam,[1] Samit Unadkat,[4] and Alexander Weller [1,5]

[1]*Departments of Radiology, Northwick Park and Central Middlesex Hospitals, London North West University Healthcare NHS Trust, Watford Road, Harrow HA1 3UJ, UK*
[2]*Departments of ENT Surgery, Northwick Park and Central Middlesex Hospitals, London North West University Healthcare NHS Trust, Watford Road, Harrow HA1 3UJ, UK*
[3]*Department of Radiology, Manchester Royal Infirmary, Oxford Road, Manchester M13 9WL, UK*
[4]*Royal National Throat, Nose and Ear Hospital, University College London Hospitals NHS Foundation Trust, 47–49 Huntley Street, London WC1E 6DG, UK*
[5]*Department of Radiology, St George's Hospital, St George's University Hospitals NHS Foundation Trust, Blackshaw Road, Tooting, London SW17 0QT, UK*

Academic Editor: André Luiz Ferreira Costa

Objectives. To evaluate the diagnostic performance of MRI compared with CT in differentiating neoplastic from infectious/inflammatory causes of complete unilateral maxillary sinus opacification (UMSO). Although MRI is increasingly used, no studies validate its utility compared to CT or nasal endoscopy in this context. *Methods.* A retrospective analysis of 49 patients presenting with complete UMSO to a tertiary referral centre was performed, investigated with both CT and MRI. Two head and neck radiologists independently reviewed each imaging modality and recorded both a final diagnosis and Likert-scale diagnostic certainty score. A consensus radiological diagnosis was determined, stratified into potentially neoplastic or infectious/inflammatory aetiology, and compared with nasal endoscopy and final diagnosis. Diagnostic performance and interoperator agreement for predicting neoplasia were calculated. *Results.* Both CT and MRI demonstrated high sensitivity and negative predictive value for neoplasm, although MRI was more specific (79%; 95% CI: 60–92%) than CT (14%; 95% CI: 4–32%), with a higher positive predictive value. MRI was more accurate (88%; 95% CI: 75–95%) than CT (49%; 95% CI: 34–64%) in diagnosing neoplasia. MRI had significantly higher diagnostic certainty Likert scores than CT ($p < 0.0001$ for both observers). Interobserver agreement was fair for CT (kappa coefficient = 0.327) and excellent for MRI (kappa coefficient = 0.918). *Conclusions.* MRI is more specific than CT in characterising UMSO, with greater diagnostic certainty and reproducibility. The additive diagnostic value of MRI complements CT, potentially reducing diagnostic delays in some cases and the need for diagnostic endoscopic sinus surgery in others. We recommend MRI incorporation into the diagnostic pathway for patients with UMSO.

1. Introduction

Sinonasal disease requiring clinical and imaging evaluation is common, affecting 5–12% of the population. The majority are due to infection or inflammation, most commonly chronic rhinosinusitis (primary or secondary). Neoplastic causes are rare, but localised disease such as unilateral maxillary sinus opacification (UMSO) is more likely to have neoplastic aetiology than diffuse bilateral disease [1, 2]. Inverted papilloma (IP) and squamous cell carcinoma are the most frequent benign and malignant lesions, respectively (Figure 1).

This is recognised in the 2020 European position paper on rhinosinusitis and nasal polyps (EPOS), which states *"isolated maxillary sinus opacification is a marker of neoplasia in 18% and malignancy in 7–10%"*...*"so clinicians*

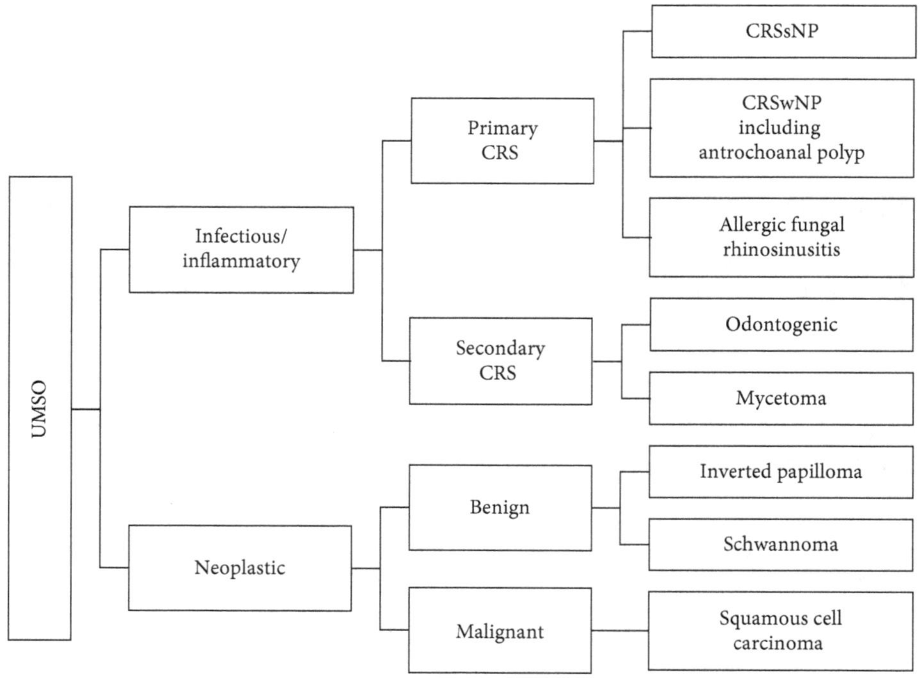

Figure 1: Causes of unilateral maxillary sinus opacification (UMSO). CRS: chronic rhinosinusitis, CRSsNP: CRS without nasal polyps, and CRSwNP: CRS with nasal polyps.

should be wary of conservative management and have a low threshold for early surgical intervention" [3].

For localised obstruction, the primary concern is to differentiate neoplasia from inflammation. However, as symptoms overlap and tumours often have superimposed inflammation, differentiation is challenging clinically [4]. In addition, due to the intricate anatomy, early- and late-stage sinonasal malignancy have vastly different prognoses, leading to considerable medicolegal costs when missed [5]. High sensitivity for neoplasia is therefore crucial, although this is at the expense of low specificity with the current standard of care of low dose CT and flexible nasal endoscopy (FNE) [6, 7].

CT forms the mainstay for sinonasal imaging, providing a low-cost technique for assessing drainage pathways, pattern of obstruction, and bony structures. However, other than inference from Hounsfield-unit densities, intralesional soft tissue characterisation is limited [6, 7]. Aggressive features such as bony erosion or fat infiltration are seen with both benign and malignant aetiologies [8] and may be absent at early stages. Thus, even when heralding malignancy, the diagnosis may be at an advanced stage [9, 10].

FNE is performed for the majority of patients referred to otolaryngology clinics with rhinological symptoms. Although able to identify meatal obstruction by nasal polyps or oedematous mucosa, its role in UMSO is limited due to restricted views of middle meatus, little to no visualisation of the maxillary ostium, sinus contents, and consequent failure to demonstrate abnormalities deep to middle meatus [3, 11, 12].

Due to the relatively high baseline risk of malignancy, a large proportion of patients with UMSO on CT require further investigation with endoscopic sinus surgery (ESS) for histological confirmation regardless of FNE findings [13]. This results in multiple surgical procedures (diagnostic and therapeutic), prolonging time to diagnosis as well as treatment.

MRI is used extensively in the head and neck and potentially provides superb soft tissue characterisation for sinonasal obstruction. It can delineate tumour from secretions and define invasion of adjacent structures, including crucially at the skull base and orbit [14]. If MRI was confirmed to have a greater diagnostic accuracy than CT in differentiating neoplastic from infectious/inflammatory causes of UMSO, it could avoid missed diagnoses of malignancy (improving patient triage to urgent ESS for histological confirmation) or increase the number of confident benign diagnoses, avoiding unnecessary ESS.

Whilst MRI is increasingly used in clinical practice prior to ESS, limited data exists comparing its diagnostic performance with CT or FNE. The aim of this study was to evaluate the diagnostic accuracy of MRI compared with CT (and FNE) in differentiating potentially neoplastic from infectious/inflammatory causes of UMSO (and by extrapolation sinonasal disease in general), to determine which patients warrant subsequent ESS. A secondary aim was to assess interobserver agreement for image interpretation between radiologists, to determine the level of diagnostic reproducibility.

2. Materials and Methods

Patients referred to a tertiary rhinology and head and neck oncology centre prior to January 2017, with complete UMSO detected on CT that proceeded to MRI ± ESS (under our standard institutional diagnostic pathway), were included. As this study comprised a retrospective analysis of data acquired for standard clinical care, ethics committee review and informed consent were waived. Data were collected on clinical, operative, and histological reports. FNE findings were categorised as potentially neoplastic (f-N) or infectious/inflammatory (f-I). For this study, "f-N" was recorded if reported in the operative notes as possibly neoplastic *or* equivocal, as both required further evaluation. To avoid missing potentially malignant sinus obstruction, "f-I" was recorded *only* if reported in the operative notes as such.

The final diagnosis was determined from findings at ESS and histology or diagnosis of CRSsNP based on clinical features and nasal swab (as per EPOS guidelines) and stratified into infective/inflammatory (c-I) or neoplastic (c-N).

2.1. CT and MRI Protocol. CT scans were acquired using Philips Ingenuity 128 (Philips Medical Systems, Eindhoven, The Netherlands) or Toshiba Aquilion 32 (Canon Medical Systems, Sussex, United Kingdom) systems with tube voltage 120 kV, current 30 mA, and patient positioned with an occlusal plane parallel to the gantry, with 500 mm field of view, from maxillary alveolus to top of the frontal sinuses. Images were reconstructed using high frequency (bone) and low frequency (soft tissue) convolution kernels to 0.9 mm slices (0.45 mm interval), with each 150–200 mm diameter reconstructed image presented in a 512 × 512 matrix.

MRI studies were performed on Siemens Avanto (Siemens AG, Erlangen, Germany) or Philips Achieva (Philips Medical Systems, Eindhoven, The Netherlands) 1.5T platforms with 6- or 8-channel phased array head and neck coils, according to departmental protocol. This included axial 3D isotropic T1-weighted (T1W) (repetition time (TR)/echo-time (TE) = 500/8.2 ms and slice thickness = 0.9 mm), axial 3D isotropic short-tau inversion recovery (STIR) SPACE (TR/TE = 2150/199 ms inversion time (TI) = 150 ms, and slice thickness = 1.1 mm), axial and coronal 2D T2-weighted (T2W) turbo spin-echo (TSE) (TR/TE = 5730/83 ms, slice thickness = 3 mm, and 0.6 mm interspace), axial 2D echo-planar diffusion-weighted imaging (TR/TE/TI = 7080/81/130 ms, slice thickness = 4 mm, 1.6 mm interspace, b-factors of 50 and 800 s/mm^2, and calculated apparent diffusion coefficient), and axial 3D isotropic contrast-enhanced T1W gradient echo fat-saturated images (TR/TE = 6/2.81 ms and slice thickness = 0.8 mm, with spectral attenuated inversion recovery (SPAIR) fat saturation) and acquired 100 seconds following gadolinium administration (Dotarem, Gerbet Pharma, Villepinte, France). Where 3D sequences were not possible or degraded by motion, our technicians reimaged with 2D T1W TSE, STIR T2W, and T1W contrast-enhanced fat-suppressed sequences, due to higher temporal resolution afforded by acquiring each slice individually.

2.2. Imaging Analysis. Anonymised images were independently analysed on a proprietary PACS system (Sectra PACS, Linkoping, Sweden), by two consultant head and neck radiologists, Observer1 and Observer2, each with a four-year subspecialty experience. CT and MRI images were evaluated independently of each other and more than 72 hours apart, so diagnoses made were based solely on each study in isolation.

Each observer recorded the overall radiological diagnosis as "infective/inflammatory," "equivocal," or "likely neoplastic." "I" diagnosis only resulted when confident of benign aetiology, with no concern for possible neoplastic or "equivocal" differential. So as not to miss malignancy, "equivocal" or "likely neoplastic" diagnoses were classified as potentially neoplastic "N," as both required further characterisation.

Imaging features were also assessed over three domains: soft tissue characterisation, localisation, and ability to evaluate secondary structures (Table 1). A 10-point Likert score for diagnostic certainty was calculated from this, where features scored "1" if defined (definitely present or absent) and "0" if indeterminate.

A consensus diagnosis was determined, where "r-I" resulted only if recorded as "I" by *both* observers. If one or both observers recorded as "equivocal" or "likely neoplastic," the consensus was graded as such (r-N), as practically further evaluation with biopsy would be required.

2.3. Statistical Analysis. Statistical analysis was performed using GraphPad Prism version 6 (GraphPad Software Inc., CA, USA) and Microsoft Excel, where all appropriate tests were two sided, using a significance level of $\alpha = 5\%$.

Sensitivity, specificity, positive (PPV), negative predictive values (NPV), and diagnostic accuracy of each modality for predicting final clinical diagnosis were calculated. The performance of CT and MRI for differentiating potentially neoplastic UMSO was represented graphically using receiver-operating-characteristic (ROC) analysis plots and the area under the curve (AUC) was calculated.

To assess the absolute difference between CT and MRI, Chi-squared analysis was performed for the diagnoses reached by each observer and consensus. Diagnostic certainty Likert scores were compared between modalities using Mann–Whitney U test.

Interobserver agreement was calculated using Cohen's Kappa coefficient (k) and was interpreted as proposed by Landis and Koch [15]: kappa value of 0 indicates no agreement, 0 to 0.2 slight agreement, 0.21 to 0.4 fair agreement, 0.41 to 0.6 moderate agreement, 0.61 to 0.80 substantial agreement, and 0.81 to 1.0 excellent agreement.

3. Results

Patient demographics and final diagnoses are recorded in Table 2. Forty-nine patients with complete UMSO on CT who also underwent MRI were identified, comprising 33 male and 16 female, with a mean age of 51 years (range 16 to 83 years). Twenty-nine (59%) patients had a final diagnosis of infective/inflammatory aetiology (c-I), of which twenty-one had a diagnosis of CRS: CRS without nasal polyps (CRSsNP) ($n = 6$) and CRS with nasal polyps (CRSwNP)

Table 1: 10-point diagnostic certainty criteria.

Lesion characterisation	Cystic/solid Polypoidal/mass Bone changes Aggressive/nonaggressive
Anatomic origin of the lesion	Maxillary ostium size Maxillary ostium opacification Maxillary origin
Involvement of secondary structures	Perineural invasion Soft tissue involvement Proximity to vessels

Each point scored as 0 (not defined) or 1 (defined).

Table 2: Final clinical diagnoses.

Final diagnosis	Number of cases (%)
Infective/inflammatory (c-I)	**29 (59.2)**
Chronic rhinosinusitis (CRS)	21 (42.9)
CRS without nasal polyps	6 (12.2)
CRS with nasal polyps (including antrochoanal polyp)	12 (24.5)
Fungal sinusitis	2 (4.1)
Mucormycosis	1 (2.0)
Mucocele	4 (8.2)
IgG4 disease	1 (2.0)
Arteriovenous malformation	1 (2.0)
Fibrous dysplasia	1 (2.0)
Pseudoepitheliomatous hyperplasia	1 (2.0)
Neoplastic (c-N)	**20 (40.8)**
Inverted papilloma	9 (18.4)
Cavernous haemangioma	1 (2.0)
Schwannoma	2 (4.1)
Malignant	8 (16.3)
Adenocarcinoma	1 (2.0)
Anaplastic carcinoma	1 (2.0)
Carcinoma (undifferentiated)	1 (2.0)
Lymphoma	1 (2.0)
Melanoma	1 (2.0)
Osteosarcoma	1 (2.0)
Sarcoma	1 (2.0)
Undifferentiated neuroblastoma	1 (2.0)

($n = 12$), noninvasive fungal sinusitis ($n = 2$), and acute invasive fungal sinusitis ($n = 1$). Odontogenic sinusitis was observed in two cases of both CRSsNP and CRSwNP and antrochoanal polyps in four cases of CRSwNP.

Twenty (41%) patients had neoplastic diagnoses (c-N), most frequently IP ($n = 9$), and malignancy ($n = 8$). Forty-four patients underwent surgery. The remaining five who underwent medical treatment alone had a diagnosis of CRSsNP.

3.1. Diagnostic Accuracy. The diagnostic accuracies of MR and CT in identifying potentially neoplastic aetiology, for Observer1, Observer2, and consensus, are recorded in Tables 3 and 4. Most importantly, all 20 cases with a final diagnosis of neoplasia were correctly classified on both CT and MRI, by both observers and at consensus. Using this threshold, both modalities had 100% sensitivity and 100% NPV for identifying neoplasia.

However, for CT, this was at the expense of low specificity (14%, 95%CI: 4–32%) and PPV (44%, 95%CI: 41–48%) at consensus, compared with specificity at MRI of 79% (95% CI: 60–92%) and PPV of 77% (95%CI: 62–87%)). This higher specificity and PPV of MRI are corroborated by the consistently higher number of cases correctly recorded at MRI as "infective/inflammatory," plus lower number of "potentially neoplastic" diagnoses, as a result of the increased diagnostic confidence afforded at MRI. Confirming this, chi-squared analyses showed a significantly higher number of "I" diagnoses and lower number of "N" diagnoses based on MRI compared with CT, for both observers and at consensus (Observer1 $p = 0.006$, Observer2 $p = 0.0002$, and consensus $p < 0.00002$).

A similar comparison between FNE and imaging showed no difference between CT and FNE ($p = 0.34$), whereas MRI correctly recorded a significantly higher number of infective/inflammatory and lower number of potentially neoplastic diagnoses, confirmed by a Chi-square statistic p value of <0.0005. Corroborating these findings, FNE had similar sensitivity for identifying potential neoplasia to both imaging modalities, with comparable specificity, PPV, and diagnostic accuracy to CT, but MRI again demonstrated higher specificity, PPV, and diagnostic accuracy (Table 4).

From Table 3, at CT, only 4 cases were confidently identified as infective/inflammatory at consensus, meaning that 25 required further characterisation. In contrast, a confident and correct diagnosis of infective/inflammatory aetiology was made at MRI for 23 cases by Observer1, 24 cases by Observer2, and 23 cases at consensus. These consensus results are represented graphically in Figure 2, where the ROC analysis AUC is greater for MRI (0.890) than CT (0.569).

Six cases were incorrectly assigned by MRI at consensus to "potentially neoplastic": two CRSwNP; one invasive fungal sinusitis; one IgG4-related disease; one mucormycosis; and one arteriovenous malformation. Apart from the two misdiagnosed CRSwNP, the remaining cases are transspatial aetiologies with aggressive imaging features (Figure 3).

Where CRS was the final diagnosis, both observers correctly recorded CRSwNP ($n = 12$) or CRSsNP ($n = 6$) in a large majority (16/18) on MRI. Both observers correctly identified IP in 6/9 cases on MRI, compared with only 1/9 and 2/9 at CT for Observer1 and Observer2, respectively.

Interobserver agreement for differentiating neoplastic (N) from inflammatory (I) aetiology was fair for CT ($\kappa = 0.327$) and excellent for MRI ($\kappa = 0.918$).

3.2. Diagnostic Certainty. The mean diagnostic certainty Likert-score was 6.6/10 for CT and 8.6/10 for MRI for Observer1 and 5.2/10 for CT and 9.4/10 for MRI for Observer2. MRI had significantly higher scores than CT for diagnostic certainty criteria for both observers (p value <0.00001).

Table 3: Potentially neoplastic (N) and infective/inflammatory (I) diagnoses on CT and MRI for Observer1, Observer2, and consensus compared to final clinical diagnoses.

	Observer1				Observer2				Consensus			
	CT		MRI		CT		MRI		CT		MRI	
Final diagnosis	N	I	N	I	N	I	N	I	r-N	r-I	r-N	r-I
c-N ($n = 20$)	18	2	19	1	20	0	20	0	20	0	20	0
c-I ($n = 29$)	20	9	6	23	22	7	5	24	25	4	6	23
Chi-square statistic (p value) for CT versus MRI	7.5 ($p = 0.006$)				13.6 ($p = 0.0002$)				18.5 ($p < 0.00002$)			

Table 4: Diagnostic performance of CT and MRI for Observer1, Observer2, consensus, and flexible nasal endoscopy.

	Observer1		Observer2	
	CT	MRI	CT	MRI
Sensitivity	90 (68–99)	95 (75–100)	100 (83–100)	100 (83–100)
Specificity	31 (15–51)	79 (60–92)	24 (10–44)	83 (64–94)
PPV	47 (40–54)	76 (61–87)	48 (43–53)	80 (64–90)
NPV	82 (52–95)	96 (77–99)	100	100
Accuracy	55 (40–69)	86 (73–94)	55 (40–69)	90 (78–97)

	Consensus		Flexible nasal endoscopy
	CT	MRI	
Sensitivity	100 (83–100)	100 (83–100)	85 (62–97)
Specificity	14 (4–32)	79 (60–92)	14 (4–32)
PPV	44 (41–48)	77 (62–87)	41 (35–46)
NPV	100	100	57 (25–84)
Accuracy	49 (34–64)	88 (75–95)	43 (29–58)

Sensitivity, specificity, positive (PPV) and negative predictive values (NPV), and accuracy for potentially neoplastic diagnoses are expressed in percentages (95% confidence interval).

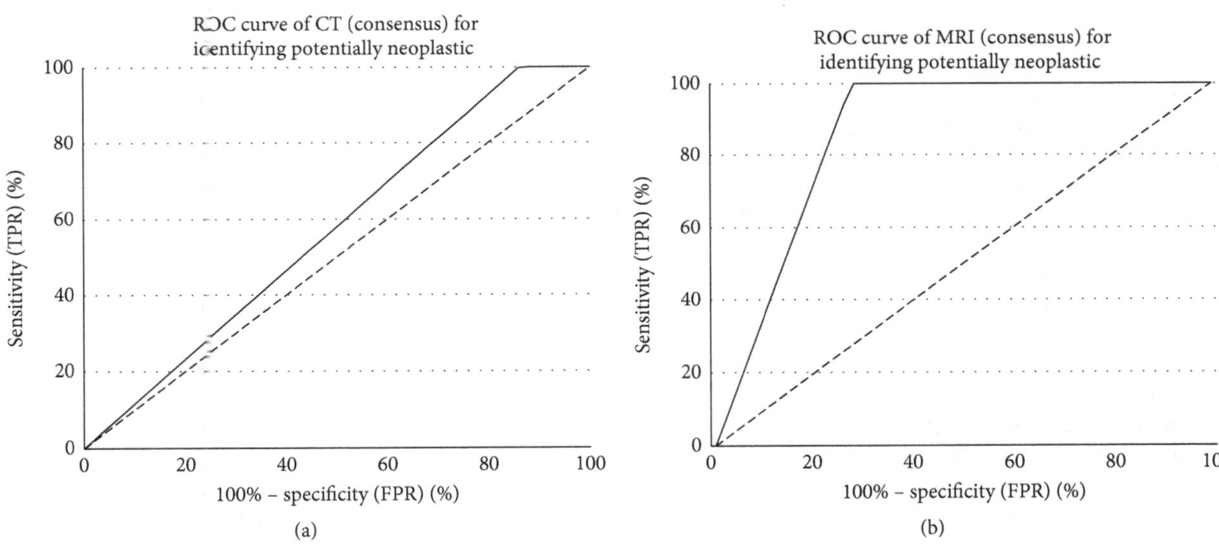

Figure 2: Receiver-operating-characteristic (ROC) curves for differentiating potentially neoplastic from infective/inflammatory causes of unilateral maxillary sinus opacification, for consensus radiological diagnoses: (a) on CT and (b) on MRI. X-axis: false positive rate (FPR), Y-axis: true positive rate (TPR).

4. Discussion

Our results demonstrate the superior diagnostic performance of MRI compared to CT and FNE in characterising UMSO, with excellent interobserver agreement for differentiating neoplasia from inflammation. These results arise from improved soft tissue characterisation, localisation (by differentiating soft tissue from obstructed sinus contents), and ability to evaluate secondary structures, as reflected by significantly higher diagnostic certainty Likert scores for MRI. To achieve this, the MRI protocol should include anatomic (T1W, T2W, and contrast-enhanced sequences) and diffusion-weighted imaging (DWI), with dynamic contrast for suspected vascular pathology. 3D GRE isotropic

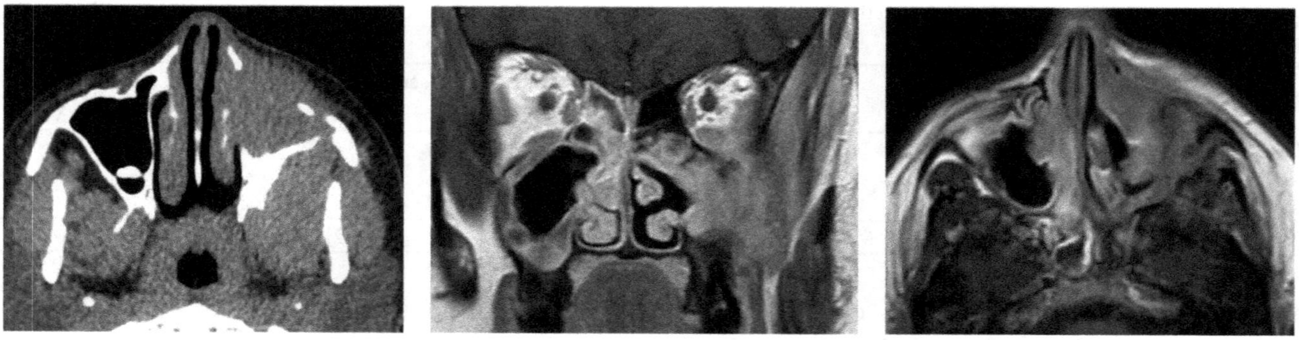

(a) (b) (c)

Figure 3: IgG4 disease. A 31-year-old female presented with epistaxis and medial-gaze diplopia. (a) Axial unenhanced CT shows soft tissue opacification of the left maxillary antrum with destruction of the antral walls and lateral pterygoid plate. (b) Coronal and (c) axial contrast-enhanced T1W demonstrates extension of the abnormally enhancing soft tissue (with restricted diffusion, not shown) into the orbit, pterygopalatine fossa, and involvement of the left infraorbital nerve.

fat-suppressed postcontrast sequences are particularly helpful due to excellent spatial resolution and opportunity for multiplanar reconstruction.

Although MRI, CT, and FNE had similar sensitivity for detecting malignancy (100%, 100%, and 85%, resp.), CT and FNE both had low specificity and high false positive rates (FPR). The smaller number of "equivocal" results at MRI yielded both (a) significantly improved specificity and PPV and (b) consistent interpretation between observers. MRI demonstrates improved specificity compared to CT (79% (95%CI: 62–87%) versus 14% (95%CI: 4–32%)) and increased diagnostic accuracy (88% (95%CI: 75–95%) versus 49% (95%CI: 34–64%)). The proportion of neoplastic and inflammatory disease in our patient cohort is comparable to that in the literature and reflects a relatively high incidence of atypical lesions in unilateral disease [2, 16]. These results demonstrate the utility of MRI in directing management, with diagnoses that are reproducible between different radiologists and therefore between institutions.

MRI correctly identified all neoplasms as equivocal or concerning for malignancy, requiring further ESS evaluation. As for CT and FNE, this confirms that MRI is an extremely safe test. Additionally, the lower FPR means that MRI is significantly able to triage patients with inflammatory aetiology to medical therapy better than CT or FNE, potentially sparing the need for general anaesthesia and ESS. Where the cause of UMSO is uncertain at CT or FNE, MRI comprises a low-cost noninvasive investigation with superior diagnostic accuracy in differentiating both (a) malignancy from benign obstruction and (b) benign neoplasms requiring urgent surgery (such as IP) from those in which medical treatment can be trialled (such as CRS). Thus, MRI has a valuable role when used in conjunction with CT for patient selection for surgical management and is routinely included in our institutional pathway in this context (Figure 4).

Whereas the current standard of care imaging with CT has high sensitivity for neoplasia, justifying its use as a "screening" investigation, the high FPR hampers patient triage as the cause of UMSO is frequently not differentiated. As illustrated in Figures 5 and 6, bony remodelling on CT is an equivocal feature observed in both infective sinusitis and malignancy [16]. By contrast, MRI differentiates secretions from inflamed mucosa, benign neoplasia [17], and malignancy [18, 19]. Most neoplasms demonstrate heterogenous internal enhancement and varying levels of restricted diffusion, whereas inflamed mucosa or polyps show thin peripheral enhancement and unrestricted diffusion [14] (Figures 5 and 6).

For a significant proportion of patients (27% in this cohort) with infectious/inflammatory UMSO that could be managed medically, the improved specificity of MRI mitigates the need for diagnostic ESS. In addition, the 5/9 cases of IP correctly identified at MRI (but not CT) could have proceeded straight to definitive surgery, without the need for diagnostic ESS and biopsy. This not only reduces the risk associated with multiple episodes of anaesthesia and surgery but reduces delay to definitive treatment and relieves service demand. As the cohort of patients with UMSO resistant to medical management is usually small, the cost of additional MRI should not generally be an issue. As elective operating capacity within hospitals can be strained due to competing demands, not least due to the impact of the COVID-19 pandemic [20], interventions that reduce the requirement for multiple surgical procedures will streamline patient pathways and reduce time to treat.

In differentiating benign neoplasms requiring urgent surgery, MRI has high accuracy for diagnosing IP, where a "convoluted cerebriform pattern" is up to 100% sensitive and 87% specific [21–23] (Figure 7). The hyperostotic "bony spur" at the IP origin requires removal [24] and whilst the sensitivity for determining this origin on CT is 63% [25], MRI is both more sensitive and specific [26, 27]. This enables surgeons to plan more extensive resections, including adequate resection of the site of origin without diagnostic ESS [28], reducing reoperation [29–31].

In differentiating benign from malignant neoplasia, overlap exists at MRI in terms of enhancement pattern and diffusion characteristics [32]. Nonetheless, both require ESS for definitive treatment or biopsy confirmation, respectively

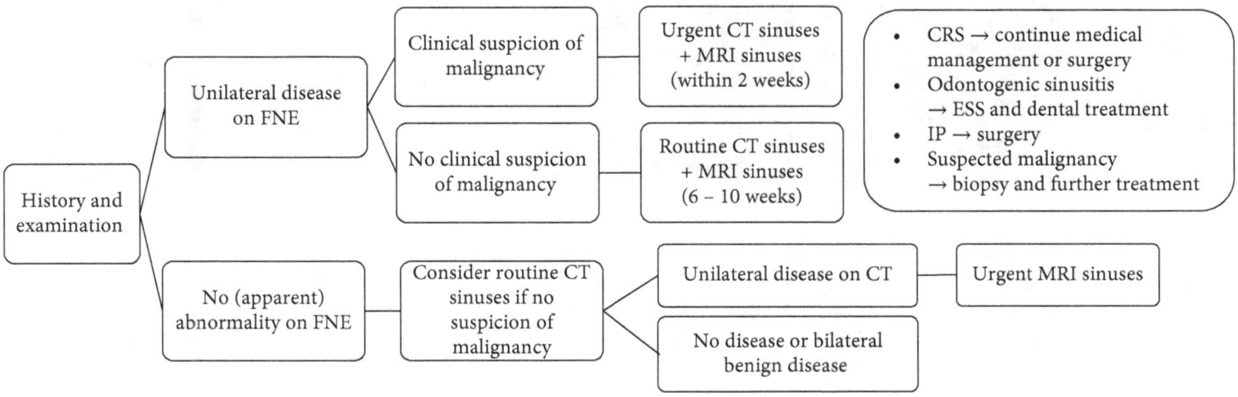

Figure 4: Example diagnostic pathway for unilateral maxillary sinus opacification. Flexible nasal endoscopy (FNE), chronic rhinosinusitis (CRS), endoscopic sinus surgery (ESS), and inverted papilloma (IP).

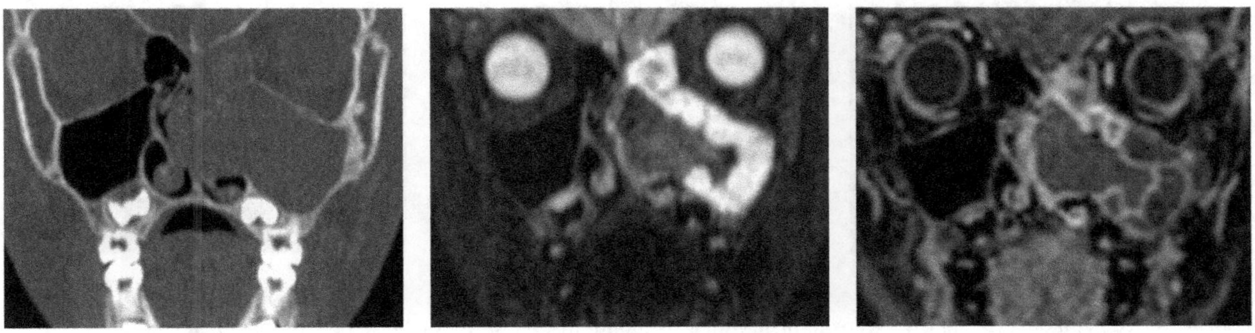

(a) (b) (c)

Figure 5: Fungal sinusitis in 7-year-old male with symptoms of nasal obstruction. (a) Coronal unenhanced CT demonstrates left ostiomeatal pattern opacification with maxillary mural osteitis plus expansion of maxillary antrum. This appearance is equivocal and could represent chronic rhinosinusitis, fungal sinusitis, or tumour. However, low signal centrally on (b) coronal STIR, surrounded by peripherally enhancing thickened mucosa on (c) coronal contrast-enhanced T1W, is consistent with a left maxillary into middle meatal mycetoma and maxillary sinusitis.

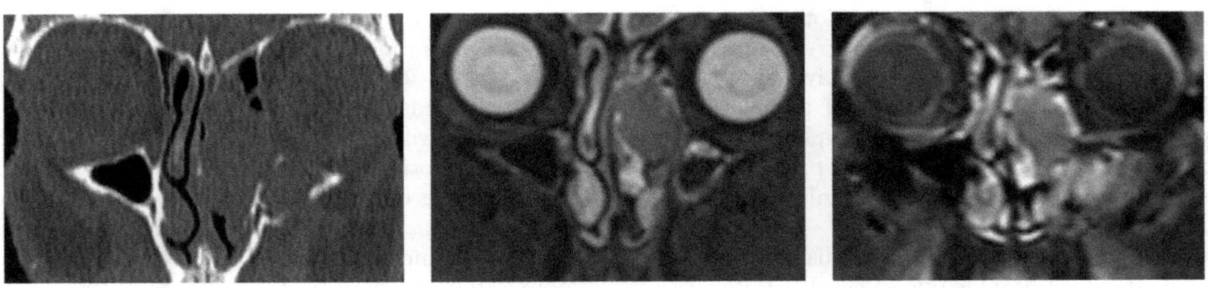

(a) (b) (c)

Figure 6: Continued.

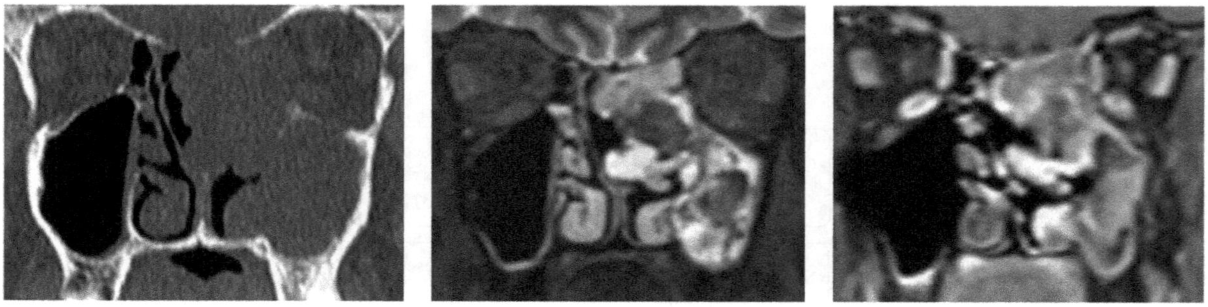

(d) (e) (f)

Figure 6: Diffuse large B-cell lymphoma in a 60-year-old male with a 4-month history of nasal blockage not responding to antibiotics. (a) Coronal unenhanced CT shows left sinonasal opacification with thinned medial maxillary sinus wall and destroyed middle turbinate. (b) Coronal STIR demonstrates a left nasal cavity lesion obstructing the maxillary sinus, which is hypointense to mucosa with heterogenous enhancement on (c) contrast-enhanced T1W. The left cribriform plate appears thinned and focally dehiscent on unenhanced CT (d); however, (e) STIR and (f) contrast-enhanced T1W show the skull base and medial orbital wall are intact.

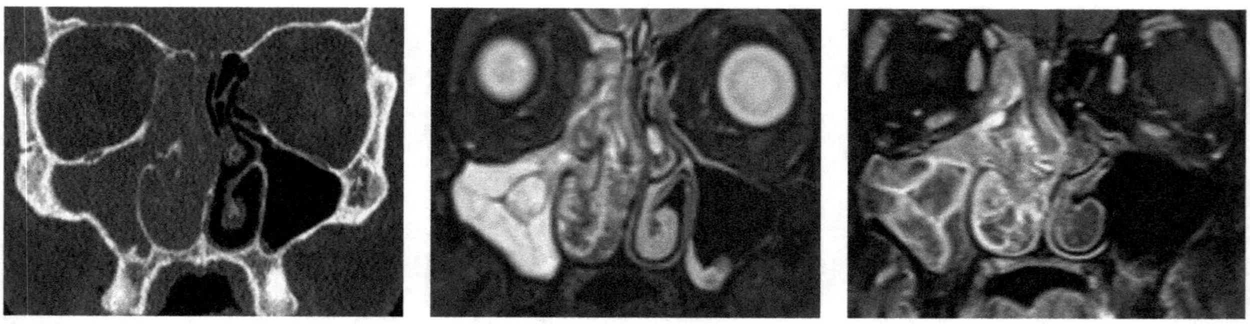

(a) (b) (c)

Figure 7: Inverted papilloma (IP) in a 32-year-old male with a 18-month history of rhinorrhoea. (a) Coronal unenhanced CT shows right unilateral maxillary sinus opacification (UMSO) with complete obstruction of the ostiomeatal unit. Bowing of the nasal septum and amorphous faint calcification could be associated with fungal disease; however, (b) coronal STIR and (c) contrast-enhanced T1W demonstrate a right nasal cavity lesion with the typical "cerebriform" appearance of IP and attachment point at the inferior orbit. Hyperintense right UMSO with mucosal enhancement indicates inspissated secretions rather than lesion extension.

[33]. Where malignancy is confirmed, the diagnostic confidence demonstrated by our results confirms the superiority of MRI over CT in delineating perineural and skull base invasion [14] or overall resection/radiotherapy margins (Figure 6).

At MRI, three of the six "false positive" cases for potential neoplasm comprised transspatial pathologies with aggressive features that overlap with neoplasia. The potentially aggressive natural history and poor prognosis of these processes justify the triage to ESS to confirm the final diagnosis (Figure 4).

No other studies have compared the diagnostic accuracy of CT with MRI for UMSO to our knowledge. Case series of UMSO have only provided qualitative descriptions of CT and MRI features in various aetiologies [16, 34–36]. Chen et al. recorded a relatively large cohort of 116 patients with UMSO but only described findings on CT. Of note, bony erosion was seen in fungal infection, benign, and malignant tumours [16]. Case series of unilateral sinonasal opacification have also presented CT findings in isolation and recommended proceeding to further investigation with biopsy [13, 37]. MRI was only utilised in a small subset of cases if neurological deficits or complications of infection were suspected [33]; thus, evaluation of its PPV for neoplastic disease was not possible.

Plain films can depict sinus opacification and air-fluid levels, but the Royal College of Radiologists has proposed that it is redundant in evaluation of sinonasal disease due to its low sensitivity and specificity [34, 38]. It is possible to diagnose rhinosinusitis on ultrasound, but the literature is not conclusive on its use in sinusitis and it plays a very limited role in characterisation of sinonasal aetiology [38]. Contrast-enhanced CT may be useful in assessment of complications of sinusitis but cannot differentiate inflammatory from malignant disease, as both can enhance [34]. Although fluorodeoxyglucose- (FDG-) PET is utilised in tumour staging and surveillance for recurrence, both tumour and inflammatory cells may demonstrate high FDG uptake, limiting its use for UMSO characterisation. Furthermore, benign tumours such as IP can have moderate FDG uptake, whilst a highly malignant tumour such as adenoid cystic carcinoma can have low FDG uptake [39].

Newer agents such as fluoro-deoxy-thymidine (FLT) have been shown to accumulate only in actively replicating cells rather than inflammatory cells, but further studies on its use in sinonasal disease are required [40].

4.1. Limitations. The main study limitation was small sample size. Although five patients were managed medically and hence no histological correlate was available, the final diagnosis was based on clinical findings and nasal swab as per EPOS guidelines [3]. Although the patient cohort may represent a sample in which CT and/or FNE was less informative than average (therefore necessitating MRI), resulting in a selection bias, our study demonstrates the additional diagnostic value of MRI in these uncertain cases.

Despite these limitations, the value of our data lies in the lack of studies validating the utility of MRI compared with CT in UMSO and in the high level of statistical significance of our results, indicating likely generalizable application between observers and across institutions.

5. Conclusions

MRI provides safe, efficient, and effective triage of patients with UMSO and by extrapolation indeterminate patterns of paranasal sinus opacification at CT. We recommend MRI evaluation in patients with complete UMSO on CT who are resistant to initial medical therapy. MRI has a higher specificity and diagnostic certainty and lower FPR for malignancy than CT, with excellent interobserver agreement. Evaluation at MRI complements CT and has the potential to reduce the need for diagnostic ESS, accelerating diagnosis and definitive management. As it informs surgical planning, it can enable better patient counselling, reduce the risk of multiple procedures, and increase cost-effectiveness of overall care. In the future, multiparametric MRI using DWI, dynamic contrast-enhanced sequences, and intravoxel incoherent motion techniques may further improve presurgical diagnostic accuracy.

References

[1] A. Whyte and R. Boeddinghaus, "Imaging of adult nasal obstruction," *Clinical Radiology*, vol. 75, no. 9, pp. 688–704, 2020.

[2] A. Eckhoff, D. Cox, L. Luk, S. Maidman, S. K. Wise, and J. M. DelGaudio, "Unilateral versus bilateral sinonasal disease: considerations in differential diagnosis and workup," *The Laryngoscope*, vol. 130, no. 4, pp. E116–E121, 2020.

[3] W. J. Fokkens, V. J. Lund, C. Hopkins et al., "European position paper on rhinosinusitis and nasal polyps 2020," *Rhinology*, vol. 58, no. Suppl S29, pp. 1–464, 2020.

[4] P. M. Som, M. S. Brandwein-Gensler, E. E. Kassel, and E. M. Genden, "Tumors and tumor-like conditions of the sinonasal cavities," *Head and Neck Imaging, 5th ed., Elsevier, St Louis, MO, USA*, pp. 253–410, 2011.

[5] D. D. Lydiatt and R. K. Sewell, "Medical malpractice and sinonasal disease," *Otolaryngology-Head and Neck Surgery*, vol. 139, no. 5, pp. 677–681, 2008.

[6] G. G. Pulickal, A. V. Navaratnam, T. Nguyen, A. D. Dragan, M. Dziedzic, and R. K. Lingam, "Imaging sinonasal disease with MRI: providing insight over and above CT," *European Journal of Radiology*, vol. 102, pp. 157–168, 2018.

[7] M. Kawaguchi, H. Kato, H. Tomita et al., "Imaging characteristics of malignant sinonasal tumors," *Journal of Clinical Medicine*, vol. 6, no. 12, p. 116, 2017.

[8] H. B. Eggesbo, "Imaging of sinonasal tumours," *Cancer Imaging*, vol. 12, no. 1, pp. 136–152, 2012.

[9] C. Thorup, L. Sebbesen, H. Danø et al., "Carcinoma of the nasal cavity and paranasal sinuses in Denmark 1995–2004," *Acta Oncologica*, vol. 49, no. 3, pp. 389–394, 2010.

[10] N. Bhattacharyya, "Factors affecting survival in maxillary sinus cancer," *Journal of Oral and Maxillofacial Surgery*, vol. 61, no. 9, pp. 1016–1021, 2003.

[11] D. H. Kim, Y. Seo, K. M. Kim, S. Lee, and S. H. Hwang, "Usefulness of nasal endoscopy for diagnosing patients with chronic rhinosinusitis: a meta-analysis," *American Journal of Rhinology & Allergy*, vol. 34, no. 2, pp. 306–314, 2020.

[12] S. S. Lohiya, S. V. Patel, A. M. Pawde, B. D. Bokare, and P. T. Sakhare, "Comparative study of diagnostic nasal endoscopy and CT paranasal sinuses in diagnosing chronic rhinosinusitis," *Indian Journal of Otolaryngology and Head & Neck Surgery*, vol. 68, no. 2, pp. 224–229, 2016.

[13] F. Ahsan, H. El-Hakim, and K. W. Ah-See, "Unilateral opacification of paranasal sinus CT scans," *Otolaryngology-Head and Neck Surgery*, vol. 133, no. 2, pp. 178–180, 2005.

[14] P. Raghavan and C. D. Phillips, "Magnetic resonance imaging of sinonasal malignancies," *Topics in Magnetic Resonance Imaging*, vol. 18, no. 4, pp. 259–267, 2007.

[15] J. R. Landis and G. G. Koch, "The measurement of observer agreement for categorical data," *Biometrics*, vol. 33, no. 1, pp. 159–174, 1977.

[16] H.-J. Chen, H.-S. Chen, Y.-L. Chang, and Y.-C. Huang, "Complete unilateral maxillary sinus opacity in computed tomography," *Journal of the Formosan Medical Association*, vol. 109, no. 10, pp. 709–715, 2010.

[17] A. Chawla, J. Shenoy, K. Chokkappan, and R. Chung, "Imaging features of sinonasal inverted papilloma: a pictorial review," *Current Problems in Diagnostic Radiology*, vol. 45, no. 5, pp. 347–353, 2016.

[18] Q. Sun, L. An, J. Zheng, and D. Zhu, "Advances in recurrence and malignant transformation of sinonasal inverted papillomas," *Oncology Letters*, vol. 13, no. 6, pp. 4585–4592, 2017.

[19] H. B. Eggesbø, S. Ringertz, O. C. Haanæs et al., "CT and MR imaging of the paranasal sinuses in cystic fibrosis," *Acta Radiologica*, vol. 40, no. 2, pp. 154–162, 1999.

[20] COVIDSurg Collaborative, "Elective surgery cancellations due to the COVID-19 pandemic: global predictive modelling to inform surgical recovery plans," *British Journal of Surgery*, vol. 107, no. 11, pp. 1440–1449, 2020.

[21] H. Ojiri, M. Ujita, S. Tada, and K. Fukuda, "Potentially distinctive features of sinonasal inverted papilloma on MR imaging," *American Journal of Roentgenology*, vol. 175, no. 2, pp. 465–468, 2000.

[22] T. Y. Jeon, H.-J. Kim, S.-K. Chung et al., "Sinonasal inverted papilloma: value of convoluted cerebriform pattern on MR imaging," *American Journal of Neuroradiology*, vol. 29, no. 8, pp. 1556–1560, 2008.

[23] R. Maroldi, D. Farina, L. Palvarini, D. Lombardi, D. Tomenzoli, and P. Nicolai, "Magnetic resonance imaging

findings of inverted papilloma: differential diagnosis with malignant sinonasal tumors," *American Journal of Rhinology*, vol. 18, no. 5, pp. 305–310, 2004.

[24] W. Lawson, B. T. Ho, C. M. Shaari, and H. F. Biller, "Inverted papilloma: a report of 112 cases," *The Laryngoscope*, vol. 105, no. 3, pp. 282–288, 1995.

[25] D. K. Lee, S. K. Chung, H. J. Dhong, H. Y. Kim, H. J. Kim, and K. H. Bok, "Focal hyperostosis on CT of sinonasal inverted papilloma as a predictor of tumor origin," *AJNR American Journal of Neuroradiology*, vol. 28, no. 4, pp. 618–621, 2007.

[26] S. Ma, M. Xian, B. Yang et al., "Pathological changes from the originating to the peripheral sites of sinonasal inverted papilloma are the underlying mechanisms of preoperative MRI-tumor origin prediction," *Rhinology Journal*, vol. 58, no. 1, pp. 59–65, 2020.

[27] G. Fang, H. Lou, W. Yu et al., "Prediction of the originating site of sinonasal inverted papilloma by preoperative magnetic resonance imaging and computed tomography," *International Forum of Allergy & Rhinology*, vol. 6, no. 12, pp. 1221–1228, 2016.

[28] J. K. Goudakos, S. Blioskas, A. Nikolaou, K. Vlachtsis, P. Karkos, and K. D. Markou, "Endoscopic resection of sinonasal inverted papilloma: systematic review and meta-analysis," *American Journal of Rhinology & Allergy*, vol. 32, no. 3, pp. 167–174, 2018.

[29] R. Landsberg, O. Cavel, Y. Segev, A. Khafif, and D. M. Fliss, "Attachment-oriented endoscopic surgical strategy for sinonasal inverted papilloma," *American Journal of Rhinology*, vol. 22, no. 6, pp. 629–634, 2008.

[30] S. Makihara, S. Kariya, T. Naito et al., "Attachment-oriented endoscopic surgical management for inverted papillomas in the nasal cavity and paranasal sinuses," *Auris Nasus Larynx*, vol. 46, no. 5, pp. 748–753, 2019.

[31] Y. Meng, G. Fang, X. Wang et al., "Origin site-based staging system of sinonasal inverted papilloma for application to endoscopic sinus surgery," *Head & Neck*, vol. 41, no. 2, pp. 440–447, 2019.

[32] A. Das, A. S. Bhalla, R. Sharma et al., "Can diffusion weighted imaging aid in differentiating benign from malignant sinonasal masses?: a useful adjunct," *Polish Journal of Radiology*, vol. 82, pp. 345–355, 2017.

[33] P. Gomes, A. Gomes, P. Salvador, C. Lombo, S. Caselhos, and R. Fonseca, Clinical assessment, diagnosis and management of patients with unilateral sinonasal disease," *Acta Otorrinolaringológica Española*, vol. 71, no. 1, pp. 16–25, 2020.

[34] M. Rudralingam, K. Jones, and T. J. Woolford, "The unilateral opaque maxillary sinus on computed tomography," *British Journal of Oral and Maxillofacial Surgery*, vol. 40, no. 6, pp. 504–507, 2002.

[35] B. A. Kaplan and S. E. Kountakis, "Diagnosis and pathology of unilateral maxillary sinus opacification with or without evidence of contralateral disease," *The Laryngoscope*, vol. 114, no. 6, pp. 981–985, 2004.

[36] G. Lehnerdt, J. Weber, and P. Dost, "Die einseitige verschattung der nasennebenhöhlen im CT oder MRT—hinweis für einen seltenen histologischen Befund12," *Laryngo-Rhino-Otologie*, vol. 80, no. 3, pp. 141–145, 2001.

[37] J. Y. Lee, "Unilateral paranasal sinus diseases: analysis of the clinical characteristics, diagnosis, pathology, and computed tomography findings," *Acta Oto-Laryngologica*, vol. 128, no. 6, pp. 621–626, 2008.

[38] H. B. Eggesbø, "Radiological imaging of inflammatory lesions in the nasal cavity and paranasal sinuses," *European Radiology*, vol. 16, no. 4, pp. 872–888, 2006.

[39] H.-S. Jeong, M. K. Chung, Y.-I. Son et al., "Role of 18F-FDG PET/CT in management of high-grade salivary gland malignancies," *Journal of Nuclear Medicine*, vol. 48, no. 8, pp. 1237–1244, 2007.

[40] G. M. Fatterpekar, B. N. Delman, and P. M. Som, "Imaging the paranasal sinuses: where we are and where we are going," *The Anatomical Record: Advances in Integrative Anatomy and Evolutionary Biology*, vol. 291, no. 11, pp. 1564–1572, 2008.

17

4DCT Scanning Technique for Primary Hyperparathyroidism: A Scoping Review

Steven Raeymaeckers,[1] **Maurizio Tosi**,[1] **and Johan De Mey**[1,2]

[1]*Universitair Ziekenhuis Brussel, Laarbeeklaan 101, Jette 1090, Belgium*
[2]*Radiology, Vrije Universiteit Brussel, Laarbeeklaan 103, Jette 1090, Belgium*

Correspondence should be addressed to Steven Raeymaeckers; steven.raeymaeckers@uzbrussel.be

Academic Editor: Lorenzo Faggioni

Objective. 4DCT for the detection of (an) enlarged parathyroid(s) is a commonly performed examination in the management of primary hyperparathyroidism. Protocols are often institution-specific; this review aims to summarize the different protocols and explore the reported sensitivity and specificity of different 4DCT protocols as well as the associated dose. *Materials and Methods.* A literature study was independently conducted by two radiologists from April 2020 until May 2020 using the Medical Literature Analysis and Retrieval System Online (MEDLINE) database. Articles were screened and assessed for eligibility. From eligible studies, data were extracted to summarize different parameters of the scanning protocol and observed diagnostic attributes. *Results.* A total of 51 articles were included and 56 scanning protocols were identified. Most protocols use three ($n = 25$) or four different phases ($n = 23$). Almost all authors include noncontrast enhanced imaging and an arterial phase. Arterial images are usually obtained 25–30 s after administration of contrast, and less agreement exists concerning the timing of the venous phase(s). A mean contrast bolus of 100 mL is administered at 3-4 mL/s. Bolus tracking is not often used ($n = 3$). A wide range of effective doses are reported, up to 28 mSv. A mean sensitivity of 81.5% and a mean specificity of 86% are reported. *Conclusion.* Many different 4DCT scanning protocols for the detection of parathyroid adenomas exist in the literature. The number of phases does not appear to affect sensitivity or specificity. A triphasic approach, however, seems preferable, as three patterns of enhancement of parathyroid adenomas are described. Bolus tracking could help to reduce the variability of enhancement. Sensitivity and specificity also do not appear to be affected by other scan parameters like tube voltage or tube current. To keep the effective dose within limits, scanning at a lower fixed tube current seems preferable. Lowering tube voltage from 120 kV to 100 kV may yield similar image contrast but would also help lower the dose.

1. Introduction

Primary hyperparathyroidism is a common endocrine disease. In the case of an asymptomatic patient over the age of 50 without end-organ complications, conservative treatment can be assumed [1, 2]. The only cure for the disease is surgery, with resection of the affected gland(s). Bilateral exploration of the neck is the historical standard for treatment. In the last decades, however, a minimally invasive surgical approach has been made possible by more effective means of preoperative imaging combined with the development of rapid parathyroid hormone determination techniques allowing for intraoperative PTH monitoring [3].

The most accessible diagnostic technique is ultrasound because it is widely available at low cost, and it presents no adverse effects [4]. As a bonus, ultrasound is the preferred method of examination for the thyroid gland. This way parathyroid lesions can be differentiated from thyroid nodules and other thyroid pathologies. The sensitivity is very operator-dependent but can be as high as 84% in hands of an experienced ultrasonographer [5]. Color Doppler can be used to differentiate parathyroid lesions from other cervical masses, such as lymph nodes and thyroid nodules [6]. Small lesions (<5 mm) can be difficult to detect. False-negative results can occur, especially in the case of ectopic glands or in the presence of a large thyroid goiter [7].

Scintigraphy has the highest sensitivity compared to the other techniques: 88–90% and even higher sensitivity when combined with SPECT/SPECT-CT, the latter providing useful anatomical detail [8]. This technique is the method of choice when an ectopic localization is suspected or in patients having undergone prior neck surgery. The procedure relies on the uptake of 99mTechnetium (99mTc)-sestamibi in the overactivated mitochondria-rich oxyphil cells of the parathyroid gland and the difference in the rate of washout of this tracer with the thyroid. To overcome false positive results deriving from the uptake of sestamibi in solid thyroid nodules, another tracer can be administered that is exclusively taken up by the thyroid tissue, thereby permitting a subtraction of the thyroid. This method is known as the double-tracer technique and can achieve a specificity of over 90% [9].

MRI also allows for the evaluation of parathyroid disease. This technique, like ultrasound, is free of ionizing radiation but it is far a less available modality (a problem also found with scintigraphy). Due to the lack of ionizing radiation, MRI can be used without hesitation to detect ectopic glands. On a 1.5 Tesla system, the reported sensitivity of this technique is 80%; assumedly a better visualization on 3 Tesla systems can be obtained [10–12].

Computed tomography (CT) of the neck without contrast is of no value since it is not possible to discern between parathyroid tissue, ectopic thyroid tissue, and lymph nodes. Four-dimensional CT (4DCT) combines three-dimensional imaging with the inclusion of time as the fourth dimension: this allows for an evaluation of the pattern of enhancement of lesions over time. By means of the evaluation of enhancement, abnormal parathyroid glands can be detected with a sensitivity of 85.7%: typical parathyroid adenomas are hypoattenuating to thyroid tissue on noncontrast enhanced imaging (NECT) and demonstrate avid arterial hyperenhancement during the arterial phase as well as rapid washout on the venous phase [13, 14]. 4DCT is also considered to be a useful technique in the case of ectopic glands or in the case of persistence/recurrence after the initial surgery.

Many different study protocols have been suggested by different authors over the past 15 years; protocols are often very institution-specific. We set out to examine the literature to review the different protocols and their reported sensitivity/specificity. The number of different phases used in a protocol as well as their timing could be a defining factor in sensitivity: as more phases are available, it could be argued that this would increase the sensitivity of the examination. Factors like tube current, tube voltage, and administration of contrast medium affect image noise and contrast and could therefore also have implications toward sensitivity. These factors also influence the effective dose, a key part to consider in multiphasic studies using ionizing radiation.

2. Materials and Methods

2.1. Research Question. This scoping review seeks to answer a multivalent research question. First, we want to establish the number of phases and their timing as used by different authors in the literature. Secondly, we wish to assess whether different protocols are associated with different sensitivity or specificity. We also look at other scanning protocol factors like tube current and tube voltage, contrast bolus volume, and timing: factors that not only can affect the sensitivity of the exam but also influence the effective dose, a key part to consider in multiphasic studies using ionizing radiation.

2.2. Search Strategy. This scoping review is reported according to the PRISMA Extension for Scoping Reviews (PRISMA-ScR) Checklist. A literature search was independently conducted by two radiologists using the MEDLINE database from April 2020 until May 2020 using the terms "4DCT" and "parathyroid."

2.3. Inclusion and Exclusion Criteria. We included all peer-reviewed literature written in English or French. There was no limitation on the publication date. Exclusion criteria were articles written in a language other than English or French.

2.4. Data Selection and Charting Process. The two investigators independently screened the MEDLINE database for relevant articles. A first selection was made based on the title and abstract. Next, each investigator screened the obtained articles for relevancy, and a second selection was made. Finally, the remaining articles underwent a final screening: only studies citing information about the number of phases used in the scanning protocol were included in the scoping review. Forty articles were not relevant. Information regarding publication details (e.g., author, publication date) and study details (e.g., study design, scanning protocol) was obtained. Data was managed in Excel (Microsoft, Redmond, USA). Several scanning protocol factors were included in this review. We checked for the presence of a NECT in the study protocol. We evaluated the number of obtained phases and their timing: we defined a subdivision in an arterial phase (earlier than 40 seconds after contrast administration), a venous phase (40 seconds–70 seconds), a delayed venous phase (70 seconds–100 seconds), and a very delayed phase (later than 100 seconds). We evaluated whether this timing was expressed in absolute or relative relation to the onset of contrast administration; we expressed (where possible) all times in absolute relation to the administration of contrast. We also checked for the use of bolus tracking, which is defined as the use of a continuous density measurement in an arterial structure (usually at the level of the aortic arch) prior to obtaining the first arterial phase.

We also included other parameters of the scanning protocol: tube current is determined by the rate at which X-rays are produced in the X-ray tube (i.e., photons per second). It is expressed in milliampere (mA). Tube voltage is a parameter in direct relation to the number of X-rays produced. It is expressed in kilovolt (kV). The volume of the contrast bolus was included, as well as the injection speed expressed in mL/s. We included the effective dose, expressed in millisievert (mSv). Lastly, we included the reported sensitivity, PPV, specificity, and other related data provided.

3. Results

3.1. Identification of Potential Studies. The searches from the MEDLINE database hit a total of 91 records that were screened after the removal of duplicates. All articles were available to us in full-text format. The full-text screening stage led to 91 potential articles relevant to our scoping review. Additional articles were excluded after full-text assessment for the reasons mentioned in "Materials and Methods". A flow chart is provided in Figure 1.

A total of 51 articles were included, as the authors of these had defined the number of phases and at least some of the parameters of the scanning protocol. These articles are listed chronologically in order of most recently published in Table 1. In the case of six studies, the authors defined two different protocols, thus amounting to 56 scanning protocols. These alternative protocols were added in Table 1 as secondary rows in relation to the first protocol.

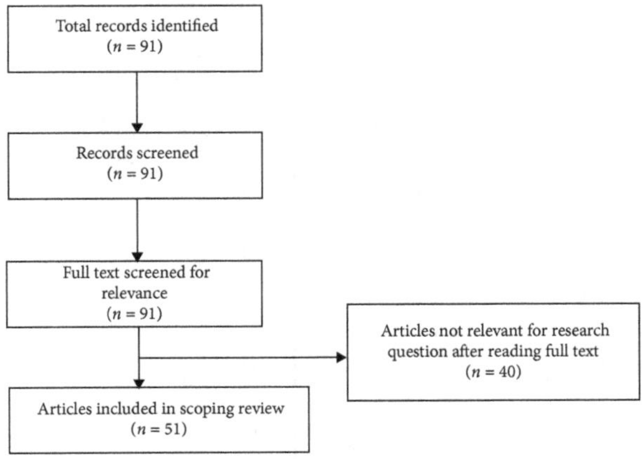

Figure 1: Flow chart of the studies' selection process.

3.2. Characteristics of the Included Studies. The peer-reviewed literature on the subject of 4DCT for the detection of parathyroid adenomas is recent: the concept of 4DCT for the detection of parathyroid adenomas was coined in 2006 by Rodgers et al. Among the included studies, 45% were published in the last five years. Most studies (76.5%) are retrospective studies.

3.3. Number of Phases. Most authors use a triphasic approach: 25 study protocols were described in this manner. A four-phasic approach is almost as prevalent; 23 study protocols were described in this manner. Far less common are biphasic studies: only 7 of these protocols could be identified. One study was unique since the authors made use of a five-phasic approach.

3.4. Use of a Noncontrast Enhanced Phase. Fifty-two out of 56 study protocols include a noncontrast enhanced phase (NECT), before administration of contrast medium. Only 4 protocols were identified in which the authors did not acquire a NECT; these protocols were all two-phasic in nature.

3.5. Contrast Phase Timing and Bolus Tracking. Only three authors use bolus tracking. All other authors opt for a fixed time interval after the start of contrast bolus administration before obtaining the first contrast phase, almost always an arterial phase.

Many authors do not provide definitions for the later phases in absolute terms (relation to the start of contrast bolus administration) and refer to relative intervals between the different phases. Since many authors do not describe pitch and rotation speed or refer to an exact scan length, the scan time of the different phases themselves is often unclear. This further complicates the definition of an exact time-frame. We expressed (where possible) all times in absolute relation to the onset of contrast administration; some error can be expected on a conversion. A graphic overview of the timing of the different phases of the selected studies is presented in Figure 2; this is in relation to the number of protocols citing these relevant time points.

3.6. Use of an Arterial Phase. Except for four studies, all cited studies choose to obtain an arterial phase. In the case of 25 different studies, the arterial images were obtained 25 s after contrast administration; in 13 studies, the authors proposed scanning after 30 s. Five other authors stated that the arterial images were obtained by scanning after 25–30 s. Forty-two protocols then perform arterial scanning after 25 to 30 s.

3.7. Use of Other Phases. The venous phase is obtained most often and can be acquired as early as 45 seconds up to 70 seconds after administration of contrast. The delayed venous phase is less popular and is usually acquired between 70 seconds and as late as 90 seconds after administration of contrast. Rarely, authors also acquire an even more delayed phase: later than 100 seconds after bolus administration and even up to 130 seconds.

3.8. Contrast Administration. Most studies define the used contrast medium, bolus volume, and injection speed. A mean volume of 100 mL contrast is administered, most commonly at 3 or 4 mL/s. Two authors define the contrast volume in function of the patient's weight.

3.9. Effective Dose. Only 24 authors present data concerning the effective dose. The described doses are wide-ranging, with the lowest dose reported at 5.5 mSv and an upper limit of 28 mSv. The mean effective dose for all relevant studies combined is calculated at 15.96 mSv. 27 authors do not discuss dose limits.

The mean effective dose for the three biphasic studies with available data is calculated at 8.1 mSv. For the three- and four-phasic studies, the mean effective dose is higher, 18.1 mSv and 15.4 mSv, respectively. The authors of the only five-phasic study report an effective dose range of 5.6–10.4 mSv.

3.10. Appraisal of Sensitivity/Specificity. All included studies were assessed for the quality of the reported findings. 74.5% of the included studies report on sensitivity and specificity.

TABLE 1: Overview of the different protocols in the literature: number and timing of different phases, tube current/voltage, contrast volume and injection speed, effective dose, and sensitivity/specificity/PPV/NPV/accuracy.

Reference	Authors	Year published	Study design	NECT	Tracking	Contrast phase timing	Number of phases	Arterial phase	Venous phase	Delayed phase	Very delayed phase	Tube current (mA)	Tube voltage (kV)	Contrast volume	Injection speed	Effective dose (mSv)	Sensitivity/specificity/PPV/NPV/accuracy
[15]	Vijayasarathi et al.	2020	Case series	Yes	Yes	Relative	3	25–30 s	60–80 s	—	—	?	?	?	?	?	
[16]	Wojtczak et al.	2020	Review	Yes	No	Relative	4	25–30 s	25–30 s	85–90 s	—	?	?	?	?	?	
[17]	Acar et al.	2020	Retrospective study	Yes	No	Absolute	4	25 s	40 s	80 s	—	?	?	0.1 mL/kg	?	?	Sensitivity 50% Specificity 100% PPV 100% NPV 85% Accuracy 86.9%
[18]	Zafereo et al.	2019	Review	Yes Yes	No No	Relative Relative	3 3	25–30 s 25–30 s	55–60 s —	— 70 s	— —	? ?	? ?	? ?	? ?	27–28 27–28	
[19]	Kedarisetty et al.	2019	Retrospective study	Yes	No	Absolute	3	25 s	—	85 s	—	?	?	75 mL	?	?	Sensitivity 80% Specificity 75% PPV 92% NPV 50% Accuracy 79%
[20]	Yeh et al.	2019	Retrospective study	Yes	No	Relative	3	30 s	60 s	—	—	?	?	75 mL	4 mL/s	22	Sensitivity 79% Specificity 96% PPV 90% NPV 90%
[21]	Amadou et al.	2019	Retrospective study	Yes	No	Absolute	3	—	45 s	70 s	—	50–100	120	120 mL	?	10–27	Sensitivity 75% Specificity 40% PPV 80% NPV 33%
[22]	Vu et al.	2019	Retrospective study	Yes	No	Absolute	4	25 s	55 s	85 s	—	220	130	120 mL	4 mL/s	17.9	
[23]	Binks et al.	2019	Retrospective study	Yes	No	Absolute	3	25–30 s	45–50 s	—	—	?	?	?	?	7.99–28	Sensitivity 85.7% PPV 94.7%
[24]	Cunha-Bezerra et al.	2018	Retrospective study	Yes	Yes	Relative	4	18–25 s	48–55 s	?	—	120–200	120	2 mL/kg max 120 mL	4-5 L/s	?	
[25]	Tian et al.	2018	Retrospective cohort study	Yes	Yes	Relative	3	Aorta: 150HU	30 s later	—	—	?	?	100 mL	4 mL/s	9.3	Sensitivity 72.9% Sensitivity 60% (persistent/recument disease) Sensitivity 67.4% (multigland disease)
[26]	Christakis et al.	2017	Retrospective study	Yes	No	Absolute	4	25 s	?	?	—	?	?	120 mL	3 mL/s	?	Sensitivity 79% Specificity 100% PPV 100% NPV 44% Accuracy 82%
[27]	Morón et al.	2017	Retrospective study	Yes	No	Absolute	2	25 s	—	—	—	150–600	120	100 mL	4 mL/s	?	Sensitivity 80% Specificity 97% PPV 89% Accuracy 92%
[28]	Goroshi et al.	2017	Retrospective study	Yes	No	Absolute	4	20 s	60 s	90 s	—	140–220	120	60 mL	4 mL/s	18.9	Left/right localization: Sensitivity 93% (hypercalcemic) Quadrant localization: Sensitivity 90% (hypercalcemic)

Table 1: Continued.

Reference	Authors	Year published	Study design	NECT	Tracking	Contrast phase timing	Number of phases	Arterial phase	Venous phase	Delayed phase	Very delayed phase	Tube current (mA)	Tube voltage (kV)	Contrast volume	Injection speed	Effective dose (mSv)	Sensitivity/specificity/ PPV/NPV/accuracy
[29]	Taywade et al.	2017	Prospective study	Yes	No	Absolute	3	25 s	—	80 s	—	?	?	75 mL	4 mL/s	11–13	
[30]	Zeina et al.	2017	Prospective study	Yes	No	Absolute	4	25 s	60 s	90 s	—	400	120	120 mL	4 mL/s	?	Accuracy 96%
[31]	Sho et al.	2016	Prospective study	Yes	No	Relative	3	25 s	55 s	—	—	230	120	100–120 mL	3-4 mL/s	?	Sensitivity: 79% (multigland disease) Specificity: 63%(multigland disease) PPV:58% (multigland disease)
[32]	Fitzgerald et al.	2017	Retrospective study	Yes	No	Absolute	3	30 s	—	90 s	—	180–600	120	75 mL	3 mL/s	10.4–28	
[33]	Rameau et al.	2017	Case series	Yes	No	Relative	3	25 s	55 s	—	—	150–300	120	100–120 mL	4 mL/s	?	Sensitivity 84.6% PPV 91.7%
[34]	Ramirez et al.	2016	Retrospective study	Yes	No	Absolute	4	25 s	55 s	85 s	-	?	?	120 mL	4 mL/s	14	Sensitivity 93% PPV:96%
				Yes	No	Absolute	2	25 s	—	—	—	?	?	120 mL	4 mL/s	6.8	Sensitivity 97% PPV:94%
[35]	Forghani et al.	2016	Retrospective study	Yes	No	Absolute	4	25 s	55 s	85 s	—	?	?	100 mL	3.5 mL/s	2.4–4.1	
[36]	Lee et al.	2016	Retrospective study	Yes	No	Absolute	4	30 s	60 s	90 s	—	140–240	120	90 mL	5 mL/s	10.9	
[37]	Hinsin et al.	2015	Case series	Yes	No	Absolute	4	30 s	—	80 s	—	?	?	75 mL	3 mL/s	13.8	Left/right localization: Sensitivity 84.2% (hypercalcemic) Left/right localization: Specificity 81.8% (hypercalcemic) Quadrant localization: Sensitivity 76.5% (hypercalcemic) Quadrant localization: Specificity 91.59% (hypercalcemic)
[38]	Bahl et al.	2015	Retrospective study	Yes	No	Absolute	3	25 s	45 s	70 s	—	100–700	120	75 mL	4 mL/s	28	Sensitivity 85% Sensitivity: 94% (single gland disease) Sensitivity: 59% (multigland disease)
[39]	Boury	2015	Review	Yes	No	Absolute	3	—	45 s	70 s	—	?	?	?	3 mL/s	?	
[40]	Hoang et al.	2015	Phantom study	Yes	No	Absolute	3	25 s	—	80 s	—	100–500	120	75 mL	4 mL/s	28	

Table 1: Continued.

Reference	Authors	Year published	Study design	NECT	Tracking	Contrast phase timing	Number of phases	Arterial phase	Venous phase	Delayed phase	Very delayed phase	Tube current (mA)	Tube voltage (kV)	Contrast volume	Injection speed	Effective dose (mSv)	Sensitivity/specificity/ PPV/NPV/accuracy
[41]	Lundstroem et al.	2016	Retrospective study	Yes	No	Absolute	5	22 s	52 s	82 s	122 s	200	120	100 mL	3.5 mL/s	5.56–10.4	Left/right localization: Sensitivity 84% (hypercalcemic) Left/right localization: Specificity 76% (hypercalcemic) Quadrant localization: Sensitivity 55% (hypercalcemic) Quadrant localization: Specificity 50% (hypercalcemic)
[42]	Seeliger et al.	2015	Prospective study	Yes	No	Absolute	4	25 s	50 s	80 s	—	250	120	120 mL	2 mL/s	?	PPV 93%
[43]	Cham et al.	2015	Retrospective study	Yes	No	Relative	3	25–34 s	55–64 s	—	—	230	120	100–120 mL	?	?	
[44]	Day et al.	2015	Retrospective study	Yes	No	Absolute	4	30 s	60 s	90 s	—	100–750	120	100,L	3 mL/s	?	Sensitivity 93% PPV 80%
[45]	Campbell et al.	2015	Retrospective study	Yes	No	Absolute	2	—	50 s	—	—	100–440	120	75–100 mL	?	5.2	Left/right localization: Sensitivity 77% (hypercalcemic) Left/right localization: Specificity 87% (hypercalcemic) Quadrant localization: Sensitivity 58% (hypercalcemic) Quadrant localization: Specificity 91% (hypercalcemic)
[46]	Sepahdari et al.	2015	Retrospective study	Yes	No	Absolute	3	25 s	55 s	—	—	230	120	100–120 mL	3–4 mL/s	?	Sensitivity 77%
				Yes	No	Absolute	3	25 s	—	80 s	—	230	120	100–120 mL	3–4 mL/s	?	Sensitivity: 95% (single gland disease) Sensitivity: 55% (multigland disease)
[47]	Suh et al.	2015	Case series	Yes	No	Absolute	4	30 s	60 s	90 s	—	140–240	120	90 mL	?	?	Sensitivity 92.1% Specificity 95.6% PPV 87.5% NPV 97.3% Accuracy 94.7%
[48]	Ginsburg et al.	2015	Retrospective study	Yes	No	Absolute	4	25 s	55 s	85 s	—	200	120	120 m	4 mL/s	?	Sensitivity 50% PPV 100% Accuracy 54.5%
[49]	Raghavan et al.	2014	Retrospective study	Yes	No	Absolute	4	25 s	50 s	80 s	—	50–400	120	120 mL	4 mL/s	?	*Accuracy, sensitivity, and specificity for localization and lateralization of the arterial phase alone were comparable with the full complement of 4 phases*

Table 1: Continued.

Reference	Authors	Year published	Study design	NECT	Tracking	Contrast phase timing	Number of phases	Arterial phase	Venous phase	Delayed phase	Very delayed phase	Tube current (mA)	Tube voltage (kV)	Contrast volume	Injection speed	Effective dose (mSv)	Sensitivity/specificity/ PPV/NPV/accuracy
[50]	Brown et al.	2015	Retrospective cohort study	Yes	No	Absolute	3	34 s	68 s	—	—	?	?	70 mL	3 mL/s	7.99 mSv (3 phases) 10.88,Sv (4 phases)	Sensitivity 92% PPV 89%
[14]	Hoang et al.	2014	Case series	Yes	No	Absolute	3	25 s	—	80 s	—	100–400	120	75 mL	4 mL/s	?	
[51]	Hunter et al.	2014	Retrospective study	Yes	No	Relative	3	30 s	60 s	—	—	180–300	140	100 mL	4 mL/s	?	Sensitivity 94% Specificity 98.3% PPV 96.7% NPV 97.1%
[52]	Bahl et al.	2014	Retrospective study	No	No	Absolute	2	20 s	70 s	—	—	100–400	120	100 mL	4 mL/s	?	
				Yes	No	Absolute	3	25 s	—	80 s	—	100–700	120	75 mL	4 mL/s	?	
[53]	Kely et al.	2014	Retrospective study	Yes	No	Relative	4	30 s	45 s	90 s	—	180–300	140	100 mL	4 mL/s	28	PPV 85.8% Accuracy 77.9%
				Yes	No	Relative	3	30 s	45 s	—	—	180–300	140	100 mL	4 mL/s	21	PPV 89% Accuracy 87.1%
[54]	Sepahdari et al.	2013	Retrospective study	Yes	No	Relative	3	25–34 s	55–84 s	—	—	230	120	100–120 mL	3–4 mL/s	2.2 mSv/ phases	*Interobserver comparison* Sensitivity 73% vs 55% Specificity 88% vs 100% PPV 91% vs 100% NPV 64% vs 52% Accuracy 78% vs 70%
[55]	Hunter et al.	2012	Retrospective study	Yes	No	Relative	4	25 s	70–73 s	—	130–133 s	240	140	120 mL	4 mL/s	21 mSv (3 phases) 27 mSv (4 phases)	Left/right localization: Accuracy 93.7% Quadrant localization: Accuracy 86.6%
[56]	Mahajan et al.	2012	?	Yes	No	Absolute	4	30 s	60 s	90 s	—	?	?	80 mL	?	10.4	
[57]	Gafton et al.	2012	Case series	No	No	Absolute	2	25 s	—	80 s	—	?	120	120 mL	3 mL/s	?	
[58]	Kutler et al.	2011	Retrospective study	Yes	No	Absolute	2	—	50 s	—	—	220–320	120	125 mL	3 mL/s	12.2	
[59]	Eichhom-Wharry et al.	2011	Retrospective study	No	No	?	2	18 s	Immediately	—	—	?	?	100 mL	?	?	Accuracy 73%
				No	No	?	2	22 s (>55y)	Immediately	—	—	?	?	100 mL	?	?	
[13]	Starker et al.	2011	Retrospective study	Yes	No	Absolute	4	30 s	60 s	—	120 s	100–750	120	100 mL	3 mL/s	?	Left/right localization: Sensitivity 93.9% Left/right localization: PPV 93.5% Quadrant localization: Sensitivity 85.7% Quadrant localization: PPV 84.9%
[60]	Beland et al.	2011	Retrospective study	Yes	No	Absolute	4	30 s	60 s	90 s	—	100–750	120	?	?	?	Sensitivity 82% Specificity 92%
[61]	Lubitz et al.	2010	Retrospective study	Yes	No	Relative	4	30 s	60 s	—	105 s	180–300	140	100 mL	?	10	Left/right localization: Sensitivity 73% Quadrant localization: Sensitivity 60%
[62]	Mortenson et al.	2008	Retrospective study	Yes	No	Relative	4	25 s	55 s	85 s	—	?	?	120 mL	4 mL/s	?	Sensitivity 88%
[63]	Rodgers et al.	2006	Mixed prospective and retrospective study	Yes	No	?	3	25 s	?	—	—	220	140	120 mL	3 mL/s	?	Sensitivity 88% Quadrant localization: Sensitivity 70%

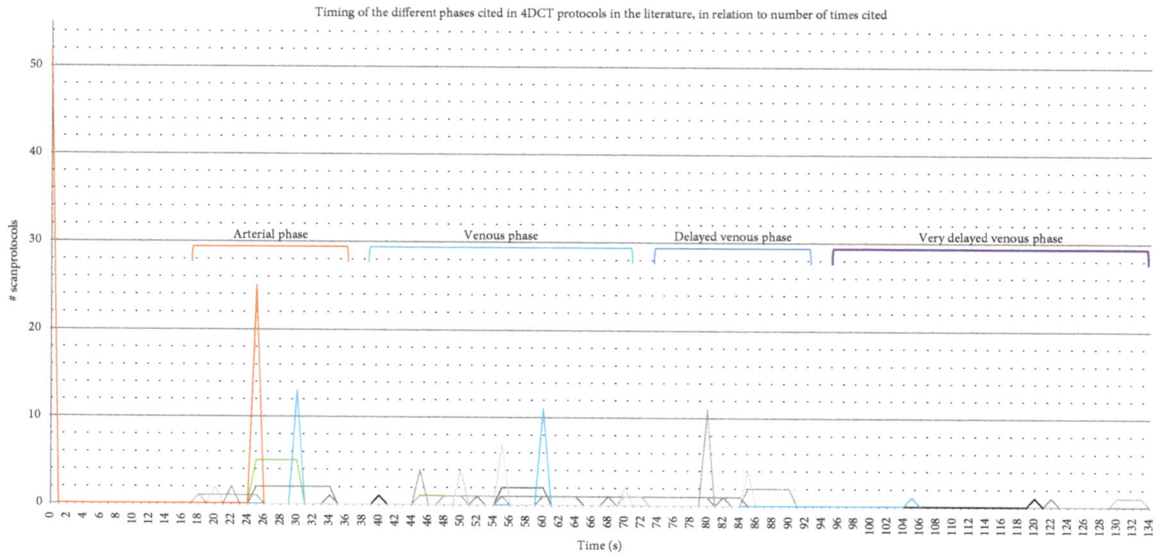

FIGURE 2: Timing of the different phases of 4DCT protocols in the literature, in relation to the number of citations for each of these relevant time points.

Some studies (14%) do not refer to general sensitivity but report on the sensitivity of lateralization or correct selection of the diseased quadrant.

We find a mean sensitivity ($n = 23$) of 81.5% for the detection of parathyroid adenomas using 4DCT. Only two studies report a lower sensitivity of 50%; both studies are four-phasic studies. We find a mean PPV ($n = 17$) of 90%. Less data is available on specificity ($n = 11$), and the mean specificity is calculated at 86%.

4. Discussion

Typical parathyroid adenomas are hypoattenuating to thyroid tissue on NECT and demonstrate avid arterial enhancement during the arterial phase as well as rapid washout on the venous phase. The arterial phase is the most important, as adenomas can be visualized as hyper-enhancing nodules in characteristic locations. In Figure 3, we provide an example of a parathyroid adenoma behaving accordingly during all three phases. Unfortunately, for approximately one-third of adenomas, the lesion will prove to be isoattenuating to the thyroid on arterial and venous phases [15].

Most authors agree to include a noncontrast enhanced phase. This phase does seem to be important in the diagnosis of parathyroid adenomas, as the study by Bahl et al. [38] identifies a type C pattern of enhancement. These lesions mimic thyroid tissue and can only be discerned by the use of noncontrast-enhanced imaging since these lesions should be lower in density compared to the thyroid on the noncontrast enhanced series. Almost all authors choose to include an arterial phase. According to Bahl et al., this is necessary to diagnose type A lesions, which demonstrate a higher peak enhancement compared to the thyroid in the arterial phase. A venous or delayed venous phase is commonly used. According to Bahl et al., this is necessary to diagnose type B lesions, which demonstrate a lower enhancement compared to the thyroid in the venous phase.

Most authors opt for a delay of 25 up to 30 seconds for the arterial phase after contrast administration. There is more variance concerning the timing of the venous phases, with some authors scanning as early as 40 seconds after administration of contrast and others no less than 50 seconds later. Other authors even prefer very delayed venous phases. We find no difference regarding the sensitivity or specificity of 4DCT in comparison to the number of phases or their timing. The two studies with the lowest sensitivity are both four-phasic studies, with numerous three-phasic studies reporting higher sensitivity.

Only three authors use bolus tracking to optimize the scanning delay, although this could easily be implemented. If the arterial peak enhancement of the adenoma should prove to be a short-lived effect, scanning at a fixed interval of time might risk missing the diagnosis. This would prove especially true in older patients with suboptimal cardiac output, as the arterial phase could be performed too early in these cases. Bolus tracking at the level of the aortic arch would allow for the arterial and later phases to be obtained at a variable time interval, with reduced variability of arterial enhancement and less risk of scanning prematurely. Bolus tracking is commonly used in clinical practice, without significant dose effect [64].

Regarding contrast administration, the variance between the reviewed studies is limited. Administered bolus volumes are situated between 75 mL and 120 mL with a mean volume of 100 mL. Injection speed varies mostly between 3 and 4 mL/s. A contrast bolus with a lower volume or at a lower injection speed may affect lesion enhancement and the timing of said enhancement. No difference regarding sensitivity or specificity of 4DCT is found, however, for different volumes or injection speeds.

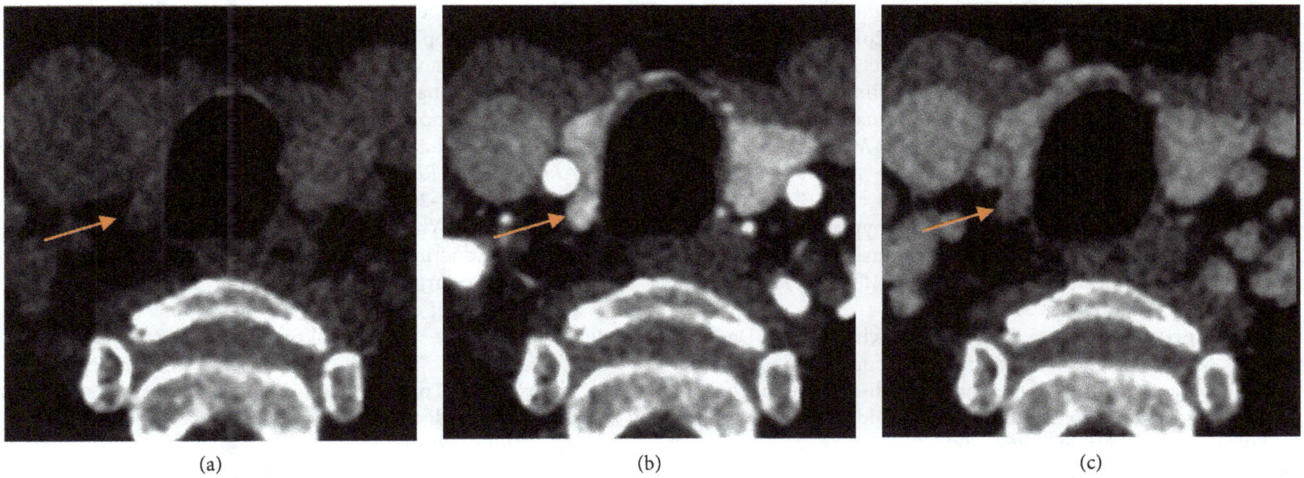

FIGURE 3: 4DCT of a small right upper parathyroid adenoma. (a) NECT with lower attenuation (b) Arterial phase with higher enhancement. (c) Venous phase with lower enhancement.

What proves striking is that 27 out of 51 authors do not mention effective dose when discussing a multiphasic CT scan of the neck. The mean effective dose for the 24 studies that do comment on patient dose is calculated at 15.96 mSv. The described dose limits are wide-ranging, with an upper limit of 28 mSv. These upper values should be considered as very high and place direct limits on the number of phases. As a limitation, it should be noted that it is difficult to calculate a correct effective organ dose. The presence of an iodinated contrast medium is a known factor that increases organ dose, yet this has not been factored into any known conversion method [65].

The mean effective dose is the lowest for biphasic studies, as could be expected. The mean effective dose for the three studies with available effective dose data is calculated at 8.1 mSv. For the more popular three- and four-phasic studies, the mean effective dose is higher, but the mean effective dose for the four-phasic studies appears lower in comparison to the three-phasic studies (15.4 mSv versus 18.1 mSv). This is probably because of lower tube current settings, an effect that can also be observed in the only five-phasic study. Here, a low mean effective dose range of 5.6–10.4 mSv is reported, probably because the authors do not use automatic tube current modulation but instead opt for a fixed tube current of 200 mA.

Changes in tube current will affect image noise: higher mA settings will result in lower noise. Changes in tube voltage will affect the amount of contrast in the resultant image: higher kV settings will result in an increase in contrast. Since increasing the tube current improves image quality by reducing noise without affecting image contrast, it can be argued that to keep the effective dose for classic 4DCT within acceptable levels, a lower fixed tube current should be preferred. Most protocols utilize a 120 kV tube voltage. Since diagnosis relies primarily on enhancement after contrast, it can be suggested that scanning at 100 kV tube voltage would yield similar image contrast, but at a lower effective dose [65]. Again, regarding tube parameters, no difference in sensitivity or specificity is found for different values.

5. Conclusion

Many different 4DCT scanning protocols for the detection of parathyroid adenomas exist in the literature. We find a mean sensitivity of 81.5% and a mean specificity of 86%. The number of phases does not appear to affect sensitivity or specificity. A triphasic approach, however, seems preferable, as three patterns of enhancement of parathyroid adenomas are described and require nonenhanced imaging as well as an arterial and a venous series. Arterial images are usually obtained 25–30 s after administration of contrast, and less agreement exists concerning the timing of the venous phase(s). A mean contrast bolus of 100 mL is administered at 3–4 mL/s. Bolus tracking is not often used but could help to reduce the variability of enhancement. Sensitivity and specificity do not appear to be affected by other scan parameters like tube voltage or tube current. To keep the effective dose within limits, scanning at a lower fixed tube current seems preferable. Lowering tube voltage from 120 kV to 100 kV may yield similar image contrast but would also help lower the dose.

Authors' Contributions

SR reviewed the literature and wrote the text. MT revised the final manuscript.

References

[1] J. P. Bilezikian, M. L. Brandi, R. Eastell et al., "Guidelines for the management of asymptomatic primary hyperparathyroidism: summary statement from the Fourth International

Workshop," *The Journal of Clinical Endocrinology & Metabolism*, vol. 99, no. 10, pp. 3561–3569, 2014.

[2] S. J. Silverberg, B. L. Clarke, M. Peacock et al., "Current issues in the presentation of asymptomatic primary hyperparathyroidism: proceedings of the Fourth International Workshop," *The Journal of Clinical Endocrinology & Metabolism*, vol. 99, no. 10, pp. 3580–3594, 2014.

[3] R. Udelsman, G. Åkerström, C. Biagini et al., "The surgical management of asymptomatic primary hyperparathyroidism: proceedings of the Fourth International Workshop," *The Journal of Clinical Endocrinology & Metabolism*, vol. 99, no. 10, pp. 3595–3606, 2014.

[4] S. Y. Morita, H. Somervell, C. B. Umbricht, A. P. B. Dackiw, and M. A. Zeiger, "Evaluation for concomitant thyroid nodules and primary hyperparathyroidism in patients undergoing parathyroidectomy or thyroidectomy," *Surgery*, vol. 144, no. 6, pp. 862–867, 2008.

[5] G. M. Vitetta, P. Neri, A. Chiecchio et al., "Role of ultrasonography in the management of patients with primary hyperparathyroidism: retrospective comparison with technetium-99m sestamibi scintigraphy," *Journal of Ultrasound*, vol. 17, no. 1, pp. 1–12, 2014.

[6] Z. Devcic, R. B. Jeffrey, A. Kamaya, and T. S. Desser, "The elusive parathyroid adenoma," *Ultrasound Quarterly*, vol. 29, no. 3, pp. 179–187, 2013.

[7] E. Berber, R. T. Parikh, N. Ballem, C. N. Garner, M. Milas, and A. E. Siperstein, "Factors contributing to negative parathyroid localization: an analysis of 1000 patients," *Surgery*, vol. 144, no. 1, pp. 74–79, 2008.

[8] C. Guerin, A. Lowery, S. Gabriel et al., "Preoperative imaging for focused parathyroidectomy: making a good strategy even better," *European Journal of Endocrinology*, vol. 172, no. 5, pp. 519–526, 2015.

[9] E. Hindié, P. Zanotti-Fregonara, A. Tabarin et al., "The role of radionuclide imaging in the surgical management of primary hyperparathyroidism," *Journal of Nuclear Medicine*, vol. 56, no. 5, pp. 737–744, 2015.

[10] E. L. Hänninen, T. J. Vogl, T. Steinmüller, J. Ricke, P. Neuhaus, and R. Felix, "Preoperative contrast-enhanced MRI of the parathyroid glands in hyperparathyroidism," *Investigative Radiology*, vol. 35, no. 7, pp. 426–430, 2000.

[11] A. M. Grayev, L. R. Gentry, M. J. Hartman, H. Chen, S. B. Perlman, and S. B. Reeder, "Presurgical localization of parathyroid adenomas with magnetic resonance imaging at 3.0 T: an adjunct method to supplement traditional imaging," *Annals of Surgical Oncology*, vol. 19, no. 3, pp. 981–989, 2012.

[12] B. Sacconi, R. Argirò, D. Diacinti et al., "MR appearance of parathyroid adenomas at 3 T in patients with primary hyperparathyroidism: what radiologists need to know for preoperative localization," *European Radiology*, vol. 26, no. 3, pp. 664–673, 2016.

[13] L. F. Starker, A. Mahajan, P. Björklund, G. Sze, R. Udelsman, and T. Carling, "4D parathyroid CT as the initial localization study for patients with de novo primary hyperparathyroidism," *Annals of Surgical Oncology*, vol. 18, no. 6, pp. 1723–1728, 2011.

[14] J. K. Hoang, W.-k. Sung, M. Bahl, and C. D. Phillips, "How to perform parathyroid 4D CT: tips and traps for technique and interpretation," *Radiology*, vol. 270, no. 1, pp. 15–24, 2014.

[15] A. Vijayasarathi, S. Karnezis, A. Azizyan, N. Salamon, and A. Sepahdari, "4D CT parathyroid for the general radiologist: a pictorial essay of illustrative cases," *Current Problems in Diagnostic Radiology*, vol. 20, pp. 30046–30053, 2020.

[16] B. Wojtczak, J. Syrycka, K. Kaliszewski, J. Rudnicki, M. Bolanowski, and M. Barczyński, "Surgical implications of recent modalities for parathyroid imaging," *Gland Surgery*, vol. 9, no. 2, pp. S86–S94, 2020.

[17] N. Acar, M. Haciyanli, M. Coskun et al., "Diagnostic value of four-dimensional computed tomography and four-dimensional magnetic resonance imaging in primary hyperparathyroidism when first-line imaging was inadequate," *The Annals of The Royal College of Surgeons of England*, vol. 102, no. 4, pp. 294–299, 2020.

[18] M. Zafereo, J. Yu, P. Angelos et al., "American head and neck society endocrine surgery section update on parathyroid imaging for surgical candidates with primary hyperparathyroidism," *Head & Neck*, vol. 41, no. 7, pp. 2398–2409, 2019.

[19] S. Kedarisetty, C. Fundakowski, K. Ramakrishnan, and S. Dadparvar, "Clinical value of Tc99m-MIBI SPECT/CT versus 4D-CT or US in management of patients with hyperparathyroidism," *Ear, Nose & Throat Journal*, vol. 98, no. 3, pp. 149–157, 2019.

[20] R. Yeh, Y.-K. D. Tay, G. Tabacco et al., "Diagnostic performance of 4D CT and sestamibi SPECT/CT in localizing parathyroid adenomas in primary hyperparathyroidism," *Radiology*, vol. 291, no. 2, pp. 469–476, 2019.

[21] C. Amadou, G. Bera, M. Ezziane et al., "18F-fluorocholine PET/CT and parathyroid 4D computed tomography for primary hyperparathyroidism: the challenge of reoperative patients," *World Journal of Surgery*, vol. 43, no. 5, pp. 1232–1242, 2019.

[22] T. H. Vu, D. Schellingerhout, N. Guha-Thakurta et al., "Solitary parathyroid adenoma localization in technetium Tc99m Sestamibi SPECT and multiphase multidetector 4D CT," *American Journal of Neuroradiology*, vol. 40, no. 1, pp. 142–149, 2019.

[23] M. Binks, D. Burrows, and D. Littlejohn, "A rural perspective on minimally invasive parathyroidectomy: optimal preoperative imaging and patient outcomes," *ANZ Journal of Surgery*, vol. 89, no. 1-2, pp. 43–47, 2019.

[24] P. Cunha-Bezerra, R. Vieira, F. Amaral, H. Cartaxo, T. Lima, and U. Montarroyos, "Better performance of four-dimension computed tomography as a localization procedure in normocalcemic primary hyperparathyroidism," *Journal of Medical Imaging and Radiation Oncology*, vol. 15, 2018.

[25] Y. Tian, S. T. Tanny, P. Einsiedel et al., "Four-dimensional computed tomography: clinical impact for patients with primary hyperparathyroidism," *Annals of Surgical Oncology*, vol. 25, no. 1, pp. 117–121, 2018.

[26] I. Christakis, T. Vu, H. H. Chuang et al., "The diagnostic accuracy of neck ultrasound, 4D-Computed tomographyand sestamibi imaging in parathyroid carcinoma," *European Journal of Radiology*, vol. 95, pp. 82–88, 2017.

[27] F. Morón, A. Delumpa, J. Chetta, D. Guffey, and D. Dunaway, "Single phase computed tomography is equivalent to dual phase method for localizing hyperfunctioning parathyroid glands in patients with primary hyperparathyroidism: a retrospective review," *PeerJ*, vol. 5, Article ID e3586, 2017.

[28] M. Goroshi, A. R. Lila, S. S. Jadhav et al., "Percentage arterial enhancement: an objective index for accurate identification of parathyroid adenoma/hyperplasia in primary hyperparathyroidism," *Clinical Endocrinology*, vol. 87, no. 6, pp. 791–798, 2017.

[29] S. K. Taywade, N. A. Damle, A Behera et al., "Comparison of 18F-fluorocholine positron emission tomography/computed tomography and four-dimensional computed tomography in the preoperative localization of parathyroid adenomas-initial results," *Indian Journal of Endocrinology and Metabolism*, vol. 21, no. 3, pp. 399–403, 2017.

[30] A. R. Zeina, H. Nakar, N Reindorp D et al., "Four-dimensional computed tomography (4DCT) for preoperative localization of parathyroid adenomas," *The Israel Medical Association Journal: IMAJ*, vol. 19, no. 4, pp. 216–220, 2017.

[31] S. Sho, M. Yilma, M. W. Yeh et al., "Prospective validation of two 4D-CT-based scoring systems for prediction of multigland disease in primary hyperparathyroidism," *American Journal of Neuroradiology*, vol. 37, no. 12, pp. 2323–2327, 2016.

[32] R. T. Fitzgerald, M. Kuruva, R. David et al., "Characterization of thyroid nodules by 4-dimensional computed tomography," *Journal of Computer Assisted Tomography*, vol. 41, no. 2, pp. 195–198, 2017.

[33] A. Rameau, S. Eng, T. Vu, R. Saket, P. Jun, and M. Friduss, "Four-dimensional computed tomography scan utility in parathyroidectomy for primary hyperparathyroidism with low baseline intact parathyroid hormone," *The Laryngoscope*, vol. 127, no. 6, pp. 1476–1482, 2017.

[34] A. G. Ramirez, A. L. Shada, A. N. Martin et al., "Clinical efficacy of 2-phase versus 4-phase computed tomography for localization in primary hyperparathyroidism," *Surgery*, vol. 160, no. 3, pp. 731–737, 2016.

[35] R. Forghani, M. Roskies, X. Liu et al., "Dual-energy CT characteristics of parathyroid adenomas on 25-and 55-second 4D-CT acquisitions," *Journal of Computer Assisted Tomography*, vol. 40, no. 5, pp. 806–814, 2016.

[36] E. K. Lee, T. J. Yun, J.-h. Kim et al., "Effect of tumor volume on the enhancement pattern of parathyroid adenoma on parathyroid four-dimensional CT," *Neuroradiology*, vol. 58, no. 5, pp. 495–501, 2016.

[37] A. M. Hinson, D. R. Lee, B. A. Hobbs, R. T. Fitzgerald, D. L. Bodenner, and B. C. Stack, "Preoperative 4D CT localization of nonlocalizing parathyroid adenomas by ultrasound and SPECT-CT," *Otolaryngology-Head and Neck Surgery*, vol. 153, no. 5, pp. 775–778, 2015.

[38] M. Bahl, A. R. Sepahdari, J. A. Sosa, and J. K. Hoang, "Parathyroid adenomas and hyperplasia on four-dimensional CT scans: three patterns of enhancement relative to the thyroid gland justify a three-phase protocol," *Radiology*, vol. 277, no. 2, pp. 454–462, 2015.

[39] S. Boury, "New methods for parathyroid imaging: sonography, 4D CT, MRI," *Annales d'Endocrinologie*, vol. 76, no. 2, pp. 148–152, 2015.

[40] J. K. Hoang, R. E. Reiman, G. B. Nguyen et al., "Lifetime attributable risk of cancer from radiation exposure during parathyroid imaging: comparison of 4D CT and parathyroid scintigraphy," *American Journal of Roentgenology*, vol. 204, no. 5, pp. W579–W585, 2015.

[41] A. K. Lundstroem, W. Trolle, C. H. Soerensen, and P. S. Myschetzky, "Preoperative localization of hyperfunctioning parathyroid glands with 4D-CT," *European Archives of Oto-Rhino-Laryngology*, vol. 273, no. 5, pp. 1253–1259, 2016.

[42] B. Seeliger, P. F. Alesina, J.-A. Koch, J. Hinrichs, B. Meier, and M. K. Walz, "Diagnostic value and clinical impact of complementary CT scan prior to surgery for non-localized primary hyperparathyroidism," *Langenbeck's Archives of Surgery*, vol. 400, no. 3, pp. 307–312, 2015.

[43] S. Cham, A. R. Sepahdari, K. E. Hall, M. W. Yeh, and A. Harari, "Dynamic parathyroid computed tomography (4DCT) facilitates reoperative parathyroidectomy and enables cure of missed hyperplasia," *Annals of Surgical Oncology*, vol. 22, no. 11, pp. 3537–3542, 2015.

[44] K. M. Day, M. Elsayed, M. D. Beland, and J. M. Monchik, "The utility of 4-dimensional computed tomography for preoperative localization of primary hyperparathyroidism in patients not localized by sestamibi or ultrasonography," *Surgery*, vol. 157, no. 3, pp. 534–539, 2015.

[45] M. J. Campbell, P. Sicuro, A. Alseidi, C. C. Blackmore, and J. A. Ryan, "Two-phase (low-dose) computed tomography is as effective as 4D-CT for identifying enlarged parathyroid glands," *International Journal of Surgery*, vol. 14, pp. 80–84, 2015.

[46] A. R. Sepahdari, M. Bahl, A. Harari, H. J. Kim, M. W. Yeh, and J. K. Hoang, "Predictors of multigland disease in primary hyperparathyroidism: a scoring system with 4D-CT imaging and biochemical markers," *American Journal of Neuroradiology*, vol. 36, no. 5, pp. 987–992, 2015.

[47] Y. J. Suh, J. Y. Choi, S.-j. Kim et al., "Comparison of 4D CT, ultrasonography, and 99mTc sestamibi SPECT/CT in localizing single-gland primary hyperparathyroidism," *Otolaryngology-Head and Neck Surgery*, vol. 152, no. 3, pp. 438–443, 2015.

[48] M. Ginsburg, G. A. Christoforidis, S. P. Zivin et al., "Adenoma localization for recurrent or persistent primary hyperparathyroidism using dynamic four-dimensional CT and venous sampling," *Journal of Vascular and Interventional Radiology*, vol. 26, no. 1, pp. 79–86, 2015.

[49] P. Raghavan, C. R. Durst, D. A. Ornan et al., "Dynamic CT for parathyroid disease: are multiple phases necessary?" *American Journal of Neuroradiology*, vol. 35, no. 10, pp. 1959–1964, 2014.

[50] S. J. Brown, J. C. Lee, J. Christie et al., "Four-dimensional computed tomography for parathyroid localization: a new imaging modality," *ANZ Journal of Surgery*, vol. 85, no. 6, pp. 483–487, 2015.

[51] G. J. Hunter, D. T. Ginat, H. R. Kelly, E. F. Halpern, and L. M. Hamberg, "Discriminating parathyroid adenoma from local mimics by using inherent tissue attenuation and vascular information obtained with four-dimensional CT: formulation of a multinomial logistic regression model," *Radiology*, vol. 270, no. 1, pp. 168–175, 2014.

[52] M. Bahl, M. Muzaffar, G. Vij, J. A. Sosa, K. R. Choudhury, and J. K. Hoang, "Prevalence of the polar vessel sign in parathyroid adenomas on the arterial phase of 4D CT," *American Journal of Neuroradiology*, vol. 35, no. 3, pp. 578–581, 2014.

[53] H. R. Kelly, L. M. Hamberg, and G. J. Hunter, "4D-CT for preoperative localization of abnormal parathyroid glands in patients with hyperparathyroidism: accuracy and ability to stratify patients by unilateral versus bilateral disease in surgery-naïve and re-exploration patients," *American Journal of Neuroradiology*, vol. 35, no. 1, pp. 176–181, 2014.

[54] A. R. Sepahdari, M. W. Yeh, D. Rodrigues, S. N. Khan, and A. Harari, "Three-phase parathyroid 4-dimensional computed tomography initial experience," *Journal of Computer Assisted Tomography*, vol. 37, no. 4, pp. 511–517, 2013.

[55] G. J. Hunter, D. Schellingerhout, T. H. Vu, N. D. Perrier, and L. M. Hamberg, "Accuracy of four-dimensional CT for the localization of abnormal parathyroid glands in patients with primary hyperparathyroidism," *Radiology*, vol. 264, no. 3, pp. 789–795, 2012.

[56] A. Mahajan, L. F. Starker, M. Ghita, R. Udelsman, J. A. Brink, and T. Carling, "Parathyroid four-dimensional computed tomography: evaluation of radiation dose exposure during preoperative localization of parathyroid tumors in primary hyperparathyroidism," *World Journal of Surgery*, vol. 36, no. 6, pp. 1335–1339, 2012.

[57] A. R. Gafton, C. M. Glastonbury, J. D. Eastwood, and J. K. Hoang, "Parathyroid lesions: characterization with dual-phase arterial and venous enhanced CT of the neck," *American Journal of Neuroradiology*, vol. 33, no. 5, pp. 949–952, 2012.

[58] D. I. Kutler, R. Moquete, E. Kazam, and W. I. Kuhel, "Parathyroid localization with modified 4D-computed tomography and ultrasonography for patients with primary hyperparathyroidism," *The Laryngoscope*, vol. 121, no. 6, pp. 1219–1224, 2011.

[59] L. I. Eichhorn-Wharry, A. M. Carlin, and G. B. Talpos, "Mild hypercalcemia: an indication to select 4-dimensional computed tomography scan for preoperative localization of parathyroid adenomas," *The American Journal of Surgery*, vol. 201, no. 3, pp. 334–338, 2011.

[60] M. D. Beland, W. W. Mayo-Smith, D. J. Grand, J. T. Machan, and J. M. Monchik, "Dynamic MDCT for localization of occult parathyroid adenomas in 26 patients with primary hyperparathyroidism," *American Journal of Roentgenology*, vol. 196, no. 1, pp. 61–65, 2011.

[61] C. C. Lubitz, G. J. Hunter, L. M. Hamberg et al., "Accuracy of 4-dimensional computed tomography in poorly localized patients with primary hyperparathyroidism," *Surgery*, vol. 148, no. 6, pp. 1129–1138, 2010.

[62] M. M. Mortenson, D. B. Evans, J. E. Lee et al., "Parathyroid exploration in the reoperative neck: improved preoperative localization with 4D-computed tomography," *Journal of the American College of Surgeons*, vol. 206, no. 5, pp. 888–895, 2008.

[63] S. E. Rodgers, G. J. Hunter, L. M. Hamberg et al., "Improved preoperative planning for directed parathyroidectomy with 4-dimensional computed tomography," *Surgery*, vol. 140, no. 6, pp. 932–941, 2006.

[64] D. P. Frush, E. B. Spencer, L. F. Donnelly, J. Y. Zheng, D. M. DeLong, and G. S. Bisset, "Optimizing contrast-enhanced abdominal CT in infants and children using bolus tracking," *American Journal of Roentgenology*, vol. 172, no. 4, pp. 1007–1013, 1999.

[65] M. Mazloumi, G. Van Gompel, V. Kersemans, J. de Mey, and N. Buls, "The presence of contrast agent increases organ radiation dose in contrast-enhanced CT," *European Radiology*, vol. 30, 2021.

[66] M. K. Gill, A. Vijayananthan, G. Kumar, K. Jayarani, K. H. Ng, and Z. Sun, "Use of 100 kV versus 120 kV in computed tomography pulmonary angiography in the detection of pulmonary embolism: effect on radiation dose and image quality," *Quantitative Imaging in Medicine and Surgery*, vol. 5, no. 4, pp. 524–533, 2015.

18

Assessment of the Local Exposure Level during Adult Chest X-Rays at the Ngaoundere Regional Hospital, Cameroon

Guiswe Gnowe,[1] Henri Paul Ekobena Fouda,[2] Mbo Amvene Jéremie,[3] Takmou Pascal,[4] and Bonaventure Babinne Graobe[1]

[1]*Higher Institute of Sciences, Health Technics and Management of Garoua, Garoua, Cameroon*
[2]*University Technological of Institute, University of Ngaoundere, Ngaoundere, Cameroon*
[3]*Faculty of Medicine and Biomedical Sciences of Garoua, Garoua, Cameroon*
[4]*General Hospital of Douala, Douala, Cameroon*

Correspondence should be addressed to Guiswe Gnowe; gnoweguiswe@gmail.com

Academic Editor: Paul Sijens

Background. The purpose of this study was to estimate the doses delivered to adult patients during chest examination for comparison with those elsewhere and to establish a local diagnostic reference level for the chest. The doses delivered in the standard X-ray examinations are not sufficiently optimized and controlled. The working protocols for the same exam given differ for similar morphotypes within the same hospital structure. *Materials and Methods.* The entrance skin dose (mGy) of the chest was evaluated on 105 adult patients with a mass of 70 ± 10 kg in accordance with the 75th percentile of the irradiation parameters. The analysis and processing of the data was carried out by Excel 2010. The entrance skin dose of the chest obtained in mGy was 0.18 ± 0.21 for the PA incidence. *Conclusion.* The present study allowed us to observe large variations at the entrance skin doses of the chest. These variations have made it possible to understand that the entrance skin doses to the chest are optimized and do not exceed the proportions of those estimated by others and standards internationally. This aspect demonstrates that the diagnostic reference levels as enumerated are dependent on the doses delivered and include not only the notions of quality of the radiographic image and the quality assurance of the radiological equipments but also the level of the manipulators trained.

1. Introduction

The medical applications of ionizing radiation have, for many years now, contributed to an improvement of medical practicals and bring a real benefit in terms of health. In radiology, dosimetry and diagnostic quality of images are inseparable. Diagnosis is a function dependent on the quality of the radiological image. Dosimetry could be defined as the measurement of ionizing radiation received or deposited in a medium [1]. Diagnostic medical examinations using ionizing radiation such as radiology, CT, and nuclear medicine lead to variable exposure of patients according to the procedure implemented, the facility of the technology, and the patient's morphotype [2]. In view of this, the reality of these risks, however, comes up against the general problem commonly referred to as the problem of low doses. As observed elsewhere, there are also wide variations in the dose for the same type of examination and the same morphotype of X-ray patients [3]. The health effects of doses delivered in radiodiagnostics are not only low but zero below an imprecise threshold [4] since the linear relationship without threshold not based on 0.6% to 3% of cancers would be attributable to radiodiagnostics.

When one is in a world structured by the important uncertainty of ionizing radiation, uncertainties remain and it is impossible as for the risks created by the ionizing radiations. Some think that the risk exists even at low doses, others think that it does not exist, and others finally think that it can be even more complicated; it is normal that knowledge from all horizons can be taken into account in the definition of protective devices. In the case of ionizing radiation, the difficulty experienced passes from the prevention of proven risks to precautionary approaches aimed at hypothetical risks. This difficulty is evident in the handling of limit values or threshold values considered useful. The radioprotection of patients in imaging appears as an emergency and a particular attention related to the practices because zero risk is hardly possible. Without compromising the effectiveness of the diagnosis or their therapeutic value, the overall goal is to reduce exposure to what is absolutely necessary. That is why any examination must be justified by its diagnostic contribution in relation with the irradiation, its realization must be optimal, that is to say, in conformity with the *ALARA* (*as low as reasonably achievable*) principle, and the doses delivered must be regularly evaluated for comparison with diagnostic reference levels, which should not be exceeded without justification [5]. Regulatory actions, if necessary, must be considered to correct any differences between dose and these irradiation parameters [6]. Moreover, the diagnosis being subordinated by the informative quality of the images may not be applicable but may substitute the DRLs which are indicators of the quality of the practices, allowing each one to situate his practice by the whole of the profession and overexposure of patients.

The use of ionizing radiation for diagnostic or therapeutic purposes is indeed incompatible with a regulatory limitation of doses: the level of irradiation is necessarily subordinate to the medical objective and imposing "a priori" impassable thresholds would be the contradiction detrimental to patients. Radiation protection for people exposed for medical reasons is therefore based exclusively on the principles of justification and optimization [7]. Diagnostic reference levels (DRLs) are defined as "dose levels in medical radiodiagnostic practices, or in the case of radiopharmaceuticals, activity levels, for standard examinations on typical patient groups or on typical ghosts, for broad categories of types of installations" [8]. The Respect for the reference levels is not, by itself, a criterion of good practice. The priority objective, inseparable from dosimetry, is the diagnostic quality of images [9]. This aspect means that the other 25% corresponding to the highest doses were made under nonoptimized conditions. For this purpose, it is necessary to initiate control and correction actions, in case of unjustified overrun of the doses delivered.

Diagnostic reference levels are tools for improving practices and optimizing doses. The Respect for the reference levels is not, by itself, a criterion of good practice. The primary and inseparable goal of dosimetry is to combine the diagnostic quality of images with the reasonably feasible low-dose processes. Recognizing that a diagnostic reference level is a level established for a standard procedure and for typical patient groups and not for individual exposures, compliance with this level does not automatically correspond to the use of good practice, as the quality of the image may be poor and this will not make a good diagnosis. Diagnostic reference levels are of diagnostic interest only if they are assigned to dosimetric quantities accessible by measurement or calculation. Characterizing the level of irradiation of an examination by a different size in conventional radiology and CT may appear as a limitation in a process of justification and optimization of radiological practices [9].

The knowledge of these doses necessarily involves in the determination of doses according to the disymmetric quantities. The determination of these values must be based on the statistical method known as the 75th percentile of the measured dose distribution [10, 11] since 75% of individuals receive doses below these values [7, 11], or the reference levels. Diagnostics are of practical interest only if they are assigned to dosimetric quantities accessible by the measurement. In conventional radiology, the entrance skin dose (ESD in mGy) and the dose area product (DAP in Gy·cm^2) were retained. The entrance skin dose (ESD) can be determined by two approaches: the indirect method, also called semiempirical method, using the exposure parameters linked to examinations and the direct method using the dosimeter thermoluminescent (TLD) for measurement. These two methods have relatively small differences. The calculation or mathematical method appears reliable and is an effective alternative for measuring the entrance skin dose [12].

The problem of dosimetry usually stems from the incorrect use of radiological equipment and the higher patient exposure required [13]. The optimization and dose determination approach must take into account the specificities associated with the standardization of procedures [14]. The factors influencing the dose delivered to patients in conventional radiology can be classified as follows [10]. Several calculation models are proposed for the evaluation of the dose at the entrance of the skin. But in our approach, we used the estimation of the output [15]. According to the manufacturers, the value of the DAP is also displayed permanently at the control room monitor or actually measured by a device installed at the output of the X-ray tube (ionization chamber) or calculated from the parameters of the exposure and the size of the irradiation field. Because of the two physical laws (inverse of the square of the distance) and geometry (Thales theorem), the value of the DAP is independent of the distance where it is measured [16].

2. Materials and Methods

Our study was monocentric and prospective and was carried out at the Radiology and Medical Imaging Department of the Regional Medical Imaging Center of Ngaoundere during the period from April to July 2016. A total of 105 adult patients weighing 70 ± 10 kg who had standard examinations during the study period were involved. The examinations were carried out on a General Electric-branded appliance, model 5192454, whose maximum voltage at the terminals is 150 kV. The studied parameters concerned the patient (age, sex, and anatomical region explored), parameters related to the procedure (focus-film-distance or FFD; focus-skin-distance or FSD; incidence), irradiation (kilovoltage or kV; milliAmperesecond or mAs), and dosimetric constants that were otherwise absent on the manipulative console (entrance skin dose or ESD; the dose area product or DAP).

The first step in calculating the entrance skin dose in standard radiography using the theoretical models is to calculate the power (output) of the ray tube. The power of the tube was estimated in our model study [16] using irradiation parameters directly involved in the achievement of the examinations.

$$\frac{O}{P}\,(\mathrm{mR}) = A \times 6.53 \times 10^{-4}\left(\frac{\mathrm{mR}}{\mathrm{mAs}}\right)\left(\mathrm{kV}^2\right)^{-1} \times \mathrm{kV}^2 \times \mathrm{mAs}, \quad (1)$$

where (O/P)mR is the power (output) of the X-ray tube; $A = 0, 8$, kV is the voltage applied to the tube, for performing the examination; mAs is the charge passing through the tube; A was an equal constant of 0.5, 0.8, and 1 for single-phase, three-phase, and high-frequency generator tubes. In our study, the X-ray tube was three-phase. The yields obtained were converted from (mR) to $\mathrm{mGy} \cdot (\mathrm{mAs})^{-1}$ by multiplication at a factor of 0.00877/mAs [17].

The entrance skin dose for each patient was calculated using the irradiation parameters of each radiographic examination following this model.

$$\mathrm{ESD}\,(\mathrm{mGy}) = A \times 6.53 \times 10^{-4}\left(\frac{\mathrm{mR}}{\mathrm{mAs}}\right)\left(\mathrm{kV}^2\right)^{-1} \times \mathrm{kV}^2 \times \mathrm{mAs} \times \left(\frac{100}{\mathrm{FSD}}\right)^2 \times \mathrm{BSF} \times 0.00877\left(\frac{\mathrm{mGy}}{\mathrm{mR}}\right), \quad (2)$$

where ESD (mGy) is the entrance skin dose, FSD (cm) is the focus-skin-distance, and BSF is the radiation backscatter factor. In the context of this work, it is equal to 1.35 for adults according to the IAEA [1].

The anthropometric data and the technical parameters used (kV, mAs, FFD, and FSD) were collected at the time of examinations. Only images of good qualities having been used for diagnosis were considered. The analysis and treatment of the data according to the 75th percentile of the irradiation parameters as well as the calculation of the entrance skin dose (ESD) of the patients were carried out by Excel 2010.

3. Results

The data relating to this examination were collected by means of a questionnaire whose items concerned the equipment, the patient, the radiological technique, the image criteria, and the dose received by the patient. These data were processed and the results obtained are presented in tabular form. Table 1 presents the distribution of sociodemographic characteristics. Table 2 shows the performance of the X-ray tube on the chest X-ray. Table 3 presents the values of the main patient exposure parameters (kV, mAs, FFD, and FSD) used during the course of this review in the study. Table 4 compares the entrance dose of the chest, the DRLs, and the values found elsewhere.

Table 1 presents the statistical distribution of the sociodemographic characteristics of the patients who participated in this study. Patient anthropometric data (sex, age, and weight) are essential for interpreting the results of radiological examination and dosimetry. Only complete data on 105 adult male and female patients were selected. The average age of men was 40.93, the standard deviation was 7.42 years, and the age range was 29–53 years. In contrast, the mean age of women was 35.58 years, the standard deviation was 10.19 years, and the age range was 23–56 years. Men were more represented than women at 52% or a sex ratio (M/F = 1.1).

Table 1: Sociodemographic data.

Radiography	Sex		Age (years)	Weight (kg)
Chest	M	55	29–53 (40.92 ± 7.42)	64–80 (70.84 ± 4.7)
	F	50	23–56 (35.58 ± 10.19)	60–78 (66.66 ± 4.71)
Total		**105**		

M: male. F: female.

Table 2: Tube yield in mR and $\mathrm{mGy} \cdot (\mathrm{mAs})^{-1}$.

Radiography	Incidence	Output (mR) Min-max	Output $\mathrm{mGy} \cdot (\mathrm{mAs})^{-1}$ Min-max
Chest	PA	75.22–81.75	0.65–0.71

PA: posteroanterior. Min: minimum. Max: maximum.

Table 2 shows the efficiency of the X-ray tube. These values are essential parameters in the process of optimizing the dose delivered and the quality of the images. They are directly a function of the high voltage (kV) and the load (mAs).

Table 3 summarizes the minimum, maximum, and mean values of the main patient exposure parameters (kV, mAs, FFD, and FSD) used during the course of this exploration in the study.

Table 4 presents a comparative state of entrance skin dose of the thorax, the DRLs, and those obtained elsewhere.

4. Discussion

We are very clearly aware of the difficulties of an evaluation without having access to the actual measurement of the dose. It is however necessary to have access to the measured dose to indicate to the user the direction towards which the technical progress is going. Indeed, if these results are closer to the reality of the actual dose, then they can contribute for the more appropriate determination of the "reference" values. From these results, we observe wide variations in the use of pulmonary chest exposure parameters (PA) for patients with similar morphotypes. This diversity of the technical protocols is at the origin of the large variations of the irradiation parameters for the same morphotype. On the contrary, despite the differences observed, our results are less than those estimated in [20], but these are similar to the DRL's for chest radiography. This aspect proves the embryonic state of radioprotection of patients in the radiology departments. These discrepancies with those obtained elsewhere and with international standards can be explained apart by the absence of dosimetric values and working protocols in the examination room.

Table 3: Technical parameters used to conduct this exam.

Radiography	Incidence	kV	mAs	FFD	FSD	ESD Min-max	ESD Max/min	3rd quartile	SD
Chest	PA	120–125 (122.8 ± 1.72)	2.5–4 (3.17 ± 0.46)	140–180 (180 ± 0.09)	160–200 (128 ± 0.20)	0.08–0.09	1.04	0.18	0.21

kV: kilovolt. mAs: milliampere second. FFD: focus-film-distance. FSD: focus-skin-distance. ESD: entrance skin dose. SD: standard deviation.

Table 4: Comparison of the entrance skin dose (mGy) with those obtained elsewhere and at DRLs.

Radiography	Incidence	Our study	IRSN (DRL)	Sudan [18]	Iran [19]	Mali [20]
Chest	PA	0.18 ± 0.21	0.3	0.53 ± 0.24	0.70 ± 0.38	3.84

On the contrary, international standards and DRLs must be used to control and optimize radiological practices. In practice, by displaying and applying these, it is possible to avoid unnecessary irradiation and the periodic evaluation of the delivered doses should become a routine activity. Consequently, the doses delivered for the realization of the thorax are not sufficiently mastered. These differences lead us to think like [5] that unlike developed countries, in sub-Saharan African countries, particularly Cameroon and Mali, legislative and regulatory frameworks are either nonexistent or implemented in a rough way. Moreover, the practice of radioprotection of patients is poorly documented in a context of constant expansion of medical imaging for a decade..

As imaging spreads to the most remote areas of the country, there is an urgent need to optimize work protocols. This optimization of doses delivered to the patients could well be effective by the setting up of a regulatory framework with the obligation of designation and training of humans competent in radioprotection which would allow not only to improve the radioprotection of the patients but also of the personnel, for the establishment of regular dosimetric control and dosimetric standards. The lack of ongoing training of personnel on radiation protection measures could be noted as potential factors of patient exposure. This finding is still very worrying, when the professional profile (nurse and caregivers) of some radiology manipulators does not correspond to their "background" because they are rather converted into radiological manipulators and a large rotation of radiology trainees who find work protocols not available and also who are often forced to produce images capable of being exploited. In view of this, they have either no idea or a rough idea of the good practice in radio-diagnostics or even radiation protection of patients. From these observations, we can affirm with [5] the low level of knowledge in radioprotection in African countries, especially those of sub-Saharan Africa, despite the existence of the laws governing radiation protection and the lack of resources forced to approximate, DRLs.

5. Conclusion

At the end of this work, it should be noted that dosimetry is a good match between the image quality and low-dose process. Far from trivializing the exposure of patients to ionizing radiation, it is important to note that the risk of irradiation increases with the nonobservance of the basic principles of radiation protection of patients. The results obtained show that the doses delivered to patients are not optimal. However, an improvement in practices, especially in relation to the technical parameters and protocols associated with strengthening the permanent radiation protection skills of radiological manipulators, could contribute to better radiological protection of patients in this radiology department. Moreover, note that the indirect method used here is a reliable alternative for measuring the entrance skin dose of the patient. This method could also serve as a means of measurement for the control and dosimetric assessment in case of dosimeter deficiency in developing countries whose scarcity of resources constrains the implementation of approximate international conventions and legislation. In radiation protection, however, corrective measures should be evaluated and undertaken, if there are excessive discrepancies between the doses delivered and those observed elsewhere. For this, the radioprotection of patients is an emergency quality in a context where quality is a global aspiration.

References

[1] Agence Internationale de l'Énergie Atomique (AIEA), "Normes fondamentales internationales de protection contre les rayonnements ionisants et de sureté des sources de rayonnements," *Collection Sécurité*, vol. 115, pp. 309–332, 1997.

[2] P. Roch, D. Celier, C. Etard, and A. Noel, *Bilan Du Recueil 2011-2012 Des Nrd Par L'irsn Et Recommandations D'évolution Du Système Par Le GPMED-ASN*, pp. 1–3, Société Française de Radioprotection, Congrès National de Radioprotection, Tours, France, 2005.

[3] J. Gray, "Reference, values-what are they?," *American Association of Physicist in Medicine*, vol. 24, pp. 9-10, 1999.

[4] A. B. de González and S. Darby, "Risk of cancer from diagnostic X-rays: estimates for the UK and 14 other countries," *The Lancet*, vol. 363, no. 9406, pp. 345–351, 2004.

[5] P. Ongolo-Zogo, C. Mpeke Mokubangele, B. Moifo, and J. Gonsu fotsin, "Évaluation de la dose patient en scanographie pédiatrique dans deux hôpitaux universitaires à yaoundé cameroun," *Radioprotection*, vol. 47, no. 4, pp. 533–542, 2012.

[6] R. Azzoz, K. M. ElShahat, R. A. MonemRezk, and R. Monem, "Evaluation of quality control systems for X-ray machines at different hospitals using patient's radiological dose assessment technology," *IOSR Journal of Applied Physics*, vol. 6, no. 5, pp. 29–34, 2014.

[7] H. Beauvais-March, M. Valero, A. Biau, N. Hocine, J.-L. Rehel, and M. Bourguignon, "L'exposition des patients en radiodiagnostic: bilan de l'étude dosimétrique réalisée en 2001–2003 dans 24 services français de radiologie," *Radioprotection*, vol. 39, no. 4, pp. 493–511, 2004.

[8] G. A. Monnehan, K. J. Anouan, D. P. Onoma et al., "Détermination des niveaux de référence diagnostiques en côte d'ivoire: cas de la radiographie Standard du thorax de face et de l'abdomen sans préparation (ASP) de face chez l'adulte dans le district d'abidjan et dans la région du sud comoé," *Revue Internationale des Sciences et Technologies*, vol. 14, pp. 45–53, 2009.

[9] Y. S. Cordoliani, P. Grenier, H. Beauvais, J. Grellet, E. Marshall-Depommier, and M. Bourguignon, "Le point sur les procédures en radiologie conventionnelle et en tomodensitométrie," *Médecine Nucléaire Imagerie Fonctionnelle et Métabolique*, vol. 26, no. 5, pp. 241–246, 2002.

[10] H. Beauvais-March, A. Biau, M. Bourguignon et al., "Les Procédures radiologiques: critères de qualité et optimisation des doses," *Office de Protection Contre les Rayonnements Ionisants-Société Française de Radiologie*, pp. 17–46, 2000.

[11] C. J. Olowookere, I. A. Babalola, N. N. Jibiri, R. I. Obed, L. Bamidele, and E. O. Ajetumobi, "A preliminary radiation dose audit in some nigerian hospitals: need for determination of national diagnostic reference levels (NDRLs)," *The Pacific Journal of Science and Technology*, vol. 13, no. 1, pp. 87–495, 2012.

[12] V. Tsapaki, I. A. Tsalafoutas, I. Chinofoti et al., "Radiation doses to patients undergoing standard radiographic examinations: a comparison between two methods," *The British Journal of Radiology*, vol. 80, no. 950, pp. 107–112, 2007.

[13] M. Gholami, N. Fazaneh, and V. Karami, "The evaluation of conventional x-ray exposure parameters including tube voltage and exposure time in private and governmental hospitals of lorestan province, Iran," *Iranian Journal of Medical Physics*, vol. 12, no. 2, pp. 85–92, 2015.

[14] M. H. Beauvais, A. Biau, M. Bourguignon, C. Challeton De Vathaire, J. F. Lacronique, and M. Valero, "Optimisation des doses délivrées aux patients en radiologie médicale," *Rapport Scientifique et Technique*, vol. 4, no. 5, pp. 143–151, 2002.

[15] S. Kothan and M. Tungjai, "An estimation of X-radiation output using mathematic model," *American Journal of Applied Sciences*, vol. 8, no. 9, pp. 923–926, 2011.

[16] M. Carlo and O. Bar, "Guide des bonnes pratiques de radioprotection du patient en cardiologie interventionnelle," *Société Française de Cardiologie*, pp. 1–54, 2015.

[17] K. Faulkner, D. A. Broadhead, and R. M. Harrison, "Patient dosimetry measurement methods," *Applied Radiation and Isotopes*, vol. 50, no. 1, pp. 113–123, 1999.

[18] A. A. Abu Khiar, A. O. Hamza, and N. A. Abbas, "Dose reference levels in radiography for the most common examinations in Sudan," *Sudan Journal of Medical Sciences*, vol. 11, no. 1, pp. 7–16, 2016.

[19] D. Khoshdel-Navi, A. Shabestani-Monfared, M. R. Deevband, R. Abdi, and M. Nabahati, "Local-reference patient dose evaluation in conventional radiography examinations in mazandaran, Iran," *Journal of Biomedical Physics and Engineering*, vol. 6, no. 2, pp. 61–70, 2016.

[20] S. Traoré, "Étude comparative de la dose patient a la dose de référence dans le service de radiologie et d'imagerie médicale de l'hôpital gabriel touré (HGT) à propos de 70 cas," Université de Bamako, Faculté de Médecine, de Pharmacie et d'Odontostomatologie (FMPOS), Bamako, Mali, Thèse de Doctorat Médecine, 2006.

19

Preprocedural Hypertension is not a Risk Factor for Postoperative Bleeding following Image-Guided Core Needle Breast Biopsy

Ninad Salastekar, Alexis Saunders, Kushal Patel, and Katherine Willer

Department of Radiology, SUNY Upstate Medical University, 750 East Adam Street, Syracuse, NY 13210, USA

Correspondence should be addressed to Ninad Salastekar; ninad.salastekar@gmail.com

Academic Editor: Alfonso Fausto

Objective. To evaluate the association between preprocedural hypertension and the risk of prolonged bleeding following image-guided core needle breast biopsy in nonpregnant/nonlactating women. *Methods.* A single institution-based, retrospective cohort study of 400 women who underwent image-guided core needle breast biopsy was conducted. Males and pregnant and lactating women were excluded. Preprocedural systolic or diastolic blood pressure greater than 140 or 90 mm of Hg, respectively, was defined as hypertension. Prolonged bleeding was defined >15 minutes of local, manual pressure required to achieve hemostasis following the biopsy. Severe bleeding complications defined as clinical significant hematoma formation, prolonged bleeding requiring an ER visit, hospitalization, or surgical intervention were also recorded. *Results.* The difference in the mean time for which manual pressure was held after biopsy for patients with and without preprocedural hypertension was not statistically significant (13 ± 7 vs. 13 ± 8 minutes, respectively, $P = 0.856$). There was no difference in the number of patients requiring manual postoperative pressure >15 minutes between those with preprocedural hypertension and the normotensive patients (13% vs. 12%, respectively, $P = 0.765$). Bivariate analysis demonstrated statistically significant association between prolonged bleeding and current antithrombotic or antiplatelet medication use ($P = 0.010$), the use of stereotactic guidance ($P = 0.019$), and a tethered vacuum-assisted device ($P = 0.045$). The use of a tethered vacuum-assisted biopsy device was the only variable associated with prolonged bleeding in the multivariate model ($P = 0.044$). *Conclusion.* Preprocedural hypertension is not a risk factor for prolonged bleeding following image-guided core needle breast biopsies in nonpregnant/nonlactating women.

1. Introduction

The lifetime risk of developing breast cancer for an average woman in the US is 12.9%, and approximately 128 new cases of breast cancer are diagnosed per 100,000 women per year [1]. Image-guided core needle breast biopsy (CNB), an accurate and cost-effective alternative to open surgical biopsy, remains the investigation of choice for further evaluation of a majority of suspicious findings discovered on breast imaging [2–4]. Core needle breast biopsies are associated with a low complication rate and are generally well tolerated by patients [2, 3]. Overall, the rate of severe complications from CNB procedure is <1% [5]. While a systematic review by Bruening et al. reported bruising, vasovagal reaction (3.0%), and pain (3.7%) as the most common minor complications, severe bleeding complications (prolonged/severe bleeding requiring treatment (0.7%) and postoperative hematoma formation (0.1%)), infections (0.15%), and severe pain (1.7%) were reported as the most common major complications following CNB [3].

While the incidence of severe bleeding complications (SBC) following CNB is low, the risk factors associated with these complications remain poorly understood. Vacuum-assisted biopsy device is associated with increased risk of SBC following CBC, while antithrombotic medication use is not [3, 6, 7]. There is insufficient evidence to demonstrate the association of patient comorbidities with the risk of SBC [3]. Particularly, systemic hypertension is a known risk factor for SBC following kidney biopsy [8, 9]. However, to the best of our knowledge, the association of systemic hypertension with severe bleeding complications following core needle breast biopsy has not been studied. In this study, we evaluate the association between systemic hypertension and the risk of SBC following CBC in women with suspicious findings on breast imaging.

2. Materials and Methods

The institutional review board approved this single institution-based, retrospective cohort study conducted at a university hospital. 400 consecutive women who underwent ultrasound (US) or stereotactic-guided core needle breast biopsy from January 2016 to June 2020 were included in this study. Exclusion criteria included concurrent pregnancy or lactation and male gender. Data were acquired through chart review.

The past medical history of the subjects was reviewed to note any hematological disorders that could affect hemostasis as well as history of systemic hypertension. Medications including antithrombotic and antiplatelet agents were noted. In accordance with currently accepted clinical guidelines, antithrombotic/antiplatelet therapy was not held prior to procedures, neither was the coagulation profile (INR/PT) acquired immediately prior to the procedure. The type of biopsy (US/Stereotactic), biopsy device (vacuum-assisted or not), number of biopsy sites, and number of biopsies per site were recorded. Preprocedural blood pressure was noted for each subject. Preprocedural systolic or diastolic blood pressure greater than 140 or 90 mm of Hg, respectively, was defined as hypertension.

The main outcome of interest was prolonged bleeding as measured by the time for which manual pressure was applied to the biopsy site to achieve hemostasis. Prolonged bleeding was defined as greater than 15 minutes of pressure required to achieve hemostasis. Severe bleeding complications defined as clinically significant hematoma formation, prolonged bleeding requiring an ER visit, hospitalization, or surgical intervention were also recorded.

3. Statistical Analysis

Analysis was conducted using R 4.0.2 and RStudio [10, 11]. Continuous variables (age and time to hemostasis) were described as mean ± standard deviation. Categorical variables were described as frequency (percentage). Bivariate analysis was conducted using the independent *T*-test/Mann–Whitney test for continuous variables and the Chi Square test/Fisher's exact test for categorical variables. Variables with P value <0.10 were included in a multivariable logistic regression model. A P value of 0.05 was considered as the threshold for statistical significance.

4. Results

The demographic and relevant clinical characteristics of the patients are described in Table 1. The average age of patients in this study was 59 ± 13 years. Approximately 2% patients had a history of hematological disorders that could potentially affect hemostasis (for example, antiphospholipid syndrome and protein C/S deficiency), 39% had a history of hypertension, and 11% had a history of current or past smoking. About 5% patients in the study were taking antithrombotic/antiplatelet medications (warfarin, direct thrombin inhibitors, and clopidogrel). 77% of all biopsies were ultrasound-guided, and the remaining were stereotactic biopsies. All stereotactic biopsies used a tethered vacuum-assisted biopsy device. Needles with ≥12 gauge were used in 68% of the biopsies. 31% of patients in this study had preprocedural hypertension, defined as a systolic or diastolic blood pressure greater than 140 or 90 mm of Hg, respectively. The distribution of patient characteristics grouped by presence of preprocedural hypertension is also described in Table 1.

A total of 137 subjects were missing information regarding bleeding outcomes and 68 were missing information regarding preprocedural blood pressure.

The distribution of the systolic and diastolic blood pressures in patients stratified by preprocedural hypertension and prolonged bleeding is shown in Table 2.

The difference in the average time for which manual pressure was held after biopsy for patients with and without preprocedural hypertension was not statistically significant (13 ± 7 vs. 13 ± 8 minutes, respectively, $P = 0.856$, Table 3). There was no difference in the number of patients requiring manual postoperative pressure >15 minutes between those with preprocedural hypertension and the normotensive patients (13% vs. 12%, respectively, $P = 0.765$, Table 1).

Bivariate analysis demonstrated statistically significant association between prolonged bleeding and current antithrombotic or antiplatelet medication use ($P = 0.010$), the use of stereotactic guidance ($P = 0.019$), and a tethered vacuum-assisted device ($P = 0.045$) (Table 3). Type of biopsy, use of tethered vacuum-assisted biopsy device, and anticoagulant use were further evaluated in a multivariate logistic regression model for association with prolonged bleeding (>15 minutes). The use of a tethered vacuum-assisted biopsy device was the only variable associated with prolonged bleeding in the multivariate model ($P = 0.044$).

A single patient required a visit to the ER for prolonged bleeding but was discharged without intervention. No clinically significant hematomas were reported.

5. Discussion

Prolonged bleeding in patients with preprocedural hypertension undergoing biopsies of the kidney has been reported [8, 9]. To the best of our knowledge, the association of systemic hypertension with severe bleeding complications following image-guided core needle breast biopsy has not been adequately evaluated.

In the current study, we found no association between preprocedural hypertension and prolonged bleeding following image-guided core needle breast biopsy (CNB). A history of systemic hypertension was also not associated with prolonged bleeding following CNB. Factors associated with prolonged bleeding, defined as >15 minutes of manual and postoperative pressure required to achieve hemostasis, were the current use of antithrombotic/antiplatelet medications, stereotactic-guided biopsies, and the use of a tethered

Table 1: Demographic and clinical characteristic of subjects by preprocedural hypertension.

	All patients ($n = 332$)	Preprocedural hypertension ($n = 104$)	Normotensive ($n = 228$)	P valueˆ
Age* (in years)	59 (13)	63 (13)	57 (12)	<0.001ˆ
History of smoking (current or past)**	37 (11%)	4 (4%)	33 (15%)	0.004ˆ
History of hypertension**	131 (39%)	55 (53%)	76 (33%)	<0.001ˆ
History of hematological disorders affecting hemostasis**	6 (2%)	1 (1%)	5 (2%)	0.435
Antithrombotic/antiplatelet medications**	17 (5%)	8 (8%)	9 (4%)	0.151
Type of biopsy**				
Ultrasound-guided	251 (77%)	79 (77%)	172 (77%)	0.895
Stereotactic	81 (24%)	24 (23%)	57 (25%)	0.690
Tethered vacuum-assisted device**	76 (23%)	25 (24%)	51 (23%)	0.768
Needle gauge ≥12**	180 (68%)	59 (71%)	121 (67%)	0.531
Bleeding after biopsy (in minutes)*	13 (8)	13 (7)	13 (8)	0.856
Prolonged postbiopsy bleeding (>15 minutes)**	32 (12%)	11 (13%)	21 (12%)	0.765

*Mean (standard deviation). **Frequency (percentage). ˆStatistically significant P value (<0.05).

Table 2: The distribution of the systolic and diastolic blood pressures stratified by preprocedural hypertension.

	Preprocedural hypertension ($n = 104$)	Normotensive ($n = 228$)	P value	Prolonged bleeding ($n = 32$)	Normal hemostasis ($n = 231$)	P value
Systolic blood pressure (mm of Hg)*	152 (14)	121 (11)	<0.001ˆ	131 (17)	131 (18)	0.944
Diastolic blood pressure (mm of Hg)*	87 (8)	77 (7)	<0.001ˆ	81 (9)	80 (9)	0.461

* Mean (standard deviation). ˆStatistically significant P value (<0.05).

Table 3: Bivariate analysis of factors affecting postbiopsy bleeding time.

	Prolonged bleeding ($n = 32$)	Normal hemostasis ($n = 231$)	P valueˆ
Age* (in years)	59 (11)	58 (14)	0.895
History of smoking (current or past)**	2 (6%)	26 (12%)	0.356
History of hypertension**	11 (34%)	87 (38%)	0.719
History of hematological disorders affecting hemostasis**	1 (3%)	5 (2%)	0.733
Antithrombotic/antiplatelet medications**	5 (16%)	10 (4%)	0.010ˆ
Type of biopsy**			
Ultrasound-guided	22 (71%)	191 (84%)	0.070ˆ
Stereotactic	11 (34%)	39 (17%)	0.019ˆ
Tethered vacuum-assisted device**	10 (31%)	38 (17%)	0.045ˆ
Needle gauge ≥12**	16 (59%)	139 (77%)	0.051
Preprocedural hypertension	11 (34%)	73 (32%)	0.765

*Mean (standard deviation). **Frequency (percentage). ˆStatistically significant Pvalue (<0.05).

vacuum-assisted device. A single patient with preprocedural hypertension (207/70 mm Hg), not anticoagulated, undergoing ultrasound-guided breast biopsy was transferred to the ER for prolonged bleeding, but was eventually discharged without the need for surgical intervention or hospitalization. There were no other reported severe bleeding complications in the study cohort (including clinically significant hematoma, ER visit/hospitalization, or surgical intervention).

The findings of prolonged postoperative bleeding in patients undergoing stereotactic biopsies/using tethered vacuum-assisted devices are similar to those reported previously [3, 5]. We report increased incidence of prolonged bleeding, defined as >15 minutes of pressure required for hemostasis, in patients taking antithrombotic/antiplatelet medications. However, none of the patients reported clinically significant postoperative hematomas or bleeding requiring intervention/hospitalization. Previous studies have used different criteria for defining bleeding complications but have also not reported clinically significant hematomas or severe bleeding complications in patients using antithrombotic medications [7]. Multivariate analysis demonstrated a significant association between prolonged bleeding and the use of a tethered vacuum-assisted device, a finding consistent with previous reports [5].

This study has several limitations. Findings from this single institution study have not been externally validated.

MRI-guided biopsies were not included. Factors that could affect bleeding such as platelet count and INR were not recorded for a majority of patients on the day of the biopsy due to absence of such a requirement in the clinical guidelines for image-guided core needle breast biopsy. Alcohol intake on the day of the procedure was not recorded may confound the bleeding time. The study could not evaluate the effect of operator experience or skill since all the biopsies were performed by attending radiologists without the involvement of residents or fellows. The type of lesion/pathology was not accounted for. However, there is no evidence in the literature that postoperative bleeding is reliably affected by the type of pathology. Data regarding the number of biopsy sites and/or the number of biopsies per site were not consistently recorded in the original reports and thus could not be included in the analysis. However, there is no evidence to suggest a differential distribution of the number of biopsies in patients with/without preprocedural hypertension, and as such, this is unlikely to affect the results. This study did not consider the effect of patient positioning which may affect postbiopsy bleeding rates. We may have missed any severe bleeding complications that were not reported to our hospital and in cases where the patients sought care elsewhere.

6. Conclusion

A history of systemic hypertension and/or preprocedural hypertension is not a risk factor for prolonged bleeding following image-guided core needle breast biopsies in nonpregnant/nonlactating women. Despite the described limitations, the findings of this study should help guide clinical management of hypertensive patients on the day of the breast biopsy, specifically avoiding unnecessary delay or postponement of the biopsy due to perceived risk of prolonged bleeding in patients with preprocedural hypertension. The findings also inform the relatively unclear literature on the patient-related risk factors for prolonged bleeding following breast biopsies.

References

[1] N. Howlader, A. Noone, M. Krapcho et al., *SEER Cancer Statistics Review*, National Cancer Institute, Bethesda, MD, USA, 2017, https://seer.cancer.gov/csr/1975_2017.

[2] S. L. Versaggi and A. De Leucio, *Breast Biopsy*, StatPearls Publishing, Treasure Island, FL, USA, 2020, http://www.ncbi.nlm.nih.gov/books/NBK559147.

[3] W. Bruening, J. Fontanarosa, K. Tipton, J. R. Treadwell, J. Launders, and K. Schoelles, "Systematic review: Comparative effectiveness of core-needle and open surgical biopsy to diagnose breast lesions," *Annals of Internal Medicine*, vol. 152, no. 4, pp. 238–246, 2010.

[4] S. Pettine, R. Place, S. Babu, W. Williard, D. Kim, and P. Carter, "Stereotactic breast biopsy is accurate, minimally invasive, and cost effective," *The American Journal of Surgery*, vol. 171, no. 5, pp. 474–476, 1996.

[5] I. J. Dahabreh, L. S. Wieland, G. P. Adam, C. Halladay, J. Lau, and T. A. Trikalinos, *Core Needle and Open Surgical Biopsy for Diagnosis of Breast Lesions: An Update to the 2009 Report*, Agency for Healthcare Research and Quality (US), Rockville. MD, USA, 2014, http://www.ncbi.nlm.nih.gov/books/NBK246878.

[6] A. L. Chetlen, C. Kasales, J. Mack, S. Schetter, and J. Zhu, "Hematoma formation during breast core needle biopsy in women taking antithrombotic therapy," *American Journal of Roentgenology*, vol. 201, no. 1, pp. 215–222, 201321.

[7] P. Somerville, P. J. Seifert, S. V. Destounis, P. F. Murphy, and W. Young, "Anticoagulation and bleeding risk after core needle biopsy," *American Journal of Roentgenology*, vol. 191, no. 4, pp. 1194–1197, 2008.

[8] M. Eiro, T. Katoh, and T. Watanabe, "Risk factors for bleeding complications in percutaneous renal biopsy," *Clinical and Experimental Nephrology*, vol. 9, no. 1, pp. 40–45, 2005.

[9] J. S. Kriegshauser, M. D. Patel, S. W. Young, F. Chen, W. G. Eversman, and Y.-H. H. Chang, "Risk of bleeding after native renal biopsy as a function of preprocedural systolic and diastolic blood pressure," *Journal of Vascular and Interventional Radiology*, vol. 26, no. 2, pp. 206–212, 2015.

[10] R Studio Team, *RStudio: Integrated Development Environment for R*, R Studio, PBC, Boston, MA, USA, 2020, http://www.rstudio.com.

[11] R Core Team, *R: A Language and Environment for Statistical Computing*, R Foundation for Statistical Computing, Vienna, Austria, 2020, https://www.R-project.org.

20

Stromal Fibrosis of the Breast: A Spectrum of Benign to Malignant Imaging Appearances

Lara Nassar,[1] Amro Baassiri,[1] Fatima Salah,[1] Andrew Barakat,[1] Elie Najem,[1] Fouad Boulos,[2] and Ghina Berjawi[1]

[1]*Department of Diagnostic Radiology, American University of Beirut Medical Center, Lebanon*
[2]*Department of Pathology, American University of Beirut Medical Center, Lebanon*

Correspondence should be addressed to Ghina Berjawi; gb02@aub.edu.lb

Academic Editor: Paul Sijens

Objectives. The aim of this study is to demonstrate the various imaging appearances of stromal fibrosis on mammography, ultrasound, and magnetic resonance imaging (MRI). *Material and Methods.* This study included 75 female patients who presented to the American University of Beirut Medical Center between January 2010 and October 2015 for breast imaging. 66 (88%) patients obtained a mammogram, 71 (95%) had an ultrasound, and 6 (8%) had an MRI. Patients included had stromal fibrosis proven on biopsy. *Results.* The most common finding on mammogram was calcifications which was present in 14 (21%) patients, while on ultrasound it was a mass which was present in 61 (86%) patients. A mass was detected on MRI in 2 (33.5%) patients. Most lesions detected had benign findings such as masses with circumscribed margins. We had a follow-up for 53 (71%) patients with an average follow-up interval of 28.5 months (range: 5 – 70). Increase in size of the index lesion was noted in only 2 patients; upon rebiopsy, pathology results read stromal fibrosis for one lesion and fibroadenoma for the other. The remaining lesions were either stable or decreased in size. The higher detection rate of a mass on ultrasound was statistically significant ($p<0.001$) in comparison to that of mammography. *Conclusion.* Stromal fibrosis can have various presentations on imaging from benign to suspicious for malignancy features. In the case of accurate targeted biopsy, when stromal fibrosis is diagnosed, the result can be considered concordant. Therefore, such lesions can be followed up by imaging to document stability and confirm benignity.

1. Introduction

Stromal fibrosis in the breast is a benign pathologic entity. It is primarily characterized by proliferation of fibrous tissue that results in the obliteration of the mammary acini and ducts [1]. The exact etiology remains unknown. However, it has been speculated that it may be related to several conditions such as estrogen related fibroblastic proliferation, end stage of inflammatory processes, or a type of breast involution [2]. In this era of screening mammography, it has become a common diagnosis in percutaneous image-guided breast biopsy. Pathologists have described this entity by various terms which include "focal fibrosis" of the breast and "fibrous mastopathy" [3]. Collectively, it has been reported to represent as high as 9% of the lesions biopsied [4].

Stromal fibrosis may present as a palpable mass or a clinically occult imaging-detected abnormality [4]. On imaging, it may present with either benign or suspicious features. The major dilemma lies in the case of radiologic-pathologic discordance, for it is one of the leading causes of missed diagnosis of breast cancer [5]. Discordance may result in a second core biopsy or even a more invasive procedure such as prompting a surgical excision of the lesion in order to avoid misdiagnosing malignant lesions [6]. Literature is almost scarce regarding the eclectic radiological features this entity may present with. It is vital for radiologists to recognize that this benign entity may present as a suspicious lesion on imaging, for it will make the assessment of concordance easier. Therefore, the aim of this study is to demonstrate the various imaging appearances of stromal fibrosis on mammography, ultrasound, and magnetic resonance imaging (MRI).

TABLE 1: Mammographic findings.

Calcification Characteristics	Number of lesions	Mass Characteristics	Number of lesions
Morphology		*Shape*	
Amorphous	9	Oval	9
Punctate	1	Round	1
Pleomorphic	1	Irregular	1
Coarse heterogeneous	1		
Round	1		
Linear	1		
Distribution		*Margin*	
Grouped	10	Circumscribed	6
Segmental	2	Obscured	3
Diffuse	1	Indistinct	2
Regional	1		
Total	*14*	*Total*	*11*

2. Materials and Methods

2.1. Patient Selection. This institutional review board (IRB) approved retrospective study included 75 female patients who presented to the American University of Beirut Medical Center (AUBMC) between January 2010 and October 2015 in which pathology examination detected only "stromal fibrosis", "focal fibrosis", or "fibrous mastopathy". Those who had multiple biopsies in the same breast at presentation where cancer was diagnosed in any of the sites biopsied were excluded. However, patients diagnosed with a contralateral breast cancer were not excluded.

2.2. Image Interpretation. A fellowship trained board certified radiologist with 5 years of experience in breast imaging and a senior resident in radiology interpreted the images by consensus. The mammograms were assessed for breast density (extremely dense, heterogeneously dense, scattered fibroglandular, and almost entirely fat), masses (shape, margin and size), calcifications (morphology and distribution), and architectural distortion. Ultrasound images were assessed for masses (shape, margin, size, echo pattern, and posterior features if any), calcifications, and special features such as intracystic mass. MRI images were assessed for masses (shape, margin, size, and internal enhancement characteristics if any), nonmass enhancements (distribution and internal enhancement characteristics if any), and kinetic curve. Changes in the lesion on follow-up images were noted. The American College of Radiology BI-RADS Atlas Fifth Edition was used as reference for image evaluation [7].

2.3. Chart Review. Patient charts were retrieved from the medical records and were reviewed for the following data: patient age, indication for presentation (screening versus diagnostic), chief complaint on presentation, family history of breast cancer, follow-up period, and pathology reports.

2.4. Statistical Analysis. Statistical analysis was performed on the SPSS software (release 23.0; SPSS Inc.) for Windows (Microsoft). Quantitative data were described as mean, range (minimum-maximum). Qualitative parameters were compared using the Chi-Square test. Results were considered statistically significant at $p \leq 0.05$ (2-sided).

3. Results

We had a total of 75 patients with a mean age of 47 years (range: 20–76 years). 33 women were presenting for their yearly screening and 42 for diagnostic purposes (palpable breast/axillary mass, bloody nipple discharge, and breast pain). 66 (88%) patients obtained a mammogram, 71 (95%) patients obtained an ultrasound, and 6 (8%) patients had a MRI. Four (5.5%) patients had all 3 imaging modalities done, 62 (82.5%) patients had a mammogram and an ultrasound, and 2 (2.5%) patients had only a mammogram and an MRI. Mammography was performed as the initial examination in women above age of 40 presenting for screening or diagnostic purposes, followed by ultrasound for evaluation of suspicious findings or for screening in dense breasts. Ultrasound was the initial exam in women younger than 40, followed by mammography if suspicious findings were present. MRI was performed in 4 high risk patients (prior personal history of breast cancer, prior radiation to the chest, or positive family history for breast cancer), in 1 patient upon her specific request and was the initial test performed in another facility in one woman presenting to our institution for a biopsy.

3.1. Mammography Findings. Mammography findings are summarized in Table 1. The frequencies of the 4 breast densities were as follows: extremely dense, 47 (71%); heterogeneously dense, 7 (10.5%); scattered fibroglandular, 7 (10.5%); almost entirely fat, 5 (7.5%).

The most common finding on mammogram was calcifications which was present in 14 (21%) patients. Amorphous calcifications were demonstrated in 9 (64%) patients. The rest of the morphologies were seen each in a single patient: punctate, pleomorphic, coarse heterogeneous, round, and linear. Concerning their distribution, calcifications were

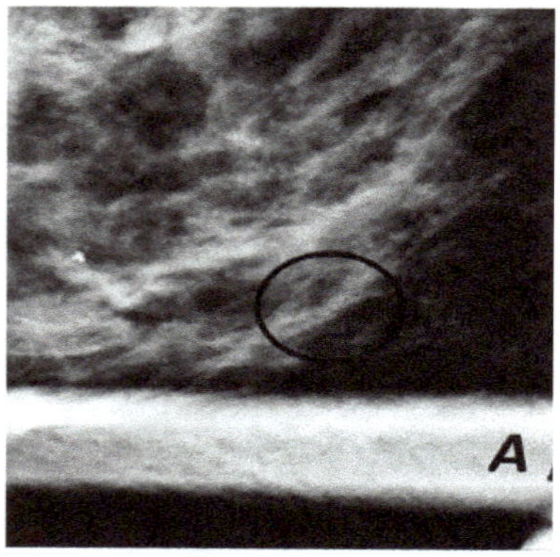

(a)

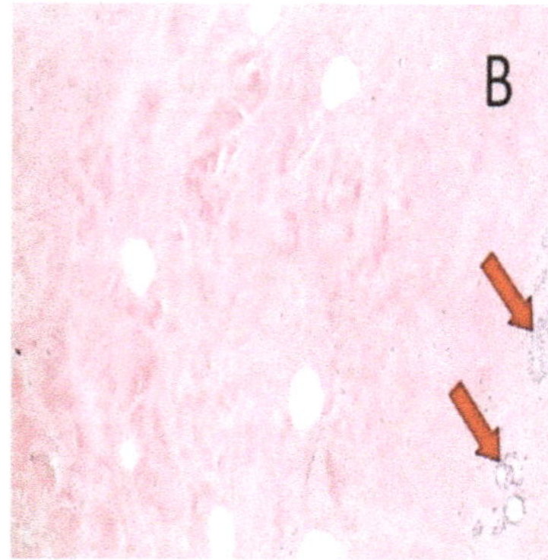

(b)

FIGURE 1: 57-year-old woman presenting for screening mammography. (a) Spot magnification view of the right breast in mediolateral position shows segmental amorphous calcifications. A follow-up mammogram was obtained 7 months following the biopsy showing stable appearance. (b) H&E stain of the biopsied tissue shows dense collagenous stroma with rare entrapped fat cells and involuted entrapped ducts (arrows).

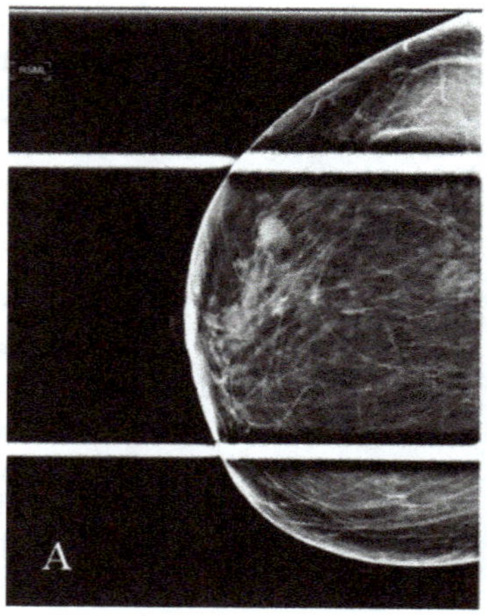

(a)

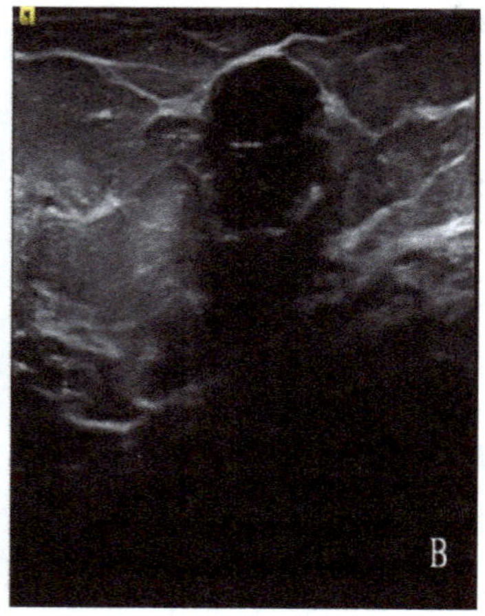

(b)

FIGURE 2: 53-year-old woman presenting for evaluation of a palpable mass. (a) Spot compression view at the site of the palpable abnormality shows an oval circumscribed equal density mass. (b) Ultrasound confirms an oval circumscribed hypoechoic mass with parallel orientation. A biopsy was recommended in view of the new palpable finding. The mass remained stable at follow-up after 18 months.

grouped in 10 (71.5%) patients, segmental in 2 (14.5%) patients (Figure 1(a)), diffuse in one patient, and regional in another. Furthermore, a mass was seen in 11 (17%) patients. The smallest mass detected had the dimensions of 8x5mm, while the largest mass was 40x44x25mm. The most common shape was an oval (Figure 2(a)), while it was irregular in one patient and round in another. Most of the masses detected were circumscribed; however, the margin of the mass was obscured in 3 (27%) patients and indistinct in 2 (18%) patients. Architectural distortion (Figure 3) was detected in 2 (3%) patients. The mammogram was negative in 39 patients.

3.2. Ultrasound Findings. The most common finding on ultrasound was a mass which was present in 61 (86%) patients (characteristics summarized in Table 2). The smallest mass detected was 3mm, while the largest mass had the dimensions of 41x44x21mm. The most common shape was oval which was seen in 33 (54%) patients. An irregular mass was seen in 24 (39%) patients (Figure 4(a)), while a round mass was seen in 4 (6.5%) patients. Most of the masses detected were circumscribed which was detected in 18 (29.5%) patients. Indistinct and irregular margins were detected in an equal number of 15 (24.5%) patients. Microlobulated margins were detected in 9 (15%) patients, while angular margins (Figure 5) were detected in 4 (6.5%) patients only. In addition, we had various echo patterns; a hypoechoic mass was the most common (Figure 2(b)). Other patterns observed were as follows: heterogeneous, isoechoic, and complex cystic-solid masses. Moreover, 2 masses were intracystic. Most masses did not have a posterior acoustic feature. However, posterior shadowing was seen in 15 (24.5%) patients and posterior enhancement was seen in 2 (3.5%) patients. Furthermore, calcifications were seen in 5 (8%) patients. The remainder of the patients had no ultrasound findings.

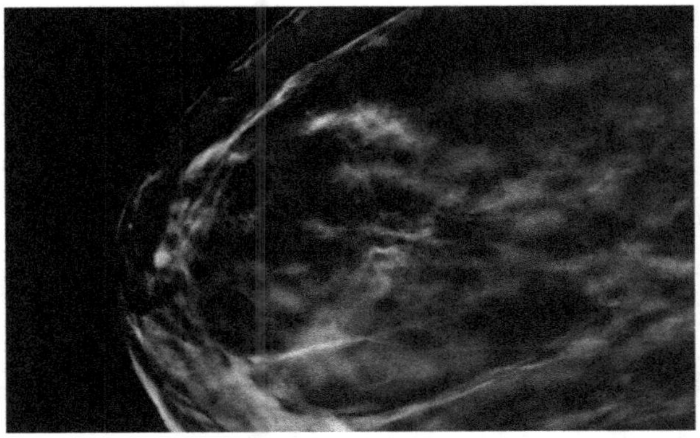

FIGURE 3: 72-year-old woman presenting for a screening mammography. Cropped image from a tomosynthesis view of the right breast in mediolateral oblique position showing an area of architectural distortion. The biopsy revealed stromal fibrosis. Surgical excision was performed and the final surgical pathology also confirmed stromal fibrosis.

TABLE 2: Mass characteristics on ultrasound.

Mass Characteristics	Number of lesions
Shape	
Oval	33
Round	4
Irregular	24
Margin	
Circumscribed	18
Indistinct	15
Irregular	15
Microlobulated	9
Angular	4
Echo Pattern	
Hypoechoic	54
Heterogeneous	4
Complex cystic	2
Isoechoic	1
Posterior Features	
Shadowing	15
Enhancement	2
None	44
Total	*61*

3.3. MRI Findings. MRI findings are summarized in Table 3. A mass was detected on MRI in 2 (33.5%) patients with dimensions of 7x4mm and 11x7mm. One mass was oval while the other was irregular in shape. Both mass margins were irregular. One mass had an enhancing rim while the other was homogenous. The last patient with a prior history of contralateral breast cancer had negative MRI finding. Clumped segmental nonmass enhancement (Figure 6) was detected in 3 (50%) patients. Three patients had kinetic curve I. Kinetic curves II and III were seen in one patient each.

3.4. Pathology Results and Follow-Up. The pathology reports read stromal fibrosis (Figures 1(b) and 4(b)) for all the patients except for one which read fibrous mastopathy. The selected cases show a similar array of histopathologic findings. These include dense stromal fibrosis (as opposed to the normal loose collagenous mammary stroma found in unaffected breast parenchyma), paucity of lobular units within the fibrous areas, and occasionally entrapped fat cells. The fibrous areas also characteristically include small capillary-sized vessels. Epithelioid fibroblasts such as the ones present in diabetic mastopathy were not seen in these cases. Also, the fibrous areas tended to interface with normal appearing breast stroma in some of the tissue-rich core biopsies. We had a follow-up for 53 (71%) patients with an average follow-up interval of 28.5 months (range: 5 – 70). 46 patients (87%) had a stable lesion with no interval history of malignancy. Four (7.5%) patients had a decrease in the size of the lesion, while 2 (4%) other patients had an increase in size. Finally, we had one patient who had a total ipsilateral mastectomy in another hospital before presenting back to us 5 months later. The indication that led the patient to undergo a surgery and the resulting pathology are unknown. As for the patients who had an increase in lesion size, their lesions were biopsied once again. The pathology report read fibroadenoma for one patient and stromal fibrosis for the other.

On chi-square test, the higher detection rate of a mass on ultrasound was statistically significant ($p<0.001$) in comparison to that of mammography. There was no significant difference in detecting calcifications ($p=1.000$) between the same imaging modalities.

4. Discussion

The pathogenesis of stromal fibrosis remains unknown. However, the theory of a hormonal role has gained support by previous studies whereby patients were almost exclusively premenopausal [3, 8]. However, similar to Taskin et al. [9] who reported a high percentage of 33% of postmenopausal women with stromal fibrosis, 25% of patients in our study were postmenopausal. This does not rule out a possible hormonal role; nevertheless, other explanations ought to be pursued. Furthermore, only 16% of the lesions detected were palpable. This is resonated in other studies where nonpalpable lesions make up 65%-100% of the cases [1, 10, 11]. This may be primarily due to increased utilization of breast ultrasound and MRI for breast cancer screening whereby lesions are being detected before they increase in size and become palpable.

The imaging features of stromal fibrosis are not specific and variable. On mammography, the most common finding in our study was calcifications followed by that of a mass although this did not reach statistical significance, unlike other studies which report mass lesion as the most common mammographic abnormality [4, 6, 9]. In fact, Harvey et al. [3] had a sample of 15 lesions where none of the lesions had calcifications. Most lesions we encountered had probably benign findings such as masses with circumscribed margins. Few lesions had findings more worrisome for malignancy such as architectural distortion, irregular masses with indistinct

TABLE 3: MRI findings.

Mass Characteristics	Number of lesions	Non-Mass Characteristics	Number of lesions
Shape		*Distribution*	
Oval	1	Segmental	3
Irregular	1		
Margin		*Internal Enhancement Pattern*	
Irregular	2	Clumped	3
Internal enhancement			
Rim enhancement	1		
Homogeneous	1		
Total	2	*Total*	3

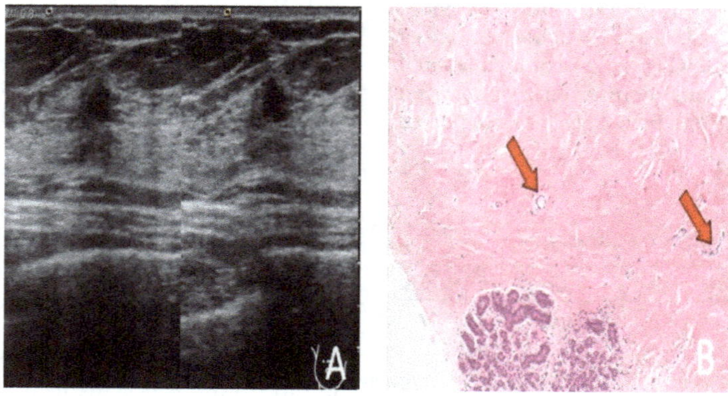

(a) (b)

FIGURE 4: 41-year-old woman presenting for screening. Mammography (not shown) demonstrated heterogeneously dense breast with no suspicious abnormality. (a) Screening ultrasound shows a hypoechoic mass with irregular shape and margin. The patient was lost to follow-up after the biopsy. (b) Dense fibrous stroma with small capillaries (arrows) and adjacent appearing lobular units.

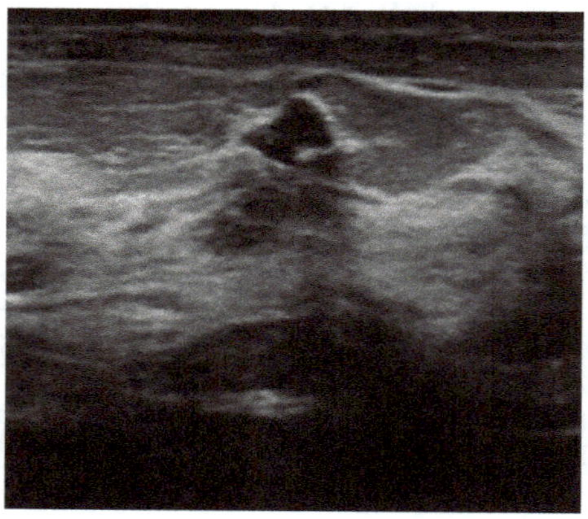

FIGURE 5: 40-year-old woman presenting for screening mammography and ultrasound. Mammography (not shown) revealed dense breasts and no focal lesions. Ultrasound showed a hypoechoic mass with angular margins. Biopsy shows stromal fibrosis. Follow-up after two years showed no malignancy.

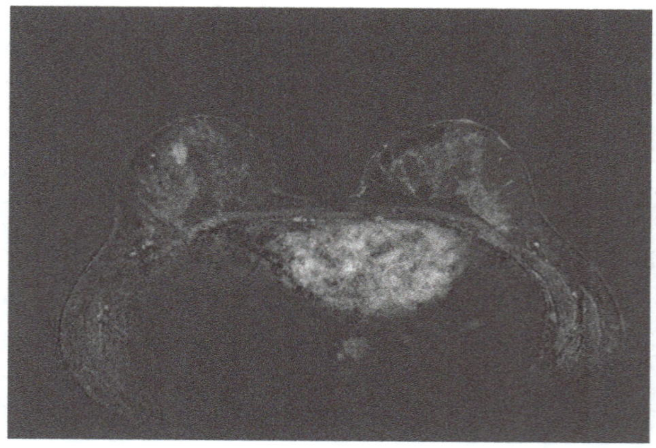

FIGURE 6: 33-year-old high risk woman (prior history of irradiation to the chest). Screening MRI shows a focal nonmass enhancement in the right breast. Biopsy shows stromal fibrosis. Initial follow-up MRI after 6 months shows stable appearance. Further screening MRI scans show slight regression in size.

margins, and pleomorphic calcifications with a segmental distribution. Other studies have documented suspicious findings such as spiculated masses more frequently within their sample [9]. On ultrasound, though a well-defined mass was the most common finding, a big proportion of lesions presented as irregular masses with irregular, microlobulated, or angular margins. The masses presented with various echo patterns, namely, hypoechoic, heterogeneous, isoechoic, and complex cystic-solid. Although most masses had no posterior acoustic features, 24.5% of the lesions had posterior shadowing. Similar ultrasound findings were reported in other studies [1, 4, 6, 9]. A higher detection rate of mass lesions on ultrasound was found to be statistically significant when compared to mammography. This could primarily be due to the fact that 81.5% of our patients had dense breasts which could limit mammography.

All lesions detected on MRI had findings suspicious for malignancy. Three lesions presented with clumped segmental nonmass enhancement. Two other mass lesions had irregular margins. One of those lesions was an irregular mass with rim enhancement. Lee et al. [11] had a larger sample of cases that had undergone MRI where most lesions presented as masses unlike our findings where nonmass enhancements were most common. However, similarly to our study, most nonmass lesions presented with clumped enhancement.

Our study has the second longest follow-up for stromal fibrosis lesions in the literature to date with a mean of 28.5 months (range: 5–70). No false negatives are to be reported. None of the patients had an interval history of malignancy. On follow-up, only 2 patients had an increase in lesion size which upon rebiopsy had pathology results that read stromal fibrosis for one and fibroadenoma for the other. Jai Kyung et al. have also demonstrated lesion size stability and/or decrease over a 2-year follow-up period with no false negatives [12]. Similarly, no false negatives were noted by Rosen et al. [4] and Harvey et al. [3] who reported rebiopsy of lesions increasing in size, proven again to be benign (focal fibrosis and fibroadenoma respectively). No false negatives were reported by Lee et al. [11] in his series of 40 cases of stromal fibrosis detected on MRI. The false negatives reported in the literature are related to either sampling error as noted by Sklair-Levy et al. [1] who describe two cases of invasive carcinoma mistakenly labeled as stromal fibrosis and to radiological-pathological discordance according to Malik et al. [13] who reported a false negative rate of 7%.

A limitation of this study is the relatively small sample size that resulted from the inclusion criteria. In addition, we had lost 22 patients to follow-up.

5. Conclusion

Although stromal fibrosis is most likely to occur as an ultrasound detected mass, this study has not identified a characteristic imaging appearance. In fact, stromal fibrosis may demonstrate a wide array of radiological phenotypes on mammography, ultrasound, and MRI, displaying features ranging from benign to suspicious for malignancy. In the case of accurate targeted biopsy, when stromal fibrosis is diagnosed, the result can be safely considered concordant. It is currently recommended that these patients undergo a follow-up ultrasound for documentation of benignity. Our study parallels several others that show no false negative results upon follow-up. In light of this reproducible finding across several studies, larger studies are needed in order to reconsider the need for short-term follow-up ultrasound after diagnosis of stromal fibrosis.

References

[1] M. Sklair-Levy, T. H. Samuels, C. Catzavelos, P. Hamilton, and R. Shumak, "Stromal fibrosis of the breast," *American Journal of Roentgenology*, vol. 177, no. 3, pp. 573–577, 2001.

[2] P. P. Rosen, *Rosen's Breast Pathology*, Lippincott-Raven, Philadelphia, PA, USA, 1997.

[3] S. C. Harvey, C. M. Denison, S. C. Lester, P. J. DiPiro, D. N. Smith, and J. E. Meyer, "Fibrous nodules found at large-core needle biopsy of the breast: Imaging features," *Radiology*, vol. 211, no. 2, pp. 535–540, 1999.

[4] E. L. Rosen, M. S. Soo, and R. C. Bentley, "Focal fibrosis: A common breast lesion diagnosed at imaging-guided core biopsy," *American Journal of Roentgenology*, vol. 173, no. 6, pp. 1657–1662, 1999.

[5] D. D. Dershaw, E. A. Morris, L. Liberman, and A. F. Abramson, "Nondiagnostic stereotaxic core breast biopsy: Results of rebiopsy," *Radiology*, vol. 198, no. 2, pp. 323–325, 1996.

[6] L. A. Venta, E. L. Wiley, H. Gabriel, and Y. T. Adler, "Imaging features of focal breast fibrosis: Mammographic-pathologic correlation of noncalcified breast lesions," *American Journal of Roentgenology*, vol. 173, no. 2, pp. 309–316, 1999.

[7] B. Bullier, G. MacGrogan, H. Bonnefoi et al., "Imaging features of sporadic breast cancer in women under 40 years old: 97 cases," *European Radiology*, vol. 23, no. 12, pp. 3237–3245, 2013.

[8] J. M. Rivera-Pomar, J. R. Vilanova, J. J. Burgos-Bretones, and G. Arocena, "Focal fibrous disease of breast," *Virchows Archiv*, vol. 386, no. 1, pp. 59–64, 1980.

[9] F. Taskin, A. Unsal, S. Ozbas, M. Erkus, and C. Karaman, "Fibrotic lesions of the breast: Radiological findings and core-neddle biopsy results," *European Journal of Radiology*, vol. 80, no. 3, pp. e231–e236, 2011.

[10] G. Revelon, M. E. Sherman, O. M. B. Gatewood, and R. F. Brem, "Focal fibrosis of the breast: imaging characteristics and histopathologic correlation," *Radiology*, vol. 216, no. 1, pp. 255–259, 2000.

[11] S.-J. Lee, M. C. Mahoney, and S. Khan, "MRI features of stromal fibrosis of the breast with histopathologic correlation," *American Journal of Roentgenology*, vol. 197, no. 3, pp. 755–762, 2011.

[12] J. K. You, E.-K. Kim, J. Y. Kwak et al., "Focal fibrosis of the breast diagnosed by a sonographically guided core biopsy of nonpalpable lesions: Imaging findings and clinical relevance," *Journal of Ultrasound in Medicine*, vol. 24, no. 10, pp. 1377–1384, 2005.

[13] N. Malik, S. Lad, J. M. Seely, and M. E. Schweitzer, "Underestimation of malignancy in biopsy-proven cases of stromal fibrosis," *British Journal of Radiology*, vol. 87, no. 1039, Article ID 20140182, 2014.

21

Ketamine Use in Hysterosalpingography (the Jimah Procedure): A Follow-Up of Bilateral Tubal Evaluation of 27 Infertile Women at a Teaching Hospital, Ghana

Bashiru Babatunde Jimah,[1] **Anthony Baffour Appiah**,[2] **Benjamin Dabo Sarkodie**,[3] **and Dorothea Anim**[4]

[1]*Department of Medical Imaging, School of Medical Sciences, University of Cape Coast, Cape Coast, Ghana*
[2]*Ghana Field Epidemiology and Laboratory Training Programme, University of Ghana, Accra, Ghana*
[3]*Department of Radiology, University of Ghana, School of Medicine Sciences, Accra, Ghana*
[4]*Department of Radiology, Korle Bu Teaching Hospital, Accra, Ghana*

Correspondence should be addressed to Bashiru Babatunde Jimah; jimah@uccsms.edu.gh

Academic Editor: Lorenzo Faggioni

Background. Pain, anxiety, and distress are common in radiological investigations including hysterosalpingogram (HSG). Studies suggest that sedation allows patients to better tolerate diagnostic imaging and image-guided procedures by relieving anxiety, discomfort, and pain. This study aimed at assessing the safety and effectiveness of ketamine use in HSG and the proportion of true positive bilateral tubal blockage during HSG using the Jimah Procedure. *Methods.* We performed repeated HSG workup under IV ketamine (20–40 mg/mL) sedation for 27 infertile women at the Cape Coast Teaching Hospital. The exclusion criteria included unilateral tubular blockage, acute infection of the vagina or cervix, active vaginal bleeding, glaucoma, and high blood pressure at the time of the study. Data were entered with Microsoft Excel and analyzed using SPSS version 21. *Results.* A total of 27 patients (age range: 25–48 years) previously diagnosed of bilateral tubal blockage or spasm were enrolled for the repeat HSG procedure. The median age was 34 years (IQR: 32–37), while secondary infertility (20) (74.1%) was the commonest indication. None of the patients reported of pain or distress during or after the procedure. Two (7.4%) women vomited after HSG. Twelve patients (44.4%) had bilateral tubal blockage (true positive), while tubal patency was seen in 15 (55.6%) patients on HSG under ketamine sedation. *Conclusion.* This study found IV ketamine sedation produces profound anesthesia and analgesia and eliminates tubal spasm. We recommend that radiologists in developing countries should consider sedating patients during HSG and documenting observations and patients' feedback to help assess safety and effectiveness in local settings.

1. Introduction

Pain, anxiety, and psychological and physical distress are likened to radiological investigations including hysterosalpingogram (HSG) [1–3]. These complications can be ameliorated by the use of sedation and analgesia [1]. Although HSG is noninvasive, patients' anxiety and psychological and physical distress might interfere with the procedure and subsequent outcome [1, 2]. However, sedation in HSG procedures is rare in low-middle-income countries (LMICs) as many radiologists consider it as noninvasive [3]. For instance, sedation under HSG recorded the lowest proportion (8.5%) compared to computed tomography (CT) (65.3%), magnetic resonance imaging (MRI) (63.6%), and interventional radiology (16.1%) practices among Nigerian radiology residents [3]. Little information exists on the use of sedation in HSG procedure in Sub-Saharan Africa and Ghana. This finding suggests that radiologists are not sedating their patients during HSG or failing to document local experience to inform practice. Studies suggest that sedation allows patients to better tolerate diagnostic imaging and image-guided procedures by relieving anxiety, discomfort, and pain [1–3].

The commonest indication for HSG is infertility, usually to examine the fallopian tubes and uterine cavities [2, 4–8]. Tubal blockage is the commonest abnormality seen during HSG [2, 4, 8]. A prior study to assess the spectrum of findings on HSG in 203 women with infertility [4] revealed that forty-four (51.3%) women with abnormalities had fallopian tube blockage including bilateral blockage, right unilateral proximal blockage, and left unilateral proximal blockage. To confirm these findings, the procedure was repeated under ketamine sedation for some patients using strict inclusion and exclusion criteria to ascertain the incidence of true bilateral tubal blockage.

Ketamine hydrochloride is a dissociative anesthetic agent. It is rapidly acting and produces profound anesthesia and analgesia [9]. The half life of ketamine is 45 minutes.

It has dissociative action and partial agonism on opiate receptors, permitting the performance of painful procedures in a consistent state of sedation and patient comfort [9]. Ketamine also relieves patients' anxiety and minor psychological and physical distress, as documented in previous studies [10, 11]. Common side effects of ketamine include nausea, vomiting, dizziness, diplopia, drowsiness, dysphoria, and confusion [9].

But World Health Organisation document reveals that chronic use of ketamine is commonly associated with slurred speech, dizziness, blurred vision, palpitations, chest pain, vomiting, and insomnia [12] and, hence, use with caution.

We hypothesized that administration of IV ketamine produces anesthesia and analgesia and relieves tubal spasm. We determined the safety and effectiveness of ketamine and the proportion of true positive bilateral tubal blockage during HSG under ketamine sedation.

2. Subjects and Methods

2.1. Study Design. This is a cross-sectional study involving 27 women (aged 25–48 years), undergoing repeated HSG under ketamine sedation for bilateral tubal blockage over 2 years (January 2018 to December 2020) at the Department of Imaging, Cape Coast Teaching Hospital, Ghana. This represents 13.3% of the 203 women who presented for the HSG procedure and were initially diagnosed with bilateral tubal blockage. The initial study [4] involving 203 women underwent the traditional method of performing HSG in Ghana, which does not include ketamine sedation. The 27 patients, thus, had the new procedure called the "Jimah procedure" which is a modified version of the traditional procedure and involves IV ketamine use.

2.2. Inclusion Criteria

(1) Diagnosis of infertility (primary or secondary)

(2) HSG diagnosis of bilateral tubal blockage

2.3. Exclusion Criteria

(1) Women with acute infection of the vagina or cervix

(2) Women with active vaginal bleeding

(3) High blood pressure at the time of the procedure

(4) Glaucoma

(5) Allergy to contrast medium or ketamine

2.4. The Jimah Procedure: "Modified Traditional HSG Procedure". Prior to the procedure, informed consent was obtained from each patient. Blood pressure, pulse, respiratory rate, and oxygen saturation were documented. Known allergies and underlying chronic conditions were documented. Patients were asked to abstain from alcohol from the start of their menstrual cycle. HSG was performed in the preovulatory phase of the menstrual cycle as an outpatient procedure between the 5th and 10th day of the menstrual cycle. The patients were placed in lithotomy position. The vulva was cleaned with antiseptic solution. Vaginal speculum was passed to visualize the cervix. Uterine sound was used to assess the patency of the cervical canal. Intravenous ketamine was administered until the patient's pulse begins to increase, at which point the patient becomes unresponsive. The dosage of ketamine and initial and final finger pulse were recorded. *It is important to visualize the cervix and assess its patency prior to sedation because, in certain situations, the cervix may not be visualised and/or there may be severe cervical canal stenosis, making it difficult to cannulate the cervical canal.* The cervical cannula was inserted after air bubbles have been expelled. Approximately 10–20 ml of water-soluble contrast medium (iopamidol) was injected manually through the cannula under fluoroscopic guidance. Two supine hysterograms were taken. The first image was obtained during the early filling of the uterus and used to evaluate any filling defects or uterine contour abnormality. The second image was taken with the uterus and fallopian tubes fully distended and free intraperitoneal spillage of contrast material seen. An oblique hysterogram was taken in uncertain cases, and no delayed images were taken. The recovery time was between 40 and 60 minutes. Patients are advised not to drive or use heavy machinery for the next twenty-four hours.

2.5. Data Analysis and Interpretation of HSG. Patient's demographic information and HSG findings were entered into Microsoft Excel and later exported with Statistical Package for the Social Sciences (IBM SPSS version 21) for the analysis. Data were summarized with descriptive statistics using median (interquartile range, IQR), frequencies, and percentages. Fisher's exact test was used to assess the association between age group of women and HSG findings at a p value <0.05.

HSG is considered normal when there is a free flow of contrast medium into the peritoneal cavity and normal uterine outline. HSG was considered abnormal when there was evidence of either unilateral or bilateral tubal obstruction or uterine cavity abnormality [4].

2.6. Ethical Considerations. This study was approved by Ethical Review Committee of the Cape Coast Teaching Hospital (CCTHERC). Written informed consent was obtained after the nature of the study was adequately explained to the clients. Clients were assured of data security and confidentiality.

3. Results

3.1. Demographic and Clinical Presentation of Women. In total, 27 patients (age range: 25–48 years) were enrolled for repeated HSG workup under 20–40 mg IV ketamine sedation with a diagnosis of bilateral tubal blockage or tubal spasm. The characteristics of the 27 patients are shown in Table 1. The median age was 34 years (IQR: 32–37). Most of them aged between 25 and 34 years 14 (51.9%), had secondary infertility 20 (74.1%), and received 20 mg of IV ketamine 18 (66.7%). The median baseline pulse rate was 65 bpm (IQR: 64–67) which increased after IV ketamine sedation (98 bpm) (IQR: 95–100). None of the patients complained of pain during or after the procedure, but 2 (7.4%) patients experienced vomiting after administering IV ketamine.

3.2. Follow-Up HSG Findings under Ketamine Sedation. In Figure 1, the distribution of tubal findings on HSG among 27 infertile women is summarized. Bilateral tubular blockage was seen in 12 (44.4%), while tubular patency was seen 15 (55.6%) on HSG under ketamine sedation.

The distribution of HSG findings by age group of infertile women is shown in Table 2. Bilateral tubal patency was commonly diagnosed among women aged 25–34 years (80%). Most women with bilateral tubal blockage were more than 35 years old (58.3%). All the uterine fibroids (3) (100.0) were seen among women aged 35 years and above. Only uterine findings were significantly associated with the age group of the women ($p = 0.041$).

The proportion of true positive bilateral tubal blockage among the 27 women was 44.4% ($n = 12$) (Table 3).

4. Discussion

Hysterosalpingography (HSG) is a frequently utilized diagnostic procedure to assess tubal patency and intrauterine anatomical defects in the infertility workup. However, tubal spasm, pain, anxiety, and distress interfere with patients' cooperation and outcome of the procedure [1–3]. This study involved twenty-seven women previously diagnosed of bilateral tubal blockage or spasm on HSG. Most of the women were within the third decade (25–34 years) (51.9%). Secondary infertility was the commonest indication (74.1%). True bilateral tubal blockage was reported among twelve (44.4%) women. None of the patients reported pain or distress during the repeat procedure, but two (7.4%) of the women experienced ketamine-induced vomiting.

There is limited literature on the safety and effectiveness of ketamine use in HSG workup in Sub-Saharan Africa. This outlines the essence of documentation and reporting of local experience of performing HSG under ketamine sedation at the Cape Coast Teaching Hospital.

The WHO 36th Expert Committee on Drug Dependence (ECDD) documented evidence on the pharmacodynamics of ketamine which showed that IV ketamine has the potential to cause changes in heart rate, cardiac output, and blood pressure [12]. The safety and effectiveness of ketamine to sedate prehospital and emergency department (ED) patients with undifferentiated agitation have been reported in a systematic review and meta-analysis [13]. Likewise, there have been several reports on ketamine use in clinical procedures and trials among children and adolescents in developed countries [11, 14–20].

In this study, intravenous ketamine sedation was generally safe and effective in alleviating pain and stress [3, 11, 13, 21, 22]. Severe pain was reported (pain score >8) in the earlier HSG procedure without ketamine sedation. None of the patient's complained of pain during the repeat with ketamine. No tubal spasm was diagnosed as compared to the previous procedure.

Nonetheless, like previous study [13], we found that two of our patients had ketamine-induced vomiting, which is a known common side effect. Previous study reported no adverse effect with ketamine use during biopsies [16]. Only few studies have reported some adverse effects of ketamine for moderate-to high-invasive procedures in children [11].

Without sedation, bilateral tubal blockage could be due to tubal spasm [6]. Similar to a previous study by Jimah et al. [4], bilateral tubal blockage was the commonest tubal abnormality seen in this study. However, injection of IV ketamine led to high incidence of tubal patency among the studied patients.

Compared with the previous study, HSG under ketamine sedation has moderate sensitivity but relatively high specificity. This was seen in the current study where the proportion of tubal patency was 55.6% (false positive) and bilateral tubal blockage was 44.4% (true positive). The false positive indicates that more than half of our patients were hitherto misdiagnosed as bilateral tubal blockage due to pain. Compared to a study done in Benin Republic, the proportion of tubal patency was twice higher [7]. Generally, this implies that sedating patients during HSG produces a more accurate fallopian tubal finding [6]. Potentially, failure to sedate patients for HSG can lead to misdiagnosis of tubal patency as blockage due to cornual spasm. These findings support the hypothesis that administration of IV ketamine reduces tubal spasm and enhances evaluation of tubal conditions. The challenge in implementing this new procedure in most developing countries is monitoring patients after procedure. Most radiology departments do not have dedicated recovery wards. However, critical assessment can identify unused spaces that can be converted to fit such a purpose.

Common limitation seen in this study is inadequate sample size, bilateral tubal blockage is rare, and only one of the tertiary hospitals in Ghana was involved. Therefore, the study findings might not be a true incident of bilateral tubal blockage among infertile women in Ghana. There is no local standard operation procedures (SOPs) on ketamine used in radiologic procedures. However, this study has provided preliminary data to inform radiology practice in the local setting and provided a new method for performing HSG in Ghana.

Table 1: Characteristics of patients undergoing ketamine sedation for HSG.

Characteristics	Frequency, $N = 27$	Percentage (%)
Age (years)		
Median (IQR)	34 (32–37)	—
25–34	14	51.9
≥35	13	48.1
Indication		
Primary infertility	7	25.9
Secondary infertility	20	74.1
Dosage of Ketamine		
Median (IQR)	20 (20–30)	—
20 mg/mL	18	66.7
30 mg/mL	4	14.8
40 mg/mL	5	18.5
Pulse rate before sedation		
Median (IQR)	65 (64–67)	—
<60 bpm	1	3.7
60–100 bpm	26	96.3
>100 bpm	0	0.0
Pulse rate when unresponsive		
Median (IQR)	98 (95–100)	—
<60 bpm	0	0.0
60–100 bpm	23	85.2
>100 bpm	4	14.8
Pain associated with first HSG		
No	0	0.0
Yes	27	100.0
Pain score associated with first HSG		
9	8	29.6
10	19	70.4
Pain associated with follow-up HSG under ketamine		
No	27	100.0
Yes	0	0.0
Complication associated with ketamine use		
None	25	92.6
Vomiting	2	7.4

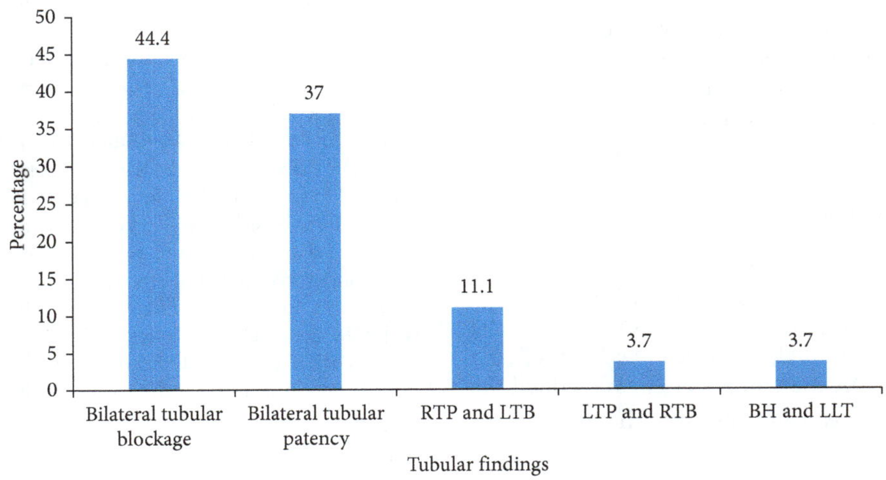

Figure 1: Distribution of tubal finding on HSG among 27 infertile women under ketamine sedation. RTP: right tubal patency; LTB: left tubal blockage; RTB: right tubal blockage; LTP: left tubal patency; BH: bilateral hydrosalpinx; LLT: leakage left tube.

Table 2: Distribution of HSG findings by the age group of infertile women under ketamine sedation.

HSG findings	Age group		Fisher's exact test
	25–34 years	≥35 years	*p* value
Tubal findings			
Bilateral tubal blockage	5 (41.7)	7 (58.3)	
Bilateral tubal patency	8 (80.0)	2 (20.0)	0.124
RTP, LTB	1 (33.3)	2 (66.7)	
LTP, RTB	0 (0.0)	1 (100.0)	
BH, LLT	0 (0.0)	1 (100.0)	
Uterine findings			
Fibroid	0 (0.0)	3 (100.0)	
Normal	14 (60.9)	9 (39.1)	0.041*
Irregular/postsurgery	0 (0.0)	1 (100.0)	

*Significant level at $p \leq 0.05$. RTP: right tubal patency; LTP: left tubal patency; LTB: left tubal blockage; RTB: right tubal blockage; BH: bilateral hydrosalpinx; LLT: leakage left tube.

Table 3: True positive HSG diagnosis (bilateral tubal blockage).

Bilateral blockage	Initial HSG (A)	Follow-up HSG (B)
Positive	27 (100.0)	12 (44.4%)#
Negative	0 (0.0)	15 (55.6%)
Total	27 (100.0)	27 (100.0)

#Proportion of true positive bilateral tubal blockage. A: HSG procedure without ketamine sedation. B: repeated HSG procedure under ketamine sedation.

5. Conclusion

This study found that intravenous ketamine sedation produces profound anesthesia and analgesia and eliminates tubal spasm. Administration of ketamine helps reveal false tubal blockage observed on HSG without sedation. Patients with true tubal blockage can undergo tubal recanalization. We recommend that radiologists in developing countries should consider sedating patients during HSG and documenting observations and patients' feedback to help assess safety and effectiveness in local settings.

Authors' Contributions

BJJ conceptualized the topic, designed the protocol, performed all the HSG procedures, interpreted HSG findings, and drafted and edited the manuscript. ABA analyzed the data and interpreted, drafted, reviewed, and edited the manuscript. BDS and DA drafted, reviewed, and edited the manuscript. All authors read and approved the final version of the manuscript.

Acknowledgments

The authors wish to acknowledge the contributions of Priscilla Laryea, Isaac Dapaah, Dr. Mohammed Owusu Ansah, Althea Mannah, Anudjo Messiah Kwame, Kortor Setor Nicholas, and Samuel Oduro for their participation in the performance of the HSG procedures.

References

[1] The Royal College of Radiologists, *Sedation, Analgesia and Anaesthesia in the Radiology Department*, The Royal College of Radiologists, London, UK, Second edition, 2018.

[2] A. O. Akintomide, D. U. Eduwem, A. A. Ikpeme, and D. E. Bassey, "Tubal assessment with hysterosalpingography following routine intravenous buscopan: a need to avoid unnecessary radiation and discomfort," *IOSR Journal of Dental and Medical Science*, vol. 15, no. 7, pp. 75–81, 2016.

[3] A. D. Omisore, A. T. Adenekan, O. O. Ayoola, A. M. Owojuyigbe, and B. I. Afolabi, "Sedation practice among Nigerian radiology residents," *Southern African Journal of Anaesthesia and Analgesia*, vol. 22, no. 5, pp. 145–150, 2016.

[4] B. B. Jimah, P. Gorleku, and A. B. Appiah, "Hysterosalpingography findings and jimah ratio of the uterine cavity in women with infertility in central region, Ghana," *Radiology Research and Practice*, vol. 2020, Article ID 6697653, 7 pages, 2020.

[5] S. Chen, X. Du, Q. Chen, and S. Chen, "Combined real-time three-dimensional hysterosalpingo-contrast sonography with B mode hysterosalpingo-contrast sonography in the evaluation of fallopian tube patency in patients undergoing infertility investigations," *BioMedical Research International*, vol. 2019, Article ID 9408141, 7 pages, 2019.

[6] G. Goynumer, G. Yetim, O. Gokcen, I. Karaaslan, L. Wetherilt, and B. Durukan, "Hysterosalpingography, laparoscopy or both in the diagnosis of tubal disease in infertility," *World Journal of Laparoscopic Surgery with DVD*, vol. 1, no. 2, pp. 23–26, 2008.

[7] M. Ogoudjobi, A. Obossou, V. King, I. Takpara, E. Alihonou, and C. Tshabu-Aguemon, "Hysterosalpingography and laparoscopy in evaluating fallopian tubes in the management of infertility in cotonou, Benin republic," *Journal of the West African College of Surgens*, vol. 4, no. 2, 2014.

[8] A. Idrisa, E. Ojiyi, and A. U. Hamidu, "Hysterosalpingography vs. laparoscopy in the evaluation of female infertility in Maiduguri, Nigeria," *Tropical Journal of Obstetrics Gynaecology*, vol. 20, no. 1, pp. 20–23, 2004.

[9] S. B. Rosenbaum, V. Gupta, and J. L. Palacios, *Ketamine*, StatPearls Publishing, Treasure Island, FL, USA, 2021.

[10] J. A. van de Bunt, S. E. Veldhoen, R. A. J. Nievelstein et al., "Effects of esketamine sedation compared to morphine analgesia on hydrostatic reduction of intussusception a case-cohort comparison study," *Pediatric Anesthesia*, vol. 27, no. 11, 2017.

[11] J. R. Grunwell, C. Travers, C. E. Mccracken et al., "Procedural sedation outside of the operating room using ketamine in 22,645 children," *Pediatric Critical Care Medicine*, vol. 17, no. 12, pp. 1109–1116, 2016.

[12] World Health Organization, "Ketamine: update review report agenda item 6.2," in *Proceedings of the Expert Committee on Drug Dependence Thirty-sixth Meeting Geneva*, pp. 1–45, World Health Organization, Geneva, Switzerland, June 2014, https://www.who.int/medicines/areas/quality_safety/6_2_Update.pdf.

[13] S. L. Mankowitz, P. Regenberg, J. Kaldan, and J. B. Cole, "Ketamine for rapid sedation of agitated patients in the prehospital and emergency department settings: a systematic review and proportional meta-analysis," *The Journal of Emergency Medicine*, vol. 55, no. 5, pp. 670–681, 2018.

[14] D. L. Reich and G. Silvay, "Ketamine: an update on the first twenty-five years of clinical experience," *Canadian Journal of Anaesthesia*, vol. 36, no. 2, pp. 186–197, 1989.

[15] S. A. Bergman, "Ketamine: review of its pharmacology and its use in pediatric anesthesia ketamnine," *Anesthesia Progress*, vol. 46, pp. 10–20, 1999.

[16] H. Padua, P. J. Fontaine, D. Zurakowski, and K. P. Mason, "Radiologist-supervised ketamine sedation for solid organ biopsies in children and adolescents," *The American Journal of Roentgenology*, vol. 192, pp. 1261–1265, 2009.

[17] J. C. Flores-González, A. Estalella-Mendoza, P. Rodríguez-Campoy, M. Saldaña-Valderas, and A. M. Lechuga-Sancho, "Topical pharyngeal lidocaine reduces respiratory adverse events during upper gastrointestinal endoscopies under ketamine sedation in children," *Pediatrics Drug*, vol. 21, 2019.

[18] K. P. Mason, E. Michna, J. A. DiNardo et al., "Evolution of a protocol for ketamine-induced sedation as an alternative to general anesthesia for interventional radiologic procedures in pediatric patients radiology," *Pediatric Imaging*, vol. 225, no. 2, 2002.

[19] H. S. Gomes, A. R. Miranda, K. A. Viana et al., "Intranasal sedation using ketamine and midazolam for pediatric dental treatment (NASO): study protocol for a randomized controlled trial," *Trials*, vol. 18, no. 1, pp. 1–15, 2017.

[20] D. A. Haas and D. G. Harper, "Ketmine: a review of its pharmacologic use in ambulatory anesthesia properties and use in ambulatory anesthesia." *Anesthia Progress*, vol. 39, pp. 61–68, 1992.

[21] J. T. Jensen, C. Hanna, S. Yao et al., "Blockade of tubal patency following transcervical administration of polidocanol foam: initial studies in rhesus macaques," *Contraception*, vol. 89, no. 6, pp. 540–549, 2014.

[22] The Royal Children's Hospital Melbourne, *Clinical Practice Guidelines Ketamine Use for Procedural Sedation*, The Royal Children's Hospital Melbourne, Parkville, Australia, 2019, https://www.rch.org.au/clinicalguide/guideline_index/Ketamine_use_for_procedural_sedation.

22

Hysterosalpingography Findings and Jimah Ratio of the Uterine Cavity in Women with Infertility in Central Region, Ghana

Bashiru Babatunde Jimah,[1] **Philip Gorleku**,[1] **and Anthony Baffour Appiah**[2]

[1]*Department of Medical Imaging, School of Medical Sciences, University of Cape Coast, Cape Coast, Ghana*
[2]*Ghana Field Epidemiology and Laboratory Training Programme, University of Ghana, Accra, Ghana*

Correspondence should be addressed to Bashiru Babatunde Jimah; jimah@uccsms.edu.gh

Academic Editor: Daniele La Forgia

Background. Infertility affects from 1.3% to 25.7% of couples worldwide and, especially, from 14.5% to 16.4% in Africa. Hysterosalpingography (HSG) is a diagnostic modality that is considered both common and efficient. It is used to investigate abnormalities of the uterine cavity and fallopian tubes. This study assessed the spectrum of findings on HSG among women with infertility in the Central Region (Ghana). *Methods.* We conducted a prospective cross-sectional study to examine 203 infertile women undergoing HSG work-up at the Cape Coast Teaching Hospital. The exclusion criteria were acute infection of the vagina or cervix and active vaginal bleeding or pregnancy. Data were entered with Microsoft Excel and analyzed using SPSS version 21. *Results.* A total of 203 women were enrolled, and eighty-five (41.87%) of the women had at least one or more abnormalities. The mean age was 32.9 years with majority of the women within 30–39 years (61.08%). More than half (50.74%) of the women presented with secondary infertility, while age of women ($p = 0.004$) and duration of infertility (0.034) were found to be in association with the type of infertility. Uterine findings were predominantly capacious uterine cavity (45.1%) and uterine fibroids (33.3%), while fallopian tube findings included bilateral blockage (24.2%), right unilateral proximal blockage (17.7%), loculated spillage (16.1%), and left unilateral proximal blockage (16.1%). The range of normal uterine cavity size, measured as ratio (*Jimah ratio*) of intercornual diameter to interiliac diameter was 0.2–0.45, with a mean of 0.36. *Conclusion.* Secondary infertility was the commonest indication for HSG in the study, and a significant proportion of infertile women had abnormalities. Abnormalities were higher in the fallopian tubes than the uterus, while capacious uterine cavity, uterine fibroid, and bilaterally blocked tubes were the top three abnormalities found.

1. Introduction

Infertility is a disease of the reproductive system defined by the failure to achieve a clinical pregnancy after 12 months or more of regular unprotected sexual intercourse [1, 2]. Generally, infertility can be primary or secondary. Primary infertility is defined as "the absence of pregnancy for a couple who desire a child after 12 months or more of regular unprotected sexual intercourse, during which they have not used any contraceptives [3]. Secondary infertility is defined as "the absence of a live birth for women who desire a child and have been in a union for at least five years since their last live birth, during which they did not use any contraceptives [3].

Infertility is a gynecological disorder with associated medical, psychological, and economic problems, and it affects 1.3% to 25.7% of couples worldwide [4, 5]. Infertility prevalence is highest in South Asia, sub-Saharan Africa, North Africa/Middle East, and Central/Eastern Europe and Central Asia [3]. Generally, the prevalence of secondary infertility is higher than primary infertility [3]. In sub-Saharan Africa, 14.5% to 16.4% of couples suffer from infertility, mostly secondary representing 52% [6, 7]. The prevalence of infertility in Ghana is 11.8% [6]. Wide range of factors have been linked to infertility [2, 8, 9], but tubal and uterine abnormalities are the most common causes of female infertility [6, 9–11]. Identified factors may be social, physical, and physiological, and these include but not limited to obesity, abuse of alcohol and tobacco, infections, history of either sexually transmitted diseases (STDs), or pregnancy complications, while orders are unexplained [2, 7–9, 12, 13].

Over the decades, the world has innovated lots of simple but effective diagnostic tools and techniques to identify the potential causes of infertility among couples. Ultrasonography (USG), computed tomography (CT), magnetic resonance imaging (MRI), hysteroscopy, laparoscopy, and hysterosalpingography (HSG) are widely used [14]. Hysterosalpingography is often the first investigation employed in female infertility. The technique uses a contrast medium to visualize the uterine cavity and fallopian tubes, hence able to infer tubal and uterine pathologies [2, 5, 15, 16].

Previous studies on HSG diagnostic outcome reported varied findings [4, 10, 11, 13, 17–22]. About 38% of Nigerian women subpopulation had tubal and uterine abnormalities, and these included tubal blockage (11.38%), uterine fibroid (5.52%), multiple myomata (1.72%), bilateral tubal adhesions (2.07%), uterine adhesions (8.28%), cervical adhesions (2.07%), cervicouterine adhesion (2.41%), hydrosalpinx with spillage (3.45%), and rotated uterus (0.69%) [17].

Another study in Nigeria revealed that 75% with tubal and uterine abnormalities, tubal occlusions (bilateral (14.0%), right (6.0%), and left (7.0%)), uterine fibroids (17.0%), and pelvic adhesion (12.0%) were the most common diagnosis [11]. A study in Iran also reported tubal abnormalities in women with primary and secondary infertility: hydrosalpinx (2.6% and 2.8%, respectively), tubal occlusion (4.7% and 9.8%, respectively), and limited passage of contrast media (2.8% and 3.6%, respectively) [23]. The only study in Ghana found 60.03% of women with various abnormalities, which includes tubal blockage (43.7%) (bilateral (20.5%), left (12.5%), and right (10.6%)) and fibroids (25.4%) [20].

The limited studies on HSG in Ghana indicate an urgent need to improve on data nationwide. This study assessed the spectrum of findings on hysterosalpingography (HSG) in women with infertility in the Central Region and proposed a method for estimating the size of the uterine cavity. The study will provide preliminary data to inform the practice of clinicians, radiologists, and other medical practitioners; add to knowledge of infertility among women in Ghana; and inform further research on infertility in women in the country.

2. Materials and Methods

2.1. Study Design. This cross-sectional study was conducted at the Department of Imaging of the Cape Coast Teaching Hospital within 8 months period (April to November 2017). Data were collected using semistructured questionnaires. HSG was performed by two radiologists.

2.2. Sample Size. A total of 300 women were estimated to attend the Department of Medical Imaging within the 8-month period. Sample size calculation was done using RAOSOFT sample size calculator, assuming minimum sample size for the study taking into consideration the holidays. We estimated 207 patients after including 5% nonrespondent rate.

2.3. Sampling Technique. We employed a consecutive sampling to enroll women attending the Department of Medical Imaging.

2.3.1. Inclusion Criteria. The inclusion criteria were as follows:

Diagnosis of infertility

2.3.2. Exclusion Criteria. The exclusion criteria were as follows:

(1) Women with acute infection of the vagina or cervix

(2) Women with active vaginal bleeding

(3) Pregnant women

2.4. Data Collection Procedure. HSG was performed in the preovulatory phase of the menstrual cycle as an outpatient procedure between the 5 and 10th day of the menstrual cycle. The suppository diclofenac (100 mg) was administered 30 minutes prior to the procedure. The patients were placed in the lithotomy position and cleaned, and vaginal speculum was passed to visualize the cervix. A cervical cannula was inserted after air bubbles have been expelled. Approximately 10–20 ml of a water-soluble contrast medium (iopamirol) was injected manually through the cannula under fluoroscopic guidance. Two supine hysterograms were taken. The first image was obtained during the early filling of the uterus and used to evaluate any filling defects or uterine contour abnormality. The second image was taken with the uterus and fallopian tubes fully distended and free intraperitoneal spillage of contrast material seen. An oblique hysterogram was taken in uncertain cases, and no delayed images were taken.

2.4.1. Data Analysis and Interpretation of HSG. Data were entered and analyzed using Statistical Package for Social Sciences (IBM SPSS version 21). We described the data in frequencies, proportions, and mean with standard deviation. Test of statistical association was done using the chi-square test and one-way analysis of variance (ANOVA). All statistical associations were considered significant at p value ≤ 0.05. HSG is considered normal when both tubes were well outlined by the free flow of contrast medium, without loculation in the peritoneal cavity and normal uterine outline. HSG was considered abnormal when there was evidence of either unilateral or bilateral tubal obstruction or uterine cavity abnormality.

2.5. Ethical Considerations. Ethical approval for this study was obtained from the Ethical Review Committee of the Cape Coast Teaching Hospital. Written informed consent was obtained after the nature of the study was adequately explained to the clients. Clients were assured of data security and confidentiality. They were also informed about the benefit of the research findings and how it will influence the way the procedure is done locally and internationally.

Participation was purely voluntary, and they had the option to terminate after been enrolled in the study.

3. Results

3.1. Demographic and Clinical Presentation of Women. A total of 203 women aged between 19 and 47 years and the mean age of 32.9 years with history of infertility were enrolled. Most of the women were within 30–39 years (61.19%). Secondary infertility (50.74%) was the most common form of infertility, and 58.62% of them have no history of live birth. The commonest duration of infertility (56.16%) was 1 to 4 years. Based on the association between age, duration of infertility, findings on HSG, and indication of HSG, women's age ($p = 0.004$) and duration of infertility ($p = 0.034$) were found to be significantly associated with the indication of HSG (Table 1).

3.2. Findings on Hysterosalpingography. Out of the 203 women studied, eighty-five (41.29%) of them were diagnosed with at least one abnormality on HSG (Table 1). Forty-four (51.3%) of the women had only fallopian tube abnormalities. The common tubal abnormalities were bilateral blockage (24.2%), right unilateral proximal blockage (17.7%), loculated spillage (16.1%), and left unilateral proximal blockage (16.1%) (Figure 1). As shown in Figure 1, 27 (31.8%) women were diagnosed with only uterine abnormality. Capacious uterine cavity (45.1%) and filling defects/fibroids (33.3%) were the common uterine abnormalities. Fourteen (16.5%) women had both fallopian tube and uterine abnormalities.

On tubal abnormalities, hydrosalpinx and left tubal patency are reported in Figure 2.

We also reported HSG image to demonstrate the bilateral tubal patency and capacious uterine cavity in a participant (Figure 3).

3.3. Complimentary Ultrasonography Findings. Forty-nine women with abnormality on HSG had complimentary ultrasound examination, and 51.1% showed abnormalities such as fibroids (78.3%), adenomyosis (4.3%), and 17.4% hydrosalpinx.

3.4. Uterine Cavity Size as a Ratio (Jimah Ratio) to the Corno-Iliac Diameter. Intercornual diameter (the diameter between the cornua of the uterus) and interiliac diameter (the diameter between lower ends of the right and left iliac bones at the level of the sacroiliac joint) were measured, and ratio (Jimah ratio) between intercornual diameter to interiliac diameter was determined. The HSG measurement of the normal uterine cavity size as a ratio (Jimah ratio) of the corno-iliac diameter is illustrated in Figure 4.

There was significant difference in the mean of intercornual diameter ($p < 0.001$), interiliac diameter ($p < 0.001$), and intercornual diameter to interiliac diameter ratio ($p < 0.001$) for all patients with normal uterine cavities (Table 2).

4. Discussion

Hysterosalpingography (HSG) is a common radiographic procedure used in the investigation of female infertility [14]. It is efficient in the detection of fallopian tube and uterine cavity pathologies including tubal occlusion and congenital uterine anomalies [2, 5, 15, 16].

In this study, two hundred and three (203) women with infertility were enrolled, and some had complimentary ultrasound scan (USG). Most of the women presented with secondary infertility (50.74%) which is similar to the findings reported by previous studies in Nigeria [8, 17, 18, 24] and Ghana [20]. On the contrary, studies from different continents reported the predominance of primary infertility in their study subjects: China [25], Iran [23], and India [26]. Our findings are consistent with the assertion that there is a higher prevalence of secondary infertility in women in developing countries compared to primary infertility in developed countries [5, 7, 20]. Previous findings also suggest that the prevalence of risk factors such as sexually transmitted infections, poor reproductive health behavior, iatrogenic health care infections, and medical neglect of precursor conditions of secondary infertility is higher in developing countries [4, 8, 16, 20].

A greater proportion of the women presented with 1 to 4 years duration of infertility, comparable to 4 years as reported by Heis et al. [10], but less than the mean years (6.7 years) as reported by Al-Jaroudi et al. [13]. In this study, age of women ($p = 0.004$) and duration of infertility ($p = 0.034$) were found to be in association with the forms of infertility. Our findings could not assign any possible reasons for this association. However, aging is likely to influence the occurrence of secondary infertility likely due to the prolonged exposure to the risk factors of infertility.

As seen in this study, eighty-five (41.87%) of the women were diagnosed with at least one or more abnormalities. This is comparable to a study in Switzerland [21] and Nigeria [17] which reported 44% and 37.6%, respectively. Our findings at the Cape Coast Teaching Hospital, Ghana, vary from those of Botwe et al. from the Korle-Bu Teaching Hospital of Ghana, who found that 60.03% of their women had abnormalities on HSG [20]. Many other studies have reported much higher proportions: 98.19% in China [25], 92% in India [26], and 85.8% and 75% in Nigeria [11, 27]. The possible explanation to the disparity in findings is likely due to exposure to infections such as sexually transmitted disease (STD) and pelvic inflammatory disease (PID).

A significant proportion (71.6%) of women who had HSG abnormalities were diagnosed with tubal pathologies. Similar proportions were reported by Aduayi et al. (66.4%) in Nigeria [18], Bhatt et al. (68.4%) in India [26], and Hong et al. (80%) in China [25]. On the contrary, our proportion is much higher than that reported by Niknezhady et al. (11.9%) in Iran [23], Eze et al. (21%) in Nigeria [11], and Schankath et al. (54.7%) in Switzerland [21]. The discrepancies between our finding and previous studies may be due to cultural disparities which predefine the exposure to premarital and

Table 1: Association between age, duration of infertility, findings on HSG, and type of infertility.

Variable	Indication						Statistical indices	
	Primary		Secondary		Total		X^2 (df)	p value
	$N = 98$	100%	$N = 103$	100%	$N = 201$	100%		
Age							10.86 (2)	0.004
<30	36	36.73	22	21.36	58	28.86		
30–39	58	59.18	65	63.11	123	61.19		
40+	4	4.08	16	15.53	20	9.95		
Duration of infertility							8.67 (3)	0.034
<1	2	2.04	5	4.85	7	3.48		
1_4	62	63.27	52	50.49	114	56.72		
5_10	33	33.67	37	35.92	70	34.83		
>10	1	1.02	9	8.74	10	4.98		
Findings on HSG							0.18 (1)	0.674
Normal	59	60.2	59	57.28	118	58.71		
Abnormal	39	39.8	44	42.72	83	41.29		

HSG, hysterosalpingography; X^2, chi-square test df-degree of freedom; significant level at $p \leq 0.05$.

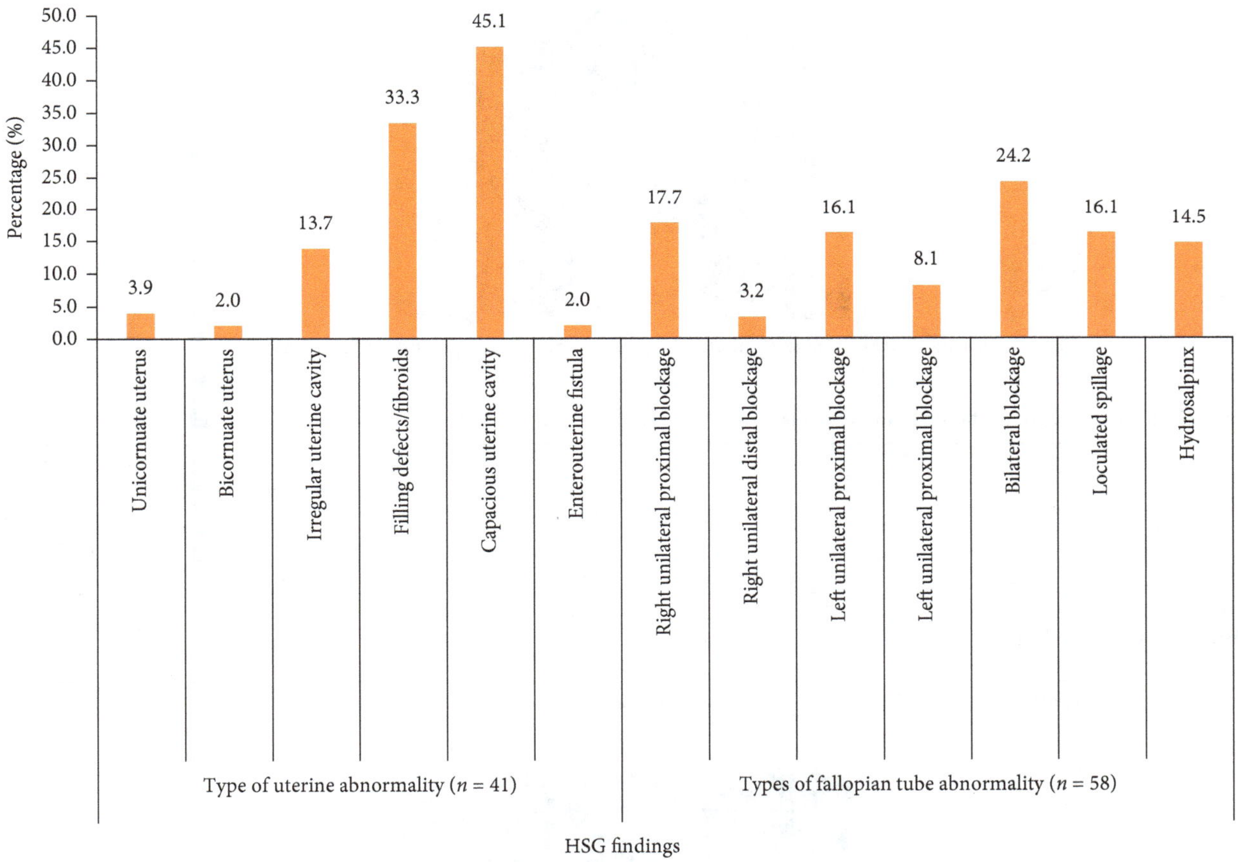

Figure 1: Hysterosalpingography findings in infertile women.

extramarital sex and its sequelae such as sexually transmitted diseases and PID [16, 17, 24].

The common tubal abnormalities found were tubal blockage which included bilateral blockage (24.2%) and right unilateral proximal blockage (17.7%), and 16.1% each had loculated spillage and left unilateral proximal blockage. A similar observation was made by Lawan et al. in Nigeria [24].

On HSG, hydrosalpinx is seen as a dilated convoluted tubular structure [27]. The fallopian tube inflammation is aggravated by STDs such as chlamydial or *tuberculosis* of the genital tract [24, 28]. Our proportion for hydrosalpinx (14.5%) among women diagnosed with tubal abnormalities was consistent with previous studies in Ghana [20] and Nigeria [23]. These proportions though low are a major

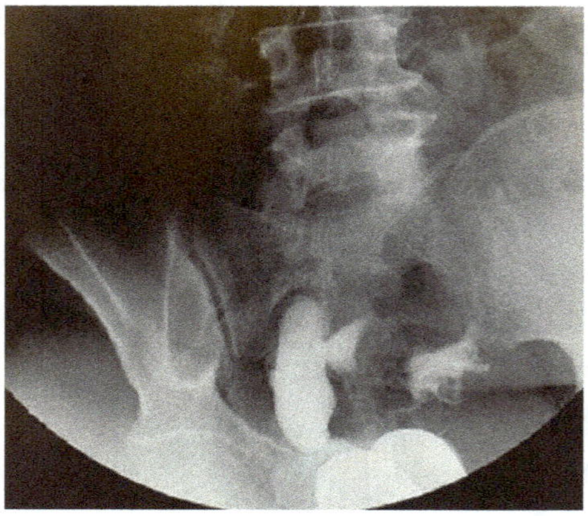

FIGURE 2: HSG image of right hydrosalpinx and left tubal patency.

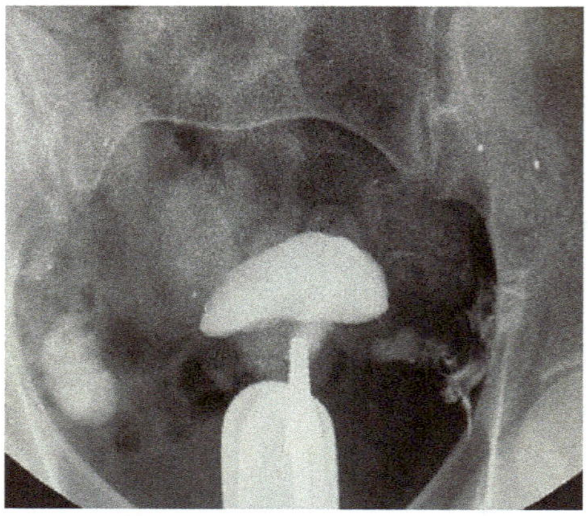

FIGURE 3: HSG image of bilateral tubal patency and capacious uterine cavity.

TABLE 2: Mean and standard deviation of intercornual diameter, interiliac diameter, and ratio of intercornual diameter to interiliac diameter.

HSG findings	Intercornual diameter ($n = 186$)		Interiliac diameter ($n = 186$)		Intercornual to interiliac ratio (Jimah ratio) ($n = 99$)	
	Mean	SD	Mean	SD	Mean	SD
Normal	29.13	4.68	80.65	10.37	0.36	0.06
Abnormal HSG without uterine abnormality	30.33	7.14	80.73	6.64	0.36	0.12
ANOVA	<0.001		<0.001		<0.001	

HSG, hysterosalpingography; SD, standard deviation; ANOVA, one-way analysis of variance; significant level at $p \leq 0.05$.

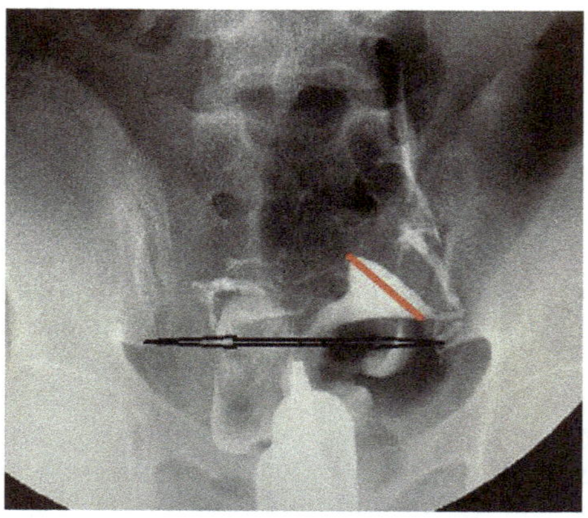

FIGURE 4: HSG image of Jimah ratio (uterine ratio) = intercornual diameter (red line)/interiliac diameter (black line).

reproductive health problem in women as PID remains a burden to developing countries [4, 8, 16, 17, 24].

Uterine factors remain the second leading cause of infertility among women [5–7, 11, 14, 17, 21, 23]. Our study indicates that almost 50% of women with HSG abnormalities had various forms of uterine pathologies. Individual studies have reported different proportions of uterine abnormalities in Nigeria (33.4% [17] and 56.10%) [27], Switzerland (34.9%) [21], and India (56.4%) [26].

Most of the uterine anomalies consist of capacious uterine cavity (45.1%) and fibroids (33.3%). A similar study in Ghana [20] reported slightly lower proportion (25.4%) of uterine fibroids. On the contrary, much lower proportions were reported by Eze et al. (17.0%) and Abubakar et al. (5.5%) in Nigeria [11, 17]. Complimentary ultrasound (USG) was done for 49 women with uterine abnormality on HSG, and it was observed that 51% had abnormalities such as uterine fibroids (78.3%)

In this study, the mean of intercornual diameter, interiliac diameter (the diameter between lower ends of the right and left iliac bones), and ratio of intercornual diameter to interiliac diameter was taken. This was done for all those with normal uterine findings on HSG, irrespective of the fallopian tube disease. Our findings showed that there was statistically significant difference in the mean of intercornual diameter ($p < 0.001$), intercornual diameter ($p < 0.001$), and the mean ratio of intercornual diameter to interiliac diameter ($p < 0.001$) between those with normal HSG findings and those with only tubal pathologies. The range of intercornual diameter to interiliac diameter ratio (otherwise known as Jimah ratio) is 0.2–0.45, for all women with a mean of 0.36 irrespective of whether there is a fallopian tube abnormality or not. The uterine cavity beyond the upper limit of normal will require further imaging to determine the cause of the enlargement.

Common limitation seen in this study is small sample size. There are five teaching hospitals and other private hospitals in Ghana with imaging departments that provide hysterosalpingography and ultrasonography services; however, this study was conducted in only one of these hospitals (Cape Coast Teaching Hospital). Therefore, the study findings could not be generalized to the entire country. However, this study has provided preliminary data to inform medical practice in our local setting and adds to the knowledge of infertility among women in Ghana.

5. Conclusion

Hysterosalpingography is an acceptable imaging modality for the investigation of the uterine cavity and fallopian tubes in infertile women. Secondary infertility was the commonest indication for HSG in the study. Our study indicated that fallopian tube abnormalities are the most common abnormal findings, while capacious uterine cavity, uterine fibroid, and bilateral tubal blockage were the top three abnormalities. The normal uterine cavity size as a ratio (Jimah ratio) of the corno-iliac diameter is 0.2–0.45 with a mean of 0.36 is documented to serve as a local reference value and adds to the existing literature We recommend further imaging research involving major referral hospitals in Ghana to better assess the spectrum of HSG abnormalities in both normal and infertile women in the country.

Authors' Contributions

BJJ conceptualized the topic, designed the protocol, performed most of the HSG procedures, interpreted the HSG findings, and drafted and edited the manuscript. PG drafted, reviewed, and edited the manuscript. ABA performed data analysis and interpretation and drafted, reviewed, and edited the manuscript. All authors read and approved the final version of the manuscript.

Acknowledgments

The authors wish to acknowledge the contributions of Priscilla Laryea, Isaac Dapaah, Dr. Mohammed Owusu Ansah, Althea Mannah, and Anudjo Messiah Kwame and Kortor Setor Nicholas and Mr. Oduro for their participation in the performance of the HSG procedures.

References

[1] F. Zegers-Hochschild, G. D. Adamson, J. D. Mouzon et al., "International committee for monitoring assisted reproductive technology (ICMART) and the world health organization (WHO) revised glossary of ART," *Fertility and Sterility*, vol. 92, no. 5, pp. 1520–1524, 2009.

[2] National Institute for Health and Clinical Excellence (NICE), *Fertility Problems: Assessment and Treatment*, National Institute for Health and Clinical Excellence (NICE), London, UK, 2018, https://www.nice.org.uk/terms-and-conditions#notice-of-rights.

[3] M. N. Mascarenhas, S. R. Flaxman, T. Boerma, S. Vanderpoel, and G. A. Stevens, "National, regional, and global trends in infertility prevalence since 1990 : a systematic analysis of 277 health surveys," *PLoS Medicine*, vol. 9, no. 12, pp. 1–12, 2012.

[4] W. Ombelet, I. Cooke, S. Dyer, G. Serour, and P. Devroey, "Infertility and the provision of infertility medical services in developing countries," *Human Reproduction Update*, vol. 14, no. 6, pp. 605–621, 2008.

[5] Royal College of Obstetricians and Gynaecologists, *Fertility: Assessment and Treatment for People with Fertility Problems Fertility: Assessment and Treatment for People with Fertility Problems*, Royal College of Obstetricians and Gynaecologists, London, UK, 2nd edition, 2013.

[6] J. Boivin, L. Bunting, J. A. Collins, and K. G. Nygren, "International estimates of infertility prevalence and treatment-seeking: potential need and demand for infertility medical care," *Human Reproduction*, vol. 22, no. 6, pp. 1506–1512, 2007.

[7] W. Cates, T. M. M. Farley, and P. J. Rowe, "Worldwide patterns of infertility: is Africa different?" *The Lancet*, vol. 326, no. 8455, pp. 596–598, 1985.

[8] I. Eo, C. Nd, P. Sd et al., "Risk factors for abnormal tubal hysterosalpingographic findings in women presenting with infertility in Jos," *Jos Journal of Medicine*, vol. 9, no. 1, pp. 47–52, 2015.

[9] J. Banu, S. Das, P. Fatima, and R. Sultana, "Association of chalamydia trachomitis infection in patients with tubal factor infertility," *Journal of Chittagong Medical College Teachers' Association*, vol. 19, no. 1, pp. 4–7, 2008.

[10] M. Heis, Z. Amarin, A. Ibrahim, N. Obeidat, B. Obeidat, and M. M. Al-Omari, "Uterine and tubal anatomical abnormalities in infertile women: diagnosis with routine hysterosalpingography prior to selective laparoscopy," *South African Journal of Radiology*, vol. 15, no. 4, pp. 120–122, 2011.

[11] C. U. Eze, C. C. Ohagwu, L. Abonyi, and J. Njoku, "A spectrum of hysterosalpingographic findings in infertile women in Benin, Nigeria," *Journal of Reproduction & Infertility*, vol. 4, no. 2, pp. 13–18, 2014.

[12] M. Niknejadi, A. Pooyan, M. Javam, and F. Niknejad, "Hysterosalpingography findings among a large sample of infertile women: a cross sectional study," *European Society of Radiology*, no. C-0851, pp. 1–7, 2015.

[13] D. Al-Jaroudi, A. A. Aldughayyim, W. S. Alshamry, A. S. Alrashidi, and A. A. Bahnassy, "Hysterosalpingogram findings among subfertile women undergoing assisted reproductive technology," *International Journal of Women's Health*, vol. 10, pp. 431–436, 2018.

[14] B. Úbeda, M. Paraira, E. Alert, and R. A. Abuin, "Hysterosalpingography," *American Journal of Roentgenology*, vol. 177, no. 1, pp. 131–135, 2001.

[15] G. Chunyan, P. Bin, Y. Ping et al., "Assessment of the influence on spontaneous pregnancy of hysterosalpingo-contrast sonography," *BioMed Research International*, vol. 2018, Article ID 4901281, 8 pages, 2018.

[16] World Health Organization, *Reproductive Health Indicators: Guidelines for Their Generation, Interpretation and Analysis for Global Monitoring*, World Health Organization, Geneva, Switzerland, 2006.

[17] M. G. Abubakar, M. Njiti, E. Mathew et al., "Evaluation of hysterosalpingography (HSG) findings among suspected infertile women at abubbakar tafawa balewa university teaching hospital (ATBUTH) bauchi," *International Journal of Research in Medical Sciences*, vol. 4, no. 3, pp. 55–59, 2016.

[18] O. Aduayi, G. Akanbi, A. Akintayo, and V. Aduayi, "Hysterosalpingography findings among women presenting for gynecological imaging in Ado-Ekiti, South western Nigeria," *International Journal of Reproduction, Contraception, Obstetrics and Gynecology*, vol. 5, no. 6, pp. 1906–1911, 2016.

[19] A. A. Olatunji, O. E. Jagun, O. O. Toyobo, O. A. Ashaolu, and O. A. Adekoya, "Hysterosalpingogram findings among women with infertility in Ogun," *Annals of Health Research*, vol. 3, no. 2, pp. 75–81, 2017.

[20] B. O. Botwe, K. Bamfo-Quaicoe, E. Hunu, and S. Anim-Sampong, "Hysterosalpingographic findings among Ghanaian women undergoing infertility work-up : a study at the Korle-Bu teaching hospital," *Fertility Research and Practice*, vol. 1, pp. 1–6, 2015.

[21] A. C. Schankath, N. Fasching, C. Urech-Ruh, M. K. Hohl, and R. A. Kubik-Huch, "Hysterosalpingography in the workup of female infertility: indications, technique and diagnostic findings," *Insights Into Imaging*, vol. 3, no. 5, pp. 475–483, 2012.

[22] C. Onwuchekwa and V. Oriji, "Hysterosalpingographic (HSG) pattern of infertility in women of reproductive age," *Journal of Human Reproductive Sciences*, vol. 10, no. 3, pp. 178–184, 2017.

[23] M. Niknezhady, M. Javam, F. Hosseyni et al., "Hysterosalpingographic assessment of tubal disorders among 3071 women with primary or secondary infertility," *European Society of Radiology*, no. no. C-1776, pp. 1–12, 2018.

[24] R. O. Lawan, P. O. Ibinaiye, P. Onwuhafua, and A. Hamidu, "Evaluation of pattern of tubo-peritoneal abnormalities potentially responsible for infertility in Zaria, Nigeria: hysterosalpingographic assessment," *Sub-Saharan African Journal of Medicine*, vol. 2, no. 3, pp. 110–116, 2015.

[25] Q. Hong, R. Cai, Q. Chen et al., "Three-dimensional HyCoSy with perfluoropropane-albumin microspheres as contrast agents and normal saline injections into the pelvic cavity for morphological assessment of the fallopian tube in infertile women," *Journal of Ultrasound in Medicine*, vol. 36, no. 4, pp. 741–748, 2017.

[26] S. Bhatt, M. Sumbul, R. Rajpal, and G. Radhakrishnan, "Value of "three dimensional multidetector CT hysterosalpingography" in infertile patients with non-contributory hysterosalpingography: a prospective study," *Journal of Reproduction & Infertility*, vol. 18, no. 3, pp. 323–332, 2017.

[27] D. U. Eduwem, A. O. Akintomide, D. E. Bassey, and M. I. Ekott, "Hysterosalpingographic patterns and relevance in the management of infertility in a Nigerian tertiary health institution," *Asian Journal of Medical Sciences*, vol. 7, no. 5, pp. 70–74, 2016.

[28] N. Bhatla, "Infection as they infect individual organs," in *Jeffcoates Principles of Gynaecology*, Butterworths: The University of Michigan, Ann Arbor, MI, USA, 6th edition, 2001.

23

Developing of a Mathematical Model to Perform Measurements of Axial Vertebral Rotation on Computer-Aided and Automated Diagnosis Systems, Using Raimondi's Method

José Hurtado-Aviles,[1] **Joaquín Roca-González**,[2,3] **Konstantsin Sergeevich Kurochka**,[4] **Jose Manuel Sanz-Mengibar**,[1] and **Fernando Santonja-Medina**[1,5]

[1]*Faculty of Medicine, University of Murcia, Murcia, Spain*
[2]*Technical University of Cartagena (UPCT), Technical School of Industrial Engineering, Cartagena, Spain*
[3]*Director of the Industrial and Medical Electronics Section of the DINTEL Research Group, Cartagena, Spain*
[4]*Head of Department of Information Technologies, P.O. Sukhoi State Technical University of Gomel, Gomel, Belarus*
[5]*V. de la Arrixaca University Hospital, Department of Traumatology, Murcia, Spain*

Correspondence should be addressed to Fernando Santonja-Medina; fernando@santonjatrauma.es

Academic Editor: André Luiz Ferreira COSTA

Introduction. Axial vertebral rotation (AVR) is a basic parameter in the study of idiopathic scoliosis and on physical two-dimensional images. Raimondi's tables are the most used method in the quantification of AVR. The development of computing technologies has enabled the creation of computer-aided or automated diagnosis systems (CADx) with which measurement on medical images can be carried out more quickly, simply, and with less intra and interobserver variabilities than manual methods. Although there are several publications dealing with the measurement of AVR in CADx systems, none of them provides information on the equation or algorithm used for the measurement applying Raimondi's method. *Goal.* The aim of this work is to perform a mathematical modelling of the data contained in Raimondi's tables that enable the Raimondi method to be used in digital medical images more precisely and in a more exact manner. *Methods.* Data from Raimondi's tables were tabulated on a first step. After this, each column of Raimondi's tables containing values corresponding to vertebral body width (D) were adjusted to a curve determined by AVR $= f(d)$. Third, representative values of each rotation divided by D were obtained through the equation of each column D. In a fourth step, a regression line was fitted to the data in each row, and from its equation, the mean value of the D/d distribution is calculated (value corresponding to the central column, $D = 45$). Finally, a curve was adjusted to the obtained data using the least squares method. *Summary and Conclusion.* Our mathematical equation allows the Raimondi method to be used in digital images of any format in a more accurate and simplified approach. This equation can be easily and freely implemented in any CADx system to quantify AVR, providing a more precise use of Raimondi's method, as well as being used in traditional manual measurement as it is performed with Raimondi tables.

1. Introduction

Axial vertebral rotation (AVR) is a basic parameter in the study of idiopathic scoliosis in adolescents [1, 2]. Its measurement is necessary to evaluate the severity of scoliosis and quantify the risk of progression [1, 3–7] for the selection of treatment [3, 4, 8, 9] and for the analysis of orthopaedic surgery [1, 6–8, 10, 11].

Two-dimensional medical images, especially anterior-posterior and lateral X-rays of the full spine when standing [12–14], continue to be the method of choice for diagnosing and monitoring scoliosis [15].

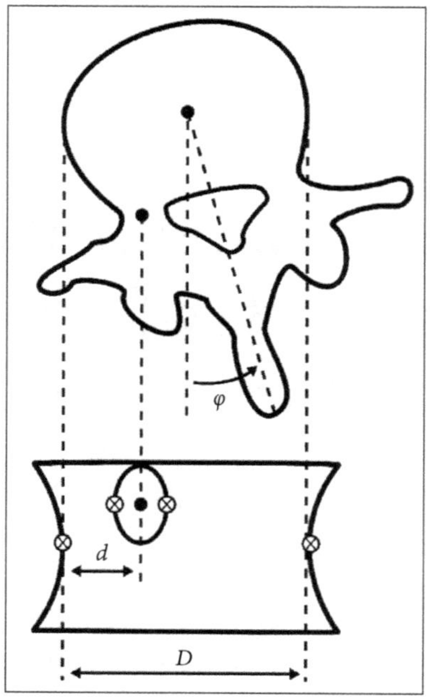

FIGURE 1: A schematic description of the anatomical references used to measure AVR in two-dimensional images.

TABLE 1: Simplified Raimondi's tables with data to obtain AVR. Modification of Raimondi. The quantification of the vertebral rotation in the scoliosis. Comparing experiences [32].

2.3	2.4	2.5	2.6	2.7	...	7.8	AVR = 2°
2.6	2.7	2.8	2.9	3	...	9	AVR = 4°
2.9	3	3.1	3.2	3.4	...	9.8	AVR = 6°
3.2	3.3	3.4	3.6	3.7	...	10.5	AVR = 8°
3.5	3.6	3.8	3.9	4.1	...	11.7	AVR = 10°
3.7	3.8	4	4.2	4.3	...	12.8	AVR = 12°
3.9	4	4.2	4.4	4.6	...	13.9	AVR = 14°
4.1	4.2	4.5	4.7	4.9	...	15	AVR = 16°
4.3	4.5	4.7	4.9	5.2	...	16	AVR = 18°
4.5	4.7	5	5.2	5.5	...	17.3	AVR = 20°
4.9	5.1	5.4	5.7	5.9	...	18.8	AVR = 22°
5.3	5.5	5.8	6.1	6.4	...	20.1	AVR = 24°
5.7	6	6.3	6.6	6.9	...	21.7	AVR = 26°
6	6.4	6.7	7	7.4	...	23.1	AVR = 28°
...	...	...	...	...	...	...	...
17.5	18.3	19.2	20	20.9	...	61.5	AVR = 60°
$D = 20$	$D = 21$	$D = 22$	$D = 23$	$D = 24$	...	$D = 70$	

On physical two-dimensional images, Raimondi's tables [16–18] are the most used method in the quantification of AVR [19–21]. This method possesses a more than acceptable degree of reproducibility between observers, and it is easy to apply [19, 21, 22].

Figure 1 shows a schematic description of the anatomical references used to measure AVR in two-dimensional images.

Based on the position of the two closest lateral faces vertebral body points and the two opposite sides of the shadow of the pedicle turned towards the centre of the vertebra in the anteroposterior projection, the software calculates the width of the vertebral body (D) and the distance from the centre of the pedicle to the side of the vertebral body (d). Adapted by permission from Nature/Springer, European Spine Journal, Vrtovec T, Pernus F, and Likar B, a review of methods was conducted for quantitative evaluation of axial vertebral rotation [7].

The development of computing technologies has enabled the creation of computer-aided or automated diagnosis systems (CADx) with which manual measurement methods on medical images (for instance, Cobb angle, distances, and wedgings) can be applied more quickly, simply, and with less intra and interobserver variabilities [23–28].

The digital X-rays require a software for the clinicians to state a precise diagnosis and treatment, as well as quantify the follow-up changes. These kinds of software are usually not designed to quantify specific AIS parameters, or they are not easily accessible due to their complex use or higher cost.

Table 2: Adjustment of data in Raimondi's tables to the function model.

D	R^2
20	0.9981
21	0.9987
22	0.9988
23	0.9989
24	0.9991
25	0.9992
26	0.9992
27	0.9994
28	0.9994
29	0.9994
30	0.9996
31	0.9996
32	0.9997
33	0.9996
34	0.9997
35	0.9997
36	0.9997
37	0.9997
38	0.9997
39	0.9997
40	0.9997
41	0.9997
42	0.9997
43	0.9997
44	0.9993
45	0.9997
46	0.9996
47	0.9997
48	0.9997
49	0.9996
50	0.9996
51	0.9996
52	0.9996
53	0.9996
54	0.9996
55	0.9996
56	0.9996
57	0.9996
58	0.9996
59	0.9995
60	0.9995
61	0.9994
62	0.9994
63	0.9994
64	0.9994
65	0.9994
66	0.9994
67	0.9994
68	0.9993
69	0.9993
70	0.9993

Although there are several publications dealing with the measurement of AVR in CADx systems, none of them provides information on the equation or algorithm used for the measurement applying Raimondi's method [3, 28–30].

The aim of this work is to perform a mathematical modelling based on the data contained in Raimondi's tables that enables them to be applied on CADx systems, allowing the Raimondi method to be used in digital medical images more precisely and in a more exact manner.

Data from Raimondi's tables were tabulated on a first step. After this, each column of Raimondi's tables containing values corresponding to vertebral body width (D) were adjusted to a curve determined by AVR $= f(d)$. In this mathematical equation, "d" represents each value of the column D. Third, representative values of each rotation divided by D were obtained through the equation of each column D. A representative value for each AVR was obtained this way. The fourth step was to adjust the data included in each row to a regression line, and this equation was used to calculate the average value of the distribution D/d (middle column value = 45). Finally, a curve was adjusted to the obtained data using the least squares method.

The novelties of our work are (a) to provide an adimentional equation to describe in a theoretically way the empirical data tabulated in Raimondi's tables with more accuracy and less precision error; (b) our mathematical equation allows the Raimondi method to be used in CADx to quantify AVR in medical images without the need for a scale; and (c) this equation can be easily and freely implemented in any CADx system, providing a more precise use of Raimondi's method than on the traditional printed X-ray.

2. Materials and Methods

In Raimondi's tables, the data pertaining to one same column correspond to a particular vertebral diameter, D, between 20 mm and 70 mm (Table 1). This value is given by the width of the vertebral body D projected on the X-ray image.

Within each column, the data correspond to the distance, d, between the centre of the shadow of the pedicle furthest from the edge of the vertebra and said edge, in millimetres.

Each pair of values (D, d) corresponds to a value of AVR between 2° and 60°.

From the distribution of empirical data in Raimondi's tables, a mathematical model that describes the information contained in them in an ideal manner is sought.

First, the data in each column are analysed separately. Using the least squares method, the equation of a curve,

$$f\left(d|_{D=x}\right) = \text{AVR}, \tag{1}$$

is pursued, such that every (d, AVR) pair is as close as possible to this curve.

Using the "Statistix 10" software by Analytical Software, a rational function in the form

$$y = \frac{a + bx}{1 + cx + dx^2}, \tag{2}$$

where a, b, and c are the constants, was chosen as the best option.

By adjusting the function model to each set of values in each column of Raimondi's tables, the adjustment values "pseudo R^2" reflected in Table 2 are obtained.

The quality of the adjustment of each curve improves as the width of the vertebra, D, increases, reaching a maximum

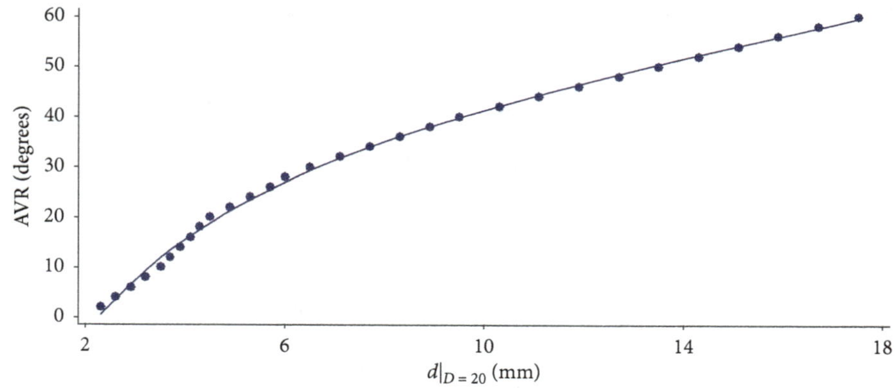

FIGURE 2: Adjustment of the data in column $D = 20$ of Raimondi's tables to the curve.

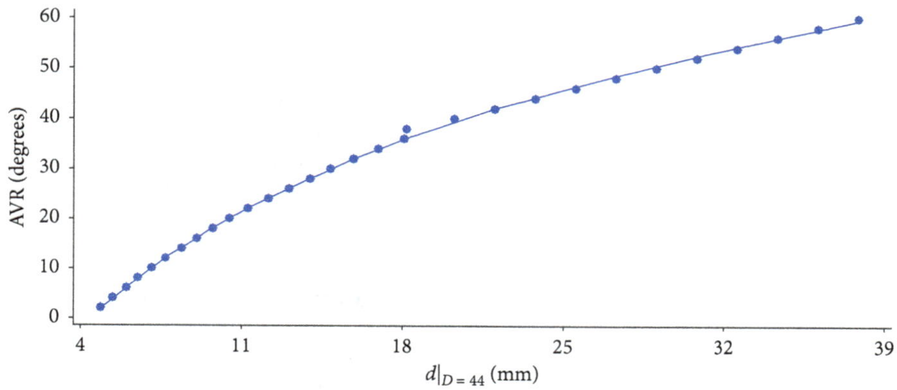

FIGURE 3: Adjustment of the data in column $D = 44$ of Raimondi's tables to the curve.

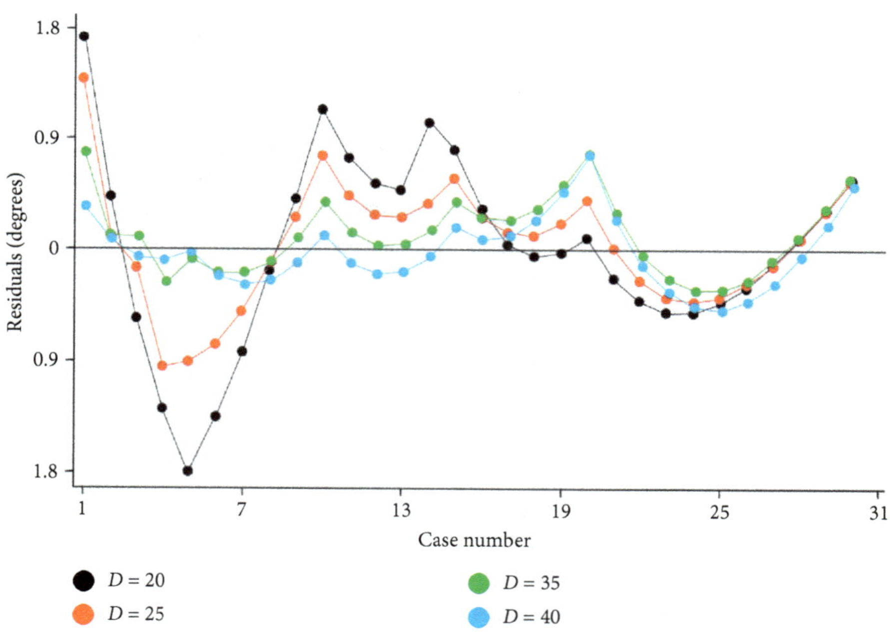

(a)

FIGURE 4: Continued.

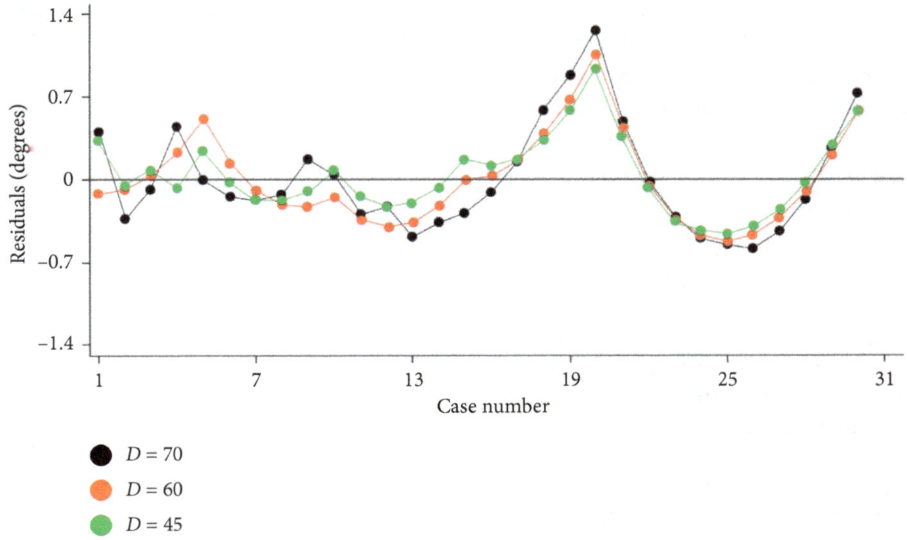

(b)

FIGURE 4: Residuals of the data of various columns from Raimondi's tables regarding their respective regression curves.

TABLE 3: Raimondi's tables completed with the results of dividing the D value of each column by the values obtained on the regression curves.

8.15408	8.27012	8.36228	8.42931	8.46827	...	8.79462	AVR = 2°
7.57368	7.68005	7.73791	7.78601	7.80927	...	7.89888	AVR = 4°
7.04025	7.13739	7.16903	7.20268	7.21409	...	7.16873	AVR = 6°
6.54855	6.637	6.64894	6.67153	6.67412	...	6.537	AVR = 8°
6.09427	6.17446	6.17198	6.18614	6.18232	...	5.98232	AVR = 10°
5.67363	5.74601	5.73329	5.74124	5.73293	...	5.49782	AVR = 12°
5.2834	5.34847	5.32888	5.33234	5.32102	...	5.06923	AVR = 14°
4.92084	4.97903	4.95525	4.95558	4.94246	...	4.69047	AVR = 16°
4.58353	4.6353	4.60946	4.60776	4.59374	...	4.34998	AVR = 18°
4.26939	4.31517	4.28895	4.28608	4.27189	...	4.04111	AVR = 20°
3.97661	4.01684	3.99152	3.98813	3.97433	...	3.76408	AVR = 22°
3.70362	3.73872	3.71525	3.71187	3.69886	...	3.51061	AVR = 24°
3.44904	3.47945	3.45849	3.4555	3.44357	...	3.2801	AVR = 26°
3.21167	3.23781	3.2198	3.21747	3.20683	...	3.06784	AVR = 28°
...	...	...	...	...	...	...	...
1.1265	1.13327	1.13167	1.13336	1.13382	...	1.11129	AVR = 60°
$20/d$	$21/d$	$22/d$	$23/d$	$24/d$	...	$70/d$	

of $R^2 = 0.9997$. The explanation for this may lie in the difficulty of performing a good measurement when this refers to very small distances (Figure 2).

From the value $D = 48$, R^2 decreases slightly until at $D = 68$, we have $R^2 = 0.9993$.

It can also be discerned that for $D = 44$, a value of R^2 outside of the collection of values described exists due to an atypical datum (Figure 3).

Residuals of the data of various columns from Raimondi's tables regarding their respective regression curves can be observed in Figures 4(a) and 4(b).

When using the Raimondi's tables on CADx systems, it is necessary for the vertebrae shown in the digital image to be of sufficient size ($20 \leq D \leq 70$) in order to be able to apply the equation [31]. In addition, the dimensions of variables D and d are given in millimetres.

All pairs of (D, d) values corresponding to a certain AVR are proportional, meaning they should produce ideally equal D/d values.

To avoid having to know the scale of the image to measure AVR, the independent variable will have the form D/d in the calculated equation, such that the value is adimensional.

To calculate the equation

$$f(D, d) = \text{AVR}, \quad (3)$$

the data in Raimondi's tables is replaced by other data obtained in the following manner (Table 3):

(i) For the set of data in each column, the nonlinear regression curve (equation (2)) is obtained

(ii) From the equation of each regression curve, the d values corresponding to the rotations 2°, 4°, 6°, ..., 60° are obtained to five decimal places

(iii) The value D/d is entered to five decimal places in each cell in the tables

In Table 3, the values of each row are very similar. To find the representative value of each rotation, a regression line is adjusted to the data in each row, and from its equation, the average D/d value of distribution is calculated (value corresponding to the central column, $D = 45$).

Figures 5–7 show that as the width of the vertebra increases, the linearity of the point cloud increases. It can also be observed how the general aspect of the data is quite regular, with the exception of those corresponding to $D = 60$ and $D = 70$, where the pattern followed loses its regularity. Consequently, each regression line is calculated by omitting some of the values as shown in the figures.

Table 4 shows the representative D/d values of each AVR calculated.

3. Results

The least squares method is used to adjust a curve to the data of Table 4. Using the "Statistix 10" software, a rational function in the form

$$y = \frac{a + bx + cx^2}{1 + dx + ex^2}, \quad (4)$$

where a, b, c, d, and e are the constants, is chosen. The adjustment obtained with this model is $R^2 = 1$.

The equation obtained is

$$\text{AVR} = \frac{20.22483 - 330.5077\,(D/d) + 33.46082\,(D/d)^2}{1 - 3.93825\,(D/d) - 1.322272\,(D/d)^2}. \quad (5)$$

Convergence criterion met after 16 iterations.

Residual SS (SSE): $9.722E-04$

Residual MS (MSE): $3.889E-05$

Standard deviation: $6.236E-03$

Degrees of freedom: 25

AICc: −294.46

Pseudo R^2: 10000

4. Discussion

AVR is a necessary parameter in being able to correctly evaluate and provide a prognosis for monitor and treat scoliosis [1–7].

Raimondi's tables are widely used on physical X-rays due to its notable reliability and ease of use in quantifying AVR [21, 32].

Table 4: Representative D/d values of each AVR.

AVR (°)	D/d
2	8.8848
4	8.0729
6	7.3639
8	6.7457
10	6.1983
12	5.7112
14	5.2751
16	4.8817
18	4.5261
20	4.2023
22	3.9068
24	3.6362
26	3.3881
28	3.1603
30	2.9495
32	2.7553
34	2.5753
36	2.4087
38	2.2544
40	2.1112
42	1.9784
44	1.8552
46	1.7409
48	1.6348
50	1.5365
52	1.4452
54	1.3607
56	1.2825
58	1.2102
60	1.1434

We are not aware that until now, a method to calculate ARV by CADx systems has been developed using the Raimondi method.

The data contained in the Raimondi's tables were obtained experimentally from thousands of measurements on educational and anatomical spines [32]. In consequence, Raimondi recognises that the measurements obtained with his method involve systematic errors [19, 32]. These errors are small in comparison with the real value of the measures made, meaning their presence will not vary the decision on the evaluation or treatment of the patient. However, these errors may propagate along with random errors due to a multitude of variables present in the measuring process such as (A) the loss of information when showing a three-dimensional structure on a flat image; (B) the characteristics of the medical image (e.g., existence of noise that hinders the legibility of the image); (C) limitations of the observer (e.g., exactitude in the identification of measurement references points, need for training, and experience); (D) the particular morphological characteristics of the vertebrae (e.g., deformations, the variability of the interpedicular distance between vertebrae); and (E) the position of the patient in the image.

On the other hand, medical images today reach the medical professional on a CD, and Raimondi's tables cannot be applied to these digital images, when they do

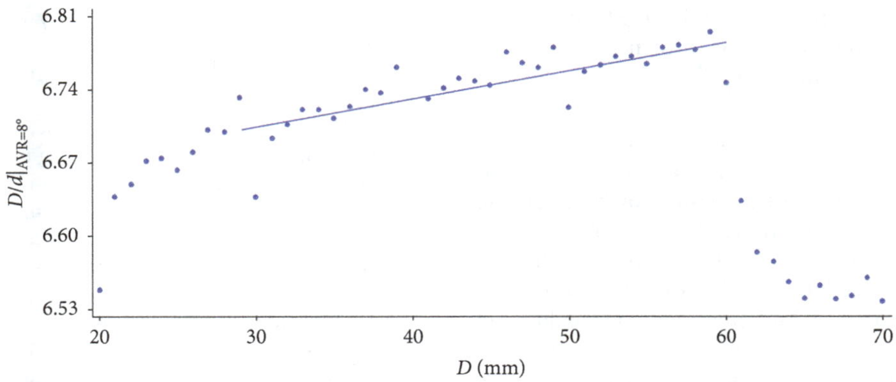

FIGURE 5: Variation of the D/d value corresponding to the AVR of 8° as D varies.

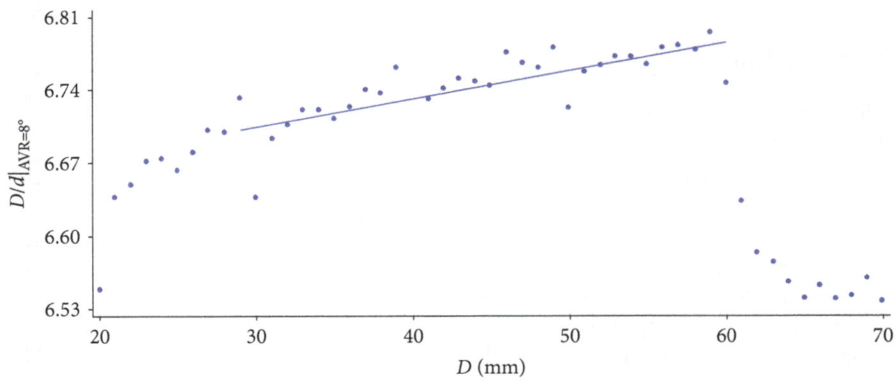

FIGURE 6: Variation of the D/d value corresponding to the AVR of 12° as D varies.

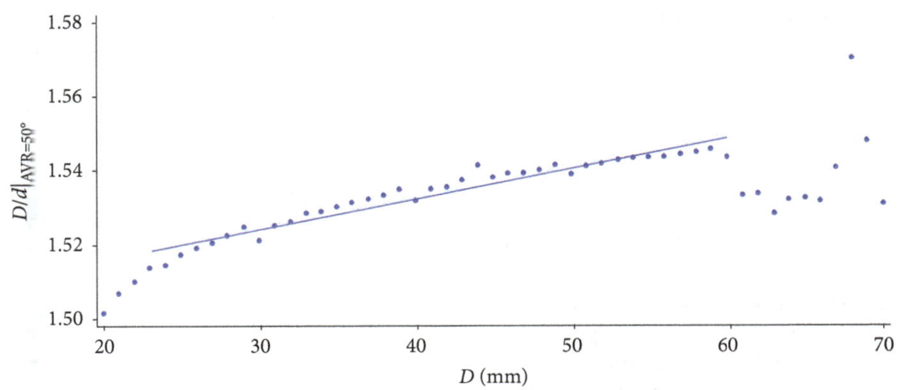

FIGURE 7: Variation of the D/d value corresponding to the AVR of 50° as D varies.

not contain information about the scale (that is, the image does not have the scale imprinted on it or the DICOM archive entry does not have this information).

The obtained equation allows the AVR measurement to be implemented in CADx systems with the Raimondi method, allowing more accurate and precise results to be obtained, due to the elimination of the systematic error contained in the Raimondi tables and the use of auxiliary tools that usually incorporate CADx systems, such as enlargement of regions of interest, application of filters, and automatic detection algorithms.

We have not found any previous work that offers an equation or an analogous algorithm to use Raimondi's method in CADx systems that show it openly. The obtained equation is available to be used freely.

The form of the equation obtained also has the advantage that allows the Raimondi method to be used in digital medical images that do not contain information about its scale (for example, images in TIFF format, in DICOM files that do not contain this information or when it is not printed on the same image).

The limitations of our study are that the programming code to implement our equation in any software is not provided. Our equation was tested using the C++ programming language and OpenCV library, so we can recommend these tools to implement the obtained equation. Also, our equation does not innovate in Raimondi's procedure but achieves a linear theoretical model based on its empirical data, improving its validity and reliability. Therefore, the highlight of our study is that this equation can be easily and freely implemented in any CADx system, allowing the use of the Raimondi method in digital medical images, whether or not they contain the scale, in a more exact and precise way.

5. Summary and Conclusion

A mathematical equation has been calculated that can be implemented in CADx systems from the mathematical modelling of the empirical data tabulated in Raimondi's tables.

This allows the Raimondi method to be used in digital images of any format more accurately, simply, and quickly, by eliminating the small systematic error existing in the discrete values of the tables and being able to use in conjunction with auxiliary tools in the CADx system such as zooming over regions of interest, algorithms for enhancing medical image structures, adjusting brightness, and contrast.

The equation can be easily and freely implemented in any CADx system.

Nomenclature

a, b, c, d, e: Constants
x: Variable
D: The value given by the width of vertebral body projected on the X-ray image, in millimetres
d: The distance between the centre of the shadow of the pedicle furthest from the edge of the vertebra and said edge, in millimetres
R^2: The value of the adjustment obtained with an equation to a set of data.

References

[1] S. P. Mohanty, M. P. Kanhangad, and A. A Gullia, "Curve severity and apical vertebral rotation and their association with curve flexibility in adolescent idiopathic scoliosis," *Musculoskeletal Surgery*, 2020.

[2] M. Mangone, P. Raimondi, M. Paoloni et al., "Vertebral rotation in adolescent idiopathic scoliosis calculated by radiograph and back surface analysis-based methods: correlation between the Raimondi method and rasterstereography," *European Spine Journal*, vol. 22, no. 2, pp. 367–37110, 2013.

[3] S. M. Eijgenraam, T. F. M. Boselie, J. M. Sieben et al., "Development and assessment of a digital X-ray software tool to determine vertebral rotation in adolescent idiopathic scoliosis," *The Spine Journal*, vol. 17, no. 2, pp. 260–265, 2017.

[4] Q. N. Vo, E. H. Lou, and L. H. Le, "Measurement of axial vertebral rotation using three-dimensional ultrasound images," *Scoliosis*, vol. 10, no. 2, p. S7, 2015.

[5] M.-L. Nault, J.-M. Mac-Thiong, M. Roy-Beaudry et al., "Three-dimensional spinal morphology can differentiate between progressive and nonprogressive patients with adolescent idiopathic scoliosis at the initial presentation," *Spine*, vol. 39, no. 10, pp. E601–E606, 2014.

[6] B. B. Carlson, D. C. Burton, and M. A. Asher, "Comparison of trunk and spine deformity in adolescent idiopathic scoliosis," *Scoliosis*, vol. 8, no. 1, p. 2, 2013.

[7] T. Vrtovec, F. Pernuš, and B. Likar, "A review of methods for quantitative evaluation of axial vertebral rotation," *European Spine Journal*, vol. 18, no. 8, pp. 1079–1090, 2009.

[8] T. R. Kuklo, B. K. Potter, and L. G. Lenke, "Vertebral rotation and thoracic torsion in adolescent idiopathic scoliosis," *Journal of Spinal Disorders & Techniques*, vol. 18, no. 2, pp. 139–147, 2005.

[9] Y. Tamura, N. Sugano, T. Sasama et al., "Surface-based registration accuracy of CT-based image-guided spine surgery," *European Spine Journal*, vol. 14, no. 3, pp. 291–297, 2005.

[10] J. Ochi, F. Zhu, L. Xu et al., "Comparison of the aorta impingement risks between thoracolumbar/lumbar curves with different convexities in adolescent idiopathic scoliosis: a computed tomography study," *European Spine Journal*, vol. 21, no. 10, pp. 2043–2049, 2012.

[11] Y. Petit, C.-É. Aubin, and H. Labelle, "Spinal shape changes resulting from scoliotic spine surgical instrumentation expressed as intervertebral rotations and centers of rotation," *Journal of Biomechanics*, vol. 37, no. 2, pp. 173–180, 2004.

[12] N. D. Fletcher and R. W. Bruce, "Early onset scoliosis: current concepts and controversies," *Current Reviews in Musculoskeletal Medicine*, vol. 5, no. 2, pp. 102–110, 2012.

[13] T. R. Kuklo, B. K. Potter, T. M. Schroeder, and M. F. O'Brien, "Comparison of manual and digital measurements in adolescent idiopathic scoliosis," *Spine*, vol. 31, no. 11, pp. 1240–1246, 2006.

[14] M. Yazici, E. R. Acaroglu, A. Alanay, V. Deviren, A. Cila, and A. Surat, "Measurement of vertebral rotation in standing versus supine position in adolescent idiopathic scoliosis," *Journal of Pediatric Orthopaedics*, vol. 21, no. 2, pp. 252–256, 2001.

[15] Sociedad Argentina de Pediatría, "Sociedad Argentina de ortopedia y traumatología infantil (saoti) y sociedad Argentina de patología de la columna vertebral (SAPCV)," *Consenso de escoliosis idiopática del adolescente. Archivos Argentinos de Pediatría*, vol. 114, no. 6, pp. 585–594, 2016.

[16] P. Raimondi, "La misurazione della rotazione vertebrale sul piano orizzontale con il Metodo Raimondi," *Scienze Motorie*, vol. 2, pp. 11–16, 2002.

[17] P. Raimondi, G. Costanzo, A. P. Santaroni, and F. Bizzarri, "Ipotesi patogenetica sul ruolo di percezione e postura nello sviluppo delle scoliosi," *Résonances Européennes du Rachis*, vol. 20, pp. 883–889, 1998.

[18] P. Raimondi, G. Costanzo, and A. P. Santaroni, "Evaluation Chiffre de la rotation vertebrale par la mèthode de Paolo Raimondi," *Kinésithérapie Scientifique*, vol. 358, pp. 19–22, 1996.

[19] V. Prosperini, P. Raimondi, E. Martinelli, and F. Bizzarri, "Misurazione della rotazione vertebrale patologica su radiografie di piccolo e grande formato con il Metodo Raimondi," *Chinesiologia*, vol. 1, pp. 23–27, 2010.

[20] S. Kadoury, F. Cheriet, M. Beauséjour, I. A. Stokes, S. Parent, and H. Labelle, "A three-dimensional retrospective analysis of the evolution of spinal instrumentation for the correction of adolescent idiopathic scoliosis," *European Spine Journal*, vol. 18, no. 1, pp. 23–37, 2009.

[21] H.-R. Weiss, "Measurement of vertebral rotation: perdriolle versus Raimondi," *European Spine Journal*, vol. 4, no. 1, pp. 34–38, 1995.

[22] H. L. A. Defino and P. H. M. de Araújo, "Comparative study of the measurements of the vertebral rotation using Nash&Moe and Raimondi methods," *Acta Ortopédica Brasileira*, vol. 3, no. 12, pp. 167–173, 2004.

[23] A. Safari, H. Parsaei, A. Zamani, and B. Pourabbas, "A semi-automatic algorithm for estimating cobb angle," *Journal of Biomedical Physics and Engineering*, vol. 9, no. 3, pp. 317–326, 2019.

[24] J. Yang, K. Zhang, H. Fan et al., "Development and validation of deep learning algorithms for scoliosis screening using back images," *Communications Biology*, vol. 2, no. 1, p. 390, 2019.

[25] Y. Pan, Q. Chen, T. Chen et al., "Evaluation of a computer-aided method for measuring the Cobb angle on chest X-rays," *European Spine Journal*, vol. 28, no. 12, pp. 3035–3043, 2019.

[26] L. Wang, Q. Xu, S. Leung, J. Chung, B. Chen, and S. Li, "Accurate automated Cobb angles estimation using multi-view extrapolation net," *Medical Image Analysis*, vol. 58, p. 101542, 2019.

[27] D. Forsberg, C. Lundström, M. Andersson, L. Vavruch, H. Tropp, and H. Knutsson, "Fully automatic measurements of axial vertebral rotation for assessment of spinal deformity in idiopathic scoliosis," *Physics in Medicine and Biology*, vol. 58, no. 5, pp. 1775–1787, 2013.

[28] T. Vrtovec, R. Vengust, B. Likar, and F. Pernuš, "Analysis of four manual and a computerized method for measuring axial vertebral rotation in computed tomography images," *Spine*, vol. 35, no. 12, pp. E535–E541, 2010.

[29] A. P. Pinheiro, M. C. Tanure, and A. S. Oliveira, "Validity and reliability of a computer method to estimate vertebral axial rotation from digital radiographs," *European Spine Journal*, vol. 19, no. 3, pp. 415–420, 2010.

[30] J. Zhang, E. Lou, D. L. Hill et al., "Computer-aided assessment of scoliosis on posteroanterior radiographs," *Medical & Biological Engineering & Computing*, vol. 48, no. 2, pp. 185–195, 2010.

[31] M. D. Rigo and M. Villagrasa, "Technical error of vertebral rotation measurement directly on the computer screen, according to Raimondi method," *Scoliosis*, vol. 5, no. S1, p. O14, 2010.

[32] P. Raimondi and V. Prosperini, "La misurazione della rotazione vertebrale nelle scoliosi," *Esperienze valutative e commento. chinesiologia n.*vol. 3, pp. 22–26, 2007.

Predicting Molecular Subtypes of Breast Cancer with Mammography and Ultrasound Findings: Introduction of Sono-Mammometry Score

Sana Shaikh[1] **and Afshan Rasheed**[2]

[1]*Radiology Department, Sindh Institute of Urology and Transplantation (SIUT), Karachi 74100, Pakistan*
[2]*Oncology Department, Sindh Institute of Urology and Transplantation (SIUT), M. A. Jinnah Road, Karachi 74100, Pakistan*

Correspondence should be addressed to Sana Shaikh; docsanashaikh@gmail.com

Academic Editor: Daniele La Forgia

We studied the correlation of sonographic and digital mammographic features with molecular classification of breast cancer. Imaging features from 313 patients with preliminary ultrasound and digital mammogram between November 2017 and May 2020 were compared with histopathology and immunohistochemical analysis for the prediction of molecular classification of breast cancer. We also devised a score called "sono-mammometry" score consisting of few simple imaging features which can easily be performed in outpatient settings. We studied that non-triple-negative breast cancers are predominantly hypoechoic and strongly correlate with the presence of irregular spiculated margins along with peripheral echogenic halo, posterior shadowing, and microcalcifications, while there is considerable variation in imaging features of TNBC as some of its imaging features overlap with those of typical benign tumors. Although imaging characteristics are helpful in the prediction of molecular classification, the prognostication value of these imaging features is still weak. There is considerable variation in imaging features which warrants vigilance towards improved diagnostic performance. To help better understand these features, our sono-mammometry score can serve as straightforward test which is assumed to be functional and productive in resource-limited settings.

1. Introduction

Breast cancer is the most common cancer in women and is the second most common cause of death from cancer in women worldwide [1]. It is a diverse group of diseases which consists of a wide range of molecular and genetic subtypes [2, 3]. During the last two decades, regrouping of breast cancer classification has been undertaken, from histopathologic subtype to the molecular categorization established by gene expression [1–4]. These subtypes exhibit significant differences in their clinical behavior and imaging pattern [2, 4]. These five different subtypes detected by immunohistochemical markers are luminal A, luminal B-1(Her-2−), B-2 (Her-2+), human epidermal growth factor receptor 2 (Her-2) enriched, and triple negative [1–5].

Breast imaging has a dominant role in the detection, staging, and follow-up of patients with breast cancer. There is a substantial effect on clinical outcome from early recognition of breast cancer [5]. Although histopathological characterization is the gold standard for classifying molecular subtypes of breast cancer after percutaneous breast mass biopsy, the trend is moving towards the development of noninvasive diagnostic procedures that can aid in easy and quick interpretation of the disease process [6]. This highlights the importance for a radiologist to have sound knowledge of these molecular subtypes of breast cancer to improve the analysis of imaging findings. The assessment of molecular subtypes of breast cancer on imaging perhaps displays intricacies as it requires the combination of imaging features on both ultrasound and mammography.

The purpose of our study is to identify the relationship of immunohistochemical markers with multimodality imaging features using mammogram and ultrasound. MRI breast was not available in our department. We also determined the association of baseline histopathological type, grade of tumor, and T and N stages of the breast cancers with each luminal classification. We also proposed a scoring system that is assumed to provide better insight into understanding imaging features of non-triple-negative breast cancer (non-TNBC) in contrast to triple-negative breast cancers (TNBC). Our hypothesis is that different sonographic and mammographic features can predict molecular classification on histopathology.

2. Materials and Methods

2.1. Study Population. Our study was conducted at the Radiology Department of Sindh Institute of Urology and Transplantation (SIUT). Our Institutional Ethics Committee waived the requirement of individual informed consent for this descriptive retrospective study. The study group was selected from both the screening and symptomatic populations. Patients with preliminary ultrasound, mammogram, and histopathological analysis done at our institution were regarded as being suitable for our study. Relevant information was gathered from ultrasound and mammogram images. Patients with incomplete records and unsatisfactory images and ductal carcinoma in situ (DCIS) were excluded from the study. Bilateral breast cancers were also excluded from the study because in our record we found only 5 such patients out of which in 3 patients we did not find satisfactory imaging. Very large inflammatory breast cancers were also excluded because these usually cause obscuration of fine details of ultrasound images of malignant masses secondary to excessive breast edema; however, locally advanced diseases in which breast edema was not present and we can comprehend ultrasound characteristics of malignant masses were included in the study. In this way, data from 313 patients with breast cancer were retrospectively collected between November 2017 and May 2020.

2.2. Ultrasound. All ultrasound examinations were done according to ACR practice parameters for the performance of a breast ultrasound examination (revised 2016) [7]. These were acquired according to the standard of care protocol as a routine practice of our breast cancer unit and these were not carried out under research study settings. For sonography, 2 scanners were used, both were Canon Xario 200, each with frequency of 14 MHz. Every sonographic examination included both breasts and was extended to involve both axillary regions.

2.3. Digital Mammography. All mammograms were performed according to ACR practice parameters for the performance of screening and diagnostic mammography (revised 2018) [8]. All mammograms were done with Selenia Dimensions 3D Digital Mammography Tomosynthesis System (Hologic, Bedford, MA, USA). Images were reviewed on high-resolution workstations at the Radiology Department of our institute. Standard 2 views (craniocaudal view and mediolateral view) were performed routinely for all patients. Supplementary views were done whenever required.

2.4. Ultrasound and Digital Mammogram Assessment. All ultrasound and mammogram images were reviewed by 1 of 2 senior consultants in breast imaging, both of whom had at least 5 years of experience in breast imaging. Both radiologists were blinded to the patient's clinical findings and histopathological results. In the case of disagreement, a consensus was reached after discussion. The sonographic and mammographic features of the breast carcinomas were assessed based on the analytical criteria of Breast Imaging Reporting and Data System (BIRADS). For ultrasound, these features include tumor size, shape, orientation, boundary, margins, echo texture, and posterior features. For the mammogram, the features that are assessed are mass shape, margins, presence or absence of suspicious microcalcifications, and architectural distortion/trabecular thickening. Additional features like T and N stages and multifocality were also assessed.

2.5. Histopathological Examination. The histopathological specimens from the core needle biopsy were formalin-fixed and paraffin-embedded tissue blocks afterwards stained with H&E (hematoxylin and eosin). These samples were assessed by an experienced pathologist for tumor type and grading. Invasive cancer was graded as grade 1 (well differentiated), grade 2 (moderately differentiated), or grade 3 (poorly differentiated) according to the Scarff–Bloom–Richardson system [9]. Subsequently, immunohistochemical analysis was done to assess ER, PR, Ki-67 index, and Her-2 neu expression. ER and PR were regarded as positive if at least 1% of the tumor nuclei were positively stained [10]. An additional fluorescence in situ hybridization (FISH) was analyzed to detect Her-2 positivity with scores of 2 or higher. Scores of 1 or 0 were defined as Her-2 negative [10]. Ki-67 index >14% was considered as high and <14% was considered as low expression [5].

2.6. Sono-Mammometry Score (Table 1). We combined ultrasound and mammogram imaging features to design a scoring system for prediction of non-TNBC and TNBC. We used bivariate Chi-square test and multivariate binary logistic analysis to select variables. Variables with p values < 0.05 were considered significant. Factors significantly associated with univariable and multivariable logistic regression analysis are listed in Tables 2–4. Results of the univariable and multivariable logistic regression analysis were shown as p values, odds ratio (OR), and corresponding 95% CI. To estimate the discriminating power of the scoring system, the receiver operator characteristic (ROC) curve (Figure 1) was created and the areas under the curves (AUCs) were calculated.

Table 1: Sono-mammometry score.

Imaging findings			
Only pleomorphic microcalcifications (without mass or focal asymmetry on mammogram or ultrasound) (0)			
Mass/focal asymmetry	Without microcalcification (+1)	With microcalcification (+2)	—
Mass shape	Round (+1)	Oval (+2)	Irregular, spiculated (+3)
Mass margins	Well circumscribed (+1)	Microlobulated (+2)	Irregular-spiculated/ill-defined/obscured (+3)
Mass boundary	Abrupt (+1)	Echogenic halo (+2)	—
Posterior shadowing	Absent (+1)	Present (+2)	—
Posterior enhancement	Absent (+1)	Present (+1)	—
Orientation	Parallel (+0)	Antiparallel (+1)	—
Max. score: 14			

Table 2: Demographic and histopathological characteristics.

Clinicoradiological features of breast cancers	Total ($n = 313$) (%)	Luminal A ($n = 62$)	Luminal B1 (Her-2-ve) ($n = 71$)	Luminal B2 (Her-2+ve) ($n = 47$)	TNBC ($n = 77$)	Her-2-neu enrich ($n = 56$)	p value
Age							
20–30	16 (5.1)	1 (1.6)	2 (2.8)	2 (4.3)	7 (9.1)	4 (7.1)	
30–50	165 (52.7)	33 (53.2)	35 (49.3)	30 (63.8)	41 (53.2)	26 (46.4)	0.3
50–80	132 (42.2)	28 (45.2)	34 (47.9)	15 (31.9)	29 (37.7)	26 (46.4)	
Side							
Right	153 (48.9)	32 (51.6)	38 (53.5)	20 (42.6)	36 (46.8)	27 (48.2)	0.79
Left	160 (51.1)	30 (48.4)	33 (46.5)	27 (57.4)	41 (53.2)	29 (51.8)	
Mammography findings							
Negative	7 (2.2)	0 (0.0)	2 (2.8)	3 (6.4)	1 (1.3)	1 (1.8)	0.232
Positive	306 (97.8)	62 (100.0)	69 (97.2)	44 (93.6)	76 (98.7)	55 (98.2)	
Ultrasound findings							
Negative	2(0.6)	0(0.0)	0(0.0)	0(0.0)	0 (0.0)	2 (3.6)	0.05
Positive	311(99.4)	62(100.0)	71(100.0)	47(100.0)	77 (100.0)	54 (96.4)	
Focality							
Unifocal	252 (80.5)	48 (77.4)	53 (74.6)	37 (78.7)	65 (84.4)	49 (87.5)	0.34
Multifocal	61 (19.5)	14 (22.6)	18 (25.4)	10 (21.3)	12 (15.6)	7 (12.5)	
T stage							
T0	2 (0.6)	0 (0.0)	0 (0.0)	0 (0.0)	0 (0.0)	2 (3.6)	
T1	30 (9.6)	3 (4.8)	8 (11.3)	9 (19.1)	4 (5.2)	6 (10.7)	
T2	112 (35.8)	26 (41.9)	31 (43.7)	15 (31.9)	27 (35.1)	13 (23.2)	0.06
T3	29 (9.3)	6 (9.7)	5 (7.0)	3 (6.4)	10 (13.0)	5 (8.9)	
T4	140 (44.7)	27 (43.5)	27 (38.0)	20 (42.6)	36 (46.8)	30 (53.6)	
N stage							
N0	93 (29.7)	16 (25.8)	23 (32.4)	11 (23.4)	26 (33.8)	17 (30.4)	
N1	131 (41.9)	27 (43.5)	28 (39.4)	22 (46.8)	34 (44.2)	20 (35.7)	0.81
N2	89 (28.4)	19 (30.6)	20 (28.2)	14 (29.8)	17 (22.1)	19 (33.9)	
Histopathology							
IDC*	273 (87.2)	47 (75.8)	62 (87.3)	44 (93.6)	66 (85.7)	54 (96.4)	
ILC*	22 (7.0)	7 (11.3)	7 (9.9)	3 (6.4)	4 (5.2)	1 (1.8)	
Metaplastic carcinoma	10 (3.2)	2 (3.2)	0 (0.0)	0 (0.0)	7 (9.1)	1 (1.8)	
Mucinous carcinoma	4 (1.3)	3 (4.8)	1 (1.4)	0 (0.0)	0 (0.0)	0 (0.0)	0.01
Invasive papillary carcinoma	3 (1.0)	2 (3.2)	1 (1.4)	0 (0.0)	0 (0.0)	0 (0.0)	
Invasive carcinoma with neuroendocrine features	1 (0.3)	1 (1.6)	0 (0.0)	0 (0.0)	0 (0.0)	0 (0.0)	
Grade							
I	34 (10.9)	14 (22.6)	9 (12.7)	5 (10.6)	2 (2.6)	4 (7.1)	
II	193(61.7)	36 (58.1)	48 (67.6)	28 (59.6)	38 (49.4)	43 (76.8)	<0.01
III	86 (27.5)	12 (19.4)	14 (19.7)	14 (29.8)	37 (48.1)	9 (16.1)	

* IDC: infiltrating ductal carcinoma, * ILC: Infiltrating lobular carcinoma, * TNBC: triple-negative breast cancer.

By multivariate logistic regression analysis, seven variables on sonography and mammogram imaging were significantly related to predict non-TNBC from TNBC and were assigned scores for the final prediction. These are summarized in Table 5. These variables were as follows:

(1) Presence of mass or focal asymmetry on mammogram or presence of mass on ultrasound: if not associated with microcalcifications (1 point); if associated with microcalcifications (2 points).
(2) Mass shape on ultrasound or mammogram: round (1 point), oval (2 points), and if irregular (3 points).
(3) Mass margins on ultrasound or mammogram: if well-circumscribed (1 point), microlobulated (2 points), and irregular-spiculated/ill-defined/obscured (3 points).
(4) Mass boundary on ultrasound: abrupt (1 point); echogenic halo (2 points).
(5) Posterior shadowing on ultrasound: absent (1 point); present (2 points).
(6) Posterior enhancement on ultrasound: absent (1 point); present (1 point).
(7) Orientation: parallel (+0); antiparallel (1 point).

This scoring system is not applicable in the absence of a sonographically and mammographically detected mass; therefore, score 0 was assigned to the presence of pleomorphic microcalcifications on mammogram without coexistent malignant mass on ultrasound and mammogram. Echogenicity was not included in the scoring system because in our study we did not find a significant difference among the echogenicity of non-TNBC and TNBC groups. The minimum and maximum scores were 6 and 14, respectively. The lower value of the score anticipates the presence of TNBC. In speculating TNBC, ROC curve analysis was performed for this sono-mammometry score, which showed significant statistical association ($p = < 0.01$). AUC was demonstrated to be 0.719 with 95% CI of 0.645–0.792. At score 10.5, sensitivity is 94%, specificity is 47%, positive predictive value is 75%, and negative predictive value is 84%.

2.7. Statistical Analysis The data was entered and analyzed in SPSS version 22.0. Mean and standard deviations were computed for continuous variables and categorical variables were presented as frequency and percentages and their comparison was done using bivariate Chi-square test. Multivariate binary logistic analysis was used to quantify the relative contribution of each imaging feature. p value <0.05 was considered as statistically significant. Odds ratios and confidence intervals were recorded for predictors of TNBC and Her-2 +ve disease. Receiver operating characteristic (ROC) analysis was performed and area under the curve (AUC) was recorded using the sono-mammometry scoring system devised for predicting imaging features for non-TNBC.

3. Results

3.1. Clinicopathological Findings (Table 2). In our data set, the median age of patients was 49.5(+−12.4 S. D), out of which the majority of cancers were detected in 30–50 years of age. Among 313 patients, the most common histopathological type was infiltrating ductal carcinoma ($n = 273$, 87.2%), among which the most common was TNBC ($n = 77$, 24.6%) followed by luminal B1 ($n = 71$, 22.7%). Out of 10 (3.2%) metaplastic carcinoma ($n = 7$, 9.1%) were TNBC. Right-sided tumors were ($n = 153$, 48.9%) and left-sided were ($n = 160$, 51.1%). Multifocality was found in 61 (19.5%). In our data, patients most commonly presented with T4 ($n = 140$, 44.7%) and N1 stages ($n = 131$, 41.9%). Patient's age, side, and focality of tumor did not show any significant correlation with molecular classification. Grade III was more frequently noted in TNBC ($n = 37$, 48.1%) vs ($n = 49$, 20.8%) in non-TNBC group.

3.2. Ultrasound Findings and Luminal Classification (Table 3). Ultrasound findings were normal in 2 (0.6%) patients, both belonging to Her-2 enriched category, which on mammogram showed only microcalcifications. The remaining 311 (99.4%) patients presented as a mass with or without calcifications. Majority of these tumors presented with irregular/spiculated margins ($n = 274$, 87.5%) ($p = 0.01$). Hormone receptor (HR) positive and Her-2+ve tumors share almost similar distribution for spiculated margins, i.e., ($n = 58$, 93.5%), ($n = 70$, 98.6%), ($n = 45$, 95.7%), and ($n = 52$, 92.9%) for luminal A, B-1, B-2, and Her-2 +ve, respectively. Although most TNBC also presented with irregular margins ($n = 36$, 46.8%) but among tumors with well-circumscribed ($n = 15$, 4.8%) or microlobulated ($n = 44$, 14.1%) margins, TNBC showed significant correlation ($n = 12$, 15.6%) and ($n = 29$, 37.7%) ($p = < 0.01$), respectively. Similarly, round- ($n = 5$, 1.6%) and oval-shaped ($n = 32$, 10.2) masses correlated well with TNBC ($p = < 0.01$). Regardless of subtype of breast cancer, most of the tumors were hypoechoic ($n = 263$, 84%) ($p = 0.03$). Only 36 (11.5%) masses appeared complex on sonography.

Triple-negative breast cancer (TNBC) exhibited a significant association with posterior acoustic enhancement. Among the tumors that were showing posterior acoustic enhancement, only almost half ($n = 39$, 50.6%) ($p = < 0.01$) were TNBC. Majority tumors with posterior acoustic shadowing only ($n = 131$, 41.9%) showed HR positivity ($n = 34$, 54.8%) for luminal A and ($n = 31$, 43.7%) and ($n = 16$, 34.0%) for luminal B-1 and B-2 ($p = 0.02$). The majority of Her-2 enriched tumors also displayed only posterior shadowing ($n = 29$, 51.8%). In ($n = 32$, 10.2%), both features were present and were most commonly seen in B-1 tumors ($n = 12$, 16.9%) ($p = 0.01$). In ($n = 73$, 23.3%) ($p = < 0.01$), both features were absent.

In our study, the majority of tumors ($n = 202$, 64.55%) showed peripheral echogenic halo, among which the most common was luminal A ($n = 56$, 90.3%) ($p = < 0.01$). With regard to orientation, the preponderance of malignant masses showed antiparallel orientation to the chest wall ($n = 297$, 94.9%) ($p = 0.03$).

3.3. Mammography Findings and Luminal Classification (Table 4). Mammography findings were normal in 7 (2.2%) patients and ($n = 7$, 2.2%) patients with focal asymmetry. In all these patients, ultrasound showed noncalcified mass. The most common mammographic feature was the presence of a mass without microcalcification ($n = 197$, 62.9%) followed by a mass with microcalcification ($n = 92$, 29.4%). Most common noncalcified tumors showed correlation with HR

TABLE 3: Ultrasound findings.

Imaging characteristics	Total (*n* = 313)	Luminal A (*n* = 62)	Luminal B1 (*n* = 71)	Luminal B2 (*n* = 47)	TNBC (*n* = 77)	Her-2 enrich (*n* = 56)	*p* value
Imaging findings							
Negative	2 (0.6)	0 (0.0)	0 (0.0)	0 (0.0)	0 (0.0)	2 (3.6)	0.05
Positive	311 (99.4)	62 (100)	71 (100)	47 (100)	77 (100)	54 (96.4)	
Mass (*n* = 311)							
Shape							
Round	5 (1.6)	0 (0)	0 (0)	1 (2.1)	4 (5.2)	0 (0)	<0.01
Oval	32 (10.2)	4 (6.5)	1 (1.4)	1 (2.1)	24 (31.2)	2 (3.6)	
Irregular	274 (87.5)	58 (93.5)	70 (98.6)	45 (95.7)	49 (63.6)	52 (92.9)	
Echogenicity							
Hypoechoic	263 (84)	51 (82.3)	65 (91.5)	42 (89.4)	59 (76.6)	46 (82.1)	0.03
Hyperechoic	1 (0.3)	0 (0)	0 (0)	1 (2.1)	0 (0)	0 (0)	
Isoechoic	11 (3.5)	4 (6.5)	1 (1.4)	1 (1.4)	2 (2.6)	2 (3.6)	
Complex	36 (11.5)	7 (11.3)	5 (1.6)	2 (4.3)	16 (5.1)	6 (10.7)	
Margins							
Well circumscribed	15 (4.8)	1 (1.6)	0 (0)	0(0)	12(15.6)	2(3.6)	<0.01
Non-well circumscribed	—	—	—	—	—	—	
Microlobulated	44 (14.1)	5 (8.1)	2 (2.8)	7 (14.9)	29 (37.7)	1 (1.8)	
Irregular/spiculated	252 (80.5)	56 (90.3)	69 (97.2)	40 (85.1)	36 (46.8)	51 (91.1)	
Orientation							
Parallel	14 (4.5)	4 (6.5)	1 (1.4)	1 (0.3)	7 (2.2)	1 (1.8)	0.03
Antiparallel	297 (94.9)	58 (93.5)	70 (98.6)	46 (97.9)	70 (90.9)	53(94.6)	
Posterior features							
Enhancement only	75 (24)	7 (11.3)	6 (8.5)	3 (6.4)	39 (50.6)	20 (35.7)	<0.01
Shadowing only	131 (41.9)	34 (54.8)	31 (43.7)	16 (34.0)	21 (27.3)	29 (51.8)	0.02
Both present	32 (10.2)	5 (8.1)	12 (16.9)	8 (17)	3 (3.9)	4 (7.1)	0.01
Both absent	73(23.3)	16 (25.8)	22 (31.0)	20 (42.6)	14 (18.2)	1 (1.8)	<0.01
Boundary							
Abrupt	109(34.8)	6 (9.7)	15 (21.1)	26 (55.3)	41 (53.2)	21 (37.5)	<0.01
Echogenic halo	202(64.5)	56 (90.3)	56 (78.9)	21 (44.7)	36 (46.8)	33 (58.9)	

*TNBC: triple-negative breast cancer.

TABLE 4: Mammographic findings.

Imaging characteristics	Total (*n* = 313)	Luminal A (*n* = 62)	Luminal B-1 (Her-2–ve) (*n* = 71)	Luminal B-2 (Her-2+ve) (*n* = 47)	TNBC (*n* = 77)	Her-2 enrich (*n* = 56)	*p* value
Findings							
Negative	7 (2.2)	0 (0.0)	2 (2.8)	3 (6.4)	1 (1.3)	1 (1.8)	<0.01
Mass only	197 (62.9)	45 (72.6)	46 (64.8)	22 (46.8)	64 (83.1)	20 (35.7)	
Microcalcifications only	10 (3.2)	1 (1.6)	1 (1.4)	4 (8.5)	0 (0.0)	4 (7.1)	
Mass with microcalcifications	92 (29.4)	15 (24.2)	19 (26.8)	17 (36.2)	12 (15.6)	29 (51.8)	
Focal asymmetry	7 (2.2)	1 (1.6)	3 (4.2)	1 (2.1)	0 (0.0)	2 (3.6)	
Mass (*n* = 289)							
Margins							
Well circumscribed	15 (4.8)	1 (1.6)	0 (0.0)	0 (0.0)	12 (15.6)	2 (3.6)	<0.01
Non-well circumscribed	—	—	—	—	—	—	
Microlobulated	40 (12.8)	5 (8.1)	1 (1.4)	5 (10.6)	28 (36.4)	1 (1.8)	
Spiculated/obscured/indistinct	234 (74.8)	54 (87.1)	64 (90.1)	34 (72.3)	36 (46.8)	46 (82.1)	
Architectural distortion/trabecular thickening							
Yes	226 (72.2)	46 (74.2)	59 (83.1)	34 (72.3)	39 (50.6)	48 (85.7)	<0.01
No	87 (27.8)	16 (25.8)	12 (16.9)	13 (27.7)	38 (49.4)	8 (14.3)	

*TNBC: triple-negative breast cancer.

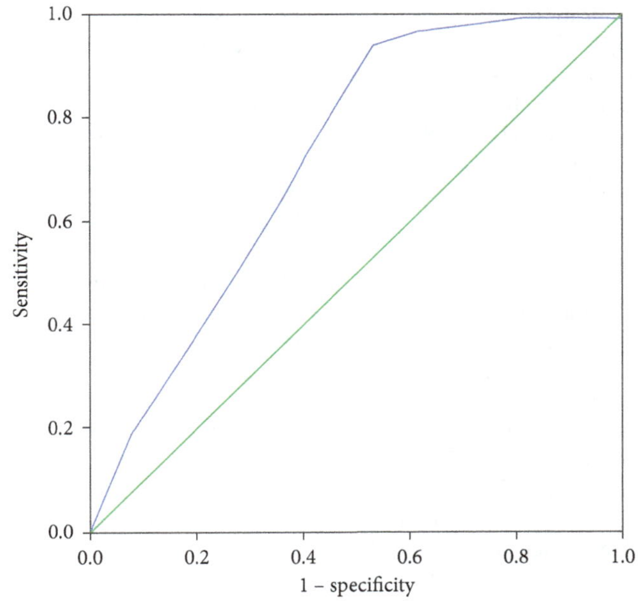

AUC	p-value	95% confidence interval
0.719	0.000	0.645–0.792

Figure 1: ROC curve.

Table 5: Multivariate analysis of ultrasound and mammographic findings.

Imaging findings	Outcome variable	p value	Odds ratio	Confidence interval
Noncalcified mass/focal asymmetry v/s mass with calcification/only microcalcifications	TNBC* v/s non-TNBC*	0.03	1.124	6.141–22.69
Mass shape round/oval v/s irregular	TNBC v/s non-TNBC	<0.01	2.443	4.836–27.382
Margins well-circumscribed/microlobulated v/s irregular spiculated	TNBC v/s non-TNBC	<0.01	2.472	1.462–6.479
Orientation parallel v/s nonparallel	TNBC v/s non-TNBC	0.03	1.176	1.100–9.562
Posterior enhancement v/s shadowing	TNBC v/s non-TNBC	<0.01	1.731	3.190–9.988
Round/oval shape + well-defined/microlobulated margins	TNBC v/s non-TNBC	<0.01	2.612	6.034–30.744
Well-circumscribed/microlobulated margins + presence of posterior enhancement + absence of posterior shadowing	TNBC v/s non-TNBC	<0.01	2.946	8.224–44.073
Tumor grade III v/s I/II	TNBC v/s Non-TNBC	<0.01	1.231	1.962–5.977
Ki-67 high (<14%) v/s low (<14%)	TNBC v/s non-TNBC	0.03	1.108	1.451–6.320
Mass with microcalcifications/only microcalcifications v/s noncalcified mass/focal asymmetry	Her-2 neu +ve v/s Her-2 neu −ve	<0.01	1.366	2.371–6.481
Irregular shape/margins v/s well-circumscribed margins	Her-2 neu +ve v/s Her-2 neu −ve	.009	.937	1.263–5.157
Mass with microcalcifications/only microcalcification + irregular margins	Her-2 neu +ve v/s Her-2 neu −ve	<0.01	1.278	2.145–6.004

*TNBC: triple-negative breast cancer. *Non-TNBC:non-triple-negative breast cancer.

negativity ($n = 64$, 83.1%) ($p = < 0.01$) followed by luminal A ($n = 45$, 72.6%). In contrast, Her-2 positive tumors (Her-2 enrich and luminal B-2) were significantly associated with microcalcifications, with ($n = 29$, 51.8%) or without associated mass ($n = 29$, 51.8%) ($p = < 0.01$).

3.4. Multivariate Analysis (Table 5). We also performed an analysis on combined imaging findings. Breast malignancies with round/oval shape and well-circumscribed/microlobulated margins were strongly associated with the absence of tumor markers—TNBC ($p = < 0.01$) (O. R = 2.612) (CI = 6.034 −30.744). Combining the presence of posterior acoustic enhancement and the absence of posterior acoustic shadowing with round/oval shape and well-circumscribed/microlobulated margins increased significantly the probability of the tumor being hormone receptor negative ($p = 0.01$) (OR = 2.946) (CI = 8.224–44.073), ($n = 24$, 31.2%). Multivariate analysis for grades and Ki-67 showed significant association of TNBC with high-grade tumors ($p < 0.01$) (OR = 1.231) (CI = 1.962–5.977) and high Ki-67 (>14%) ($p = 0.03$) (O. R = 1.108) (CI =

1.451–6.320). Presence of microcalcification with or without mass showed significant relationship with Her-2 positive tumors ($p = < 0.01$) (O. R = 1.366) (CI = 2.371–6.481). Combining irregular margins and shape with the presence of microcalcifications with or without mass also displayed a significant relationship with Her-2 positivity ($p = < 0.01$) (OR = 1.278) (CI = 2.145–6.004).

4. Discussion

We studied the correlation of sonographic and digital mammographic features with molecular classification of breast cancer and also devised a score called sono-mammometry score to anticipate the presence of non-TNBC tumors. We also determined the association of baseline histopathological type, grade of tumor, Ki-67, and T and N stages of the breast cancers with each luminal classification. We used the term "Her-2 enrich" for tumors that are hormone receptor negative and Her-2 neu +ve, while the term "Her-2 +ve" is used to indicate both luminal B-2 and Her-2 enrich tumors collectively.

We studied that non-triple-negative breast cancers are predominantly hypoechoic, less commonly complex in the echo pattern. These tumors strongly correlate with the presence of irregular spiculated margins along with peripheral echogenic halo and presence of posterior acoustic shadowing. Architectural distortion and trabecular thickening are also found frequently in this same subset. Presence of microcalcifications also correlates significantly with non-TNBC.

Spiculations in the margin are established criteria in the diagnosis of malignancy. Spiculated margins are generally secondary to drawing in of Cooper's ligaments into a tumor mass or the invasion of tumor cells into the neighboring breast tissues [11]. These irregular margins are believed to be associated with slow multiplication of tumor cells, which gives enough time for stromal interactions and induces fibrosis surrounding the invasive edge [11, 12]. Liu et al. [11] reported that masses with spiculated margins were significantly more common in patients with luminal A breast cancer than in those with other subtypes; however, we studied that HR-positive tumors (all non-TNBC) including Her-2 +ve luminal B and Her-2 enrich cancers presented with predominantly spiculated margins and we also deduced that because of this same reason non-TNBC tumor more often causes architectural distortion/trabecular thickening as secondary sign of malignancy. In our study, multivariate logistic regression analysis also determined the convincing association of irregular spiculated margins with Her-2 positivity. This is opposed to Liu et al.'s study [11] which determined that Her-2 overexpressing cancer almost never presents as spiculated masses. On the contrary, this is similar to the studies done by Lee et al. [3], Cho [4], and Elias et al. [13] who stated that circumscribed margins decreased the chance of HER-2 overexpression.

Lacroix et al. [14] determined that grade 1 and grade 2 tumors result in spicules and perilesional hyperechogenic halo. Our study supports this finding because, as discussed above, irregular margins were frequently associated with non-TNBC and this is the same subgroup that is more often related to low-grade (grade I and II) tumors. We also assume that peripheral echogenic halo which dictates the presence of desmoplastic reaction [10] can also be found routinely in this same luminal A, B and Her-2 enriched subgroups.

In invasive carcinomas, the unregulated and disorganized growth of malignant cells generates different tissue layers with variable acoustic impedance, which in turn causes an increase in the attenuation of the sound beams. This, along with fibrosis secondary to stromal interaction, results in posterior acoustic shadowing in sonographic images [10, 12]. We found a significant correlation of both HR-positive and Her-2 enriched tumors with the presence of posterior acoustic shadowing (Figures 2(a)–2(c)).

It is imperative that the presence of microcalcifications at mammography is not definite for any breast cancer subtype [3]. These are more likely encountered in Her-2 +ve and HR-positive tumors [3]. In our study, we have divided luminal B cancers into two subgroups to scrutinize the impact of Her-2 positive status on imaging features. Multivariate logistic regression analysis demonstrates a convincing interconnection of microcalcifications (with or without the presence of a malignant mass) with Her-2 +ve disease. Cen et al. [15] stated that Her-2 enriched tumors were more expected to have heterogeneous and pleomorphic microcalcifications on mammogram. Likewise, Elias et al. [13] and Lee et al. [16] found that fine, pleomorphic or fine linear branching calcifications are the most characteristics findings for Her-2 +ve cancers. It is noteworthy that Her-2 +ve tumors belong to the subgroup that can be missed with ultrasound because of the presence of microcalcifications only [5]. In our study, two cases, in which ultrasound did not show any mass, had microcalcifications on mammogram and belong to Her-2 +ve subset (Figures 3(a)–3(c) and Figures 4(a)–4(c)).

TNBC has been known to be associated with considerable differences in clinical, radiological, and pathological features compared with its counterpart [12, 17]. This is the subtype most discussed in the literature and it is the most commonly identified subgroup in our study. TNBC are also hypoechoic or show a complex echo pattern. We studied that TNBC can less commonly share imaging features similar to non-TNBC, i.e., mass with irregular margins and posterior shadowing. Imaging features that are distinctive to TNBC are similar to those that are also peculiar to benign tumors like noncalcified masses with well-circumscribed or microlobulated margins with posterior acoustic enhancement and more often with an abrupt boundary. Our findings were supported by studies by Lee et al. [3] and Lin et al. [12] who determined that benign "pseudofibroadenoma" type features can often be seen in TNBC. On sonography, the smooth well-circumscribed and microlobulated margin in TNBC is termed as "pushing border" microscopically and is considered secondary to rapid growth and high proliferation rate of malignant cells which leads to the lack of both stromal interaction and fibrosis. Cooper ligaments are believed to be displaced and not disrupted significantly in TNBC [10,12]. Identical to the benign masses, orderly and nestled growth of tumor cells in TNBC create fewer layers that lead to improved enhanced through transmission [10]. In addition,

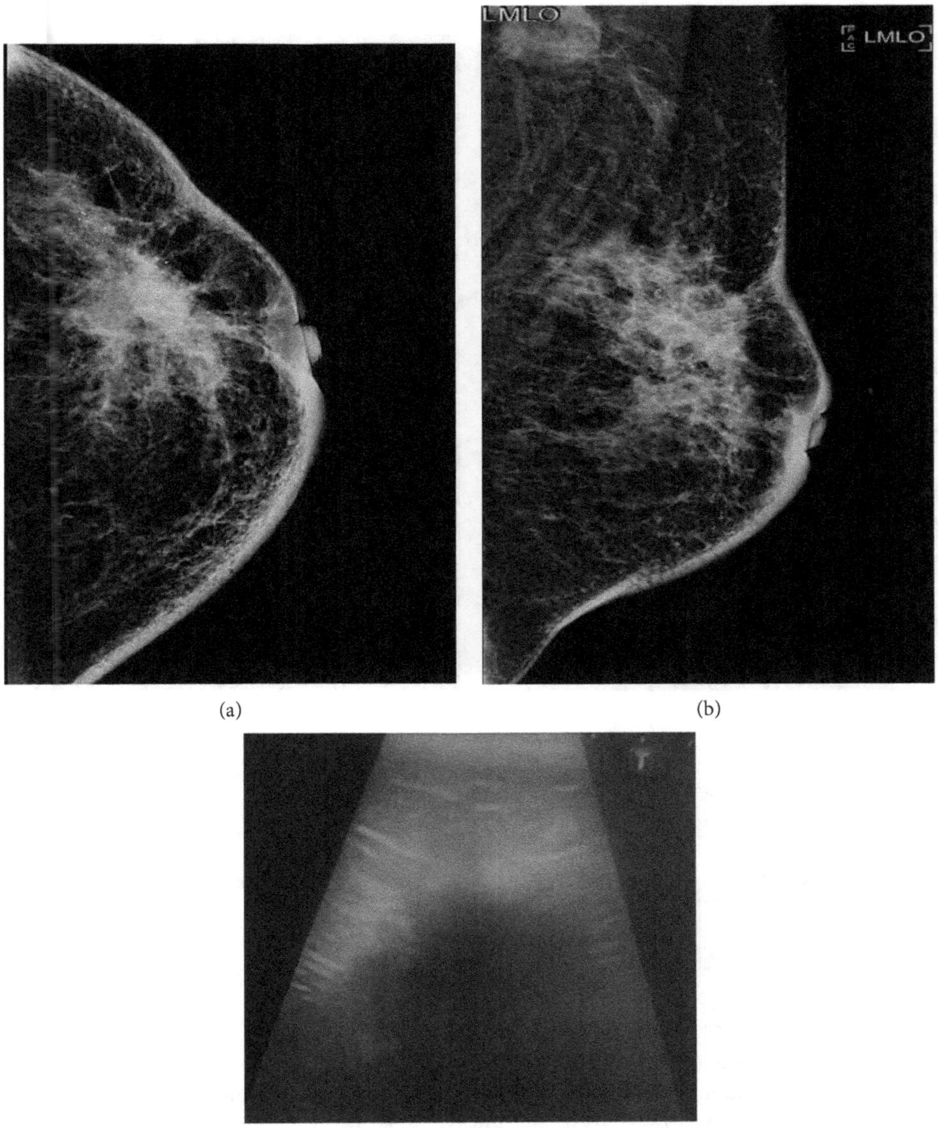

(a) (b) (c)

FIGURE 2: CC and MLO views of left breast: biopsy-proven hormone receptor +ve tumor (grade II). (a) A high-density mass is seen in upper-outer quadrant extending to retroareolar region. Irregular spiculated margins are seen with secondary signs of architectural distortion and trabecular thickening. (b) Overlying skin shows thickening and dimpling. Clustered microcalcifications are also seen within the mass. We can also see large malignant looking nodal mass in ipsilateral axilla. (c) Ultrasound of the same patient: there is a hypoechoic mass with irregular spiculated margins. Dense posterior acoustic shadowing is also seen obscuring posterior extent of the mass. We can also appreciate antiparallel orientation and peripheral echogenic halo. Sono-mammometry score = 14.

these tumors show a tendency towards being high grade and are more cellular and therefore display posterior acoustic enhancement more frequently than non-TNBC [12, 17]. Peripheral echogenic halo is believed to be less often found in TNBC. Our findings were also supported by studies done by Lacroix et al. [14] and Wojcinski et al. [10] who also found abrupt tumor parenchyma interface more frequently in these tumors. TNBC are also known to lack the presence of suspicious microcalcifications on mammogram [3, 18] (Figures 5(a)–5(c)). However, Lin et al. [12] believed that there are wide variations in imaging features for TNBC. In our study, we postulate that close resemblance of its imaging features with benign tumors warrants improving diagnostic performance for early suspicion and recognition of malignancy, particularly in outpatient clinics where prompt and precise decisions are required.

Although there are some characteristics imaging features that can be attributed to each luminal category, overall there is considerable overlap in imaging features of these 5 groups. Therefore, based on our results, we divided these cancers into two groups, non-TNBC and TNBC, and devised a score called "sono-mammometry" score (Table 5) consisting of simple sonological and mammographic features for prediction of non-TNBC and TNBC which can be easily

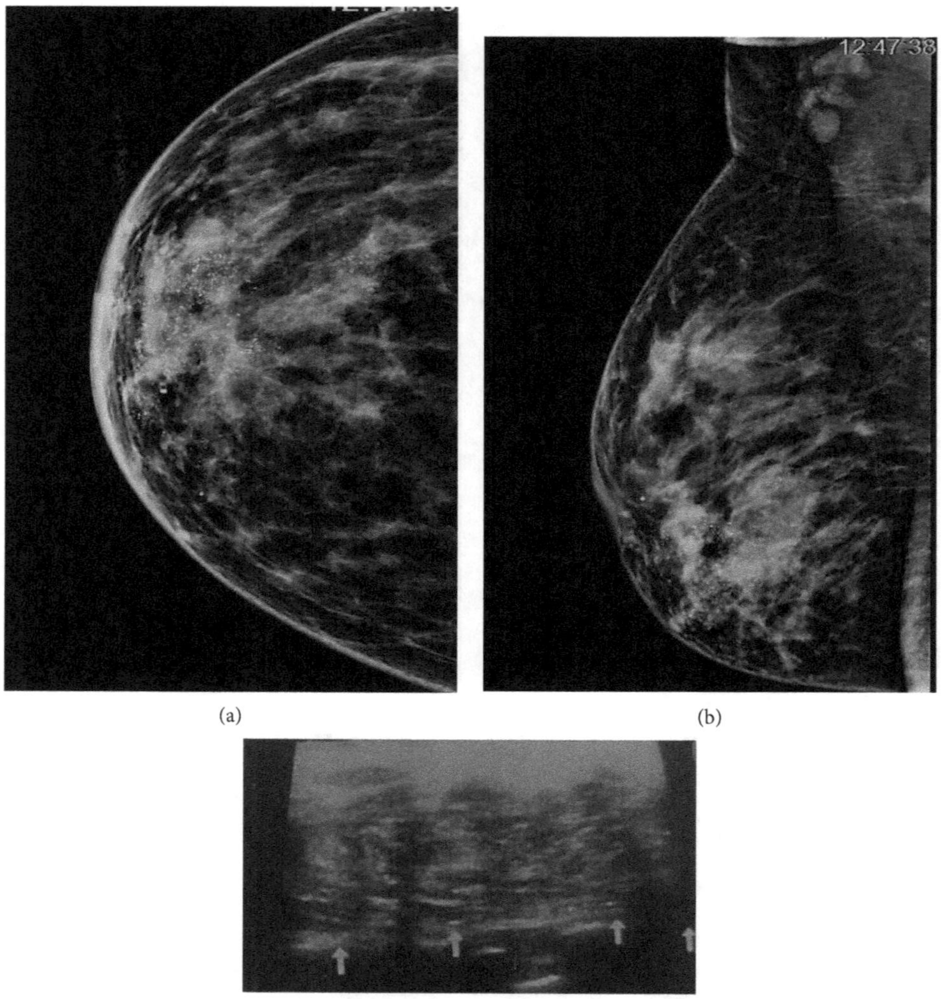

(a) (b) (c)

Figure 3: CC and MLO views of right breast. (a) Biopsy-proven infiltrating ductal carcinoma Her-2 enrich tumor (grade I). There is a high-density mass in retroareolar region extending to the lower quadrant. Irregular spiculated margins are seen along with visualization of extensive microcalcification within the mass. (b) Overlying skin thickening is also seen. Suspicious axillary lymph nodes are also there. (c) Ultrasound of the same patient shows a complex mass with partly ill-defined and partly irregular anterior margins. Abrupt boundary is seen with parallel orientation of this mass with the chest wall (wider than taller). No posterior features. Sono-mammometry score: 11.

performed in outpatient settings. Score of 10.5 shows sensitivity of 94%. Its low specificity of 47% is a limitation which warrants validation of this score on a larger number of patients before future implication. However, this score is still useful, particularly in a developing country where resources are limited. Although histopathological diagnosis providing us with indispensable information regarding tumor biology and histological interpretation cannot be ignored, all laboratory tests have the incidence of false results [11]. It highlights the importance of a radiologist to be well-aware of common and uncommon imaging features, so a question can be raised in the matter of conflicting lab results and perhaps it may be beneficial to repeat testing of the immunohistochemical receptors.

It is worthwhile to discuss the advancement of artificial intelligence with regard to medical imaging. In our study, human readers are involved in anticipating results with the help of simple features on mammogram and ultrasound; however, there are studies which have incorporated newer imaging techniques, e.g., Dilorenzo et al. [19] has shown the potential role of background parenchymal enhancement in MRI breast in discriminating different breast cancer subtypes. Fusion of ultrasound and MRI images also proved to provide information about additional occult breast lesions [20]. State-of-the-art techniques assimilate radiomics in discerning benign and malignant breast lesions on mammography [21, 22]. Different variety of machine learning techniques has also been developed and integrated for early detection of breast cancer through textural analysis of microcalcification on mammogram and for further classification of breast cancers [23–25]. Contrast-enhanced spectral mammography is a recently introduced mammographic method in which Forgia et al. have

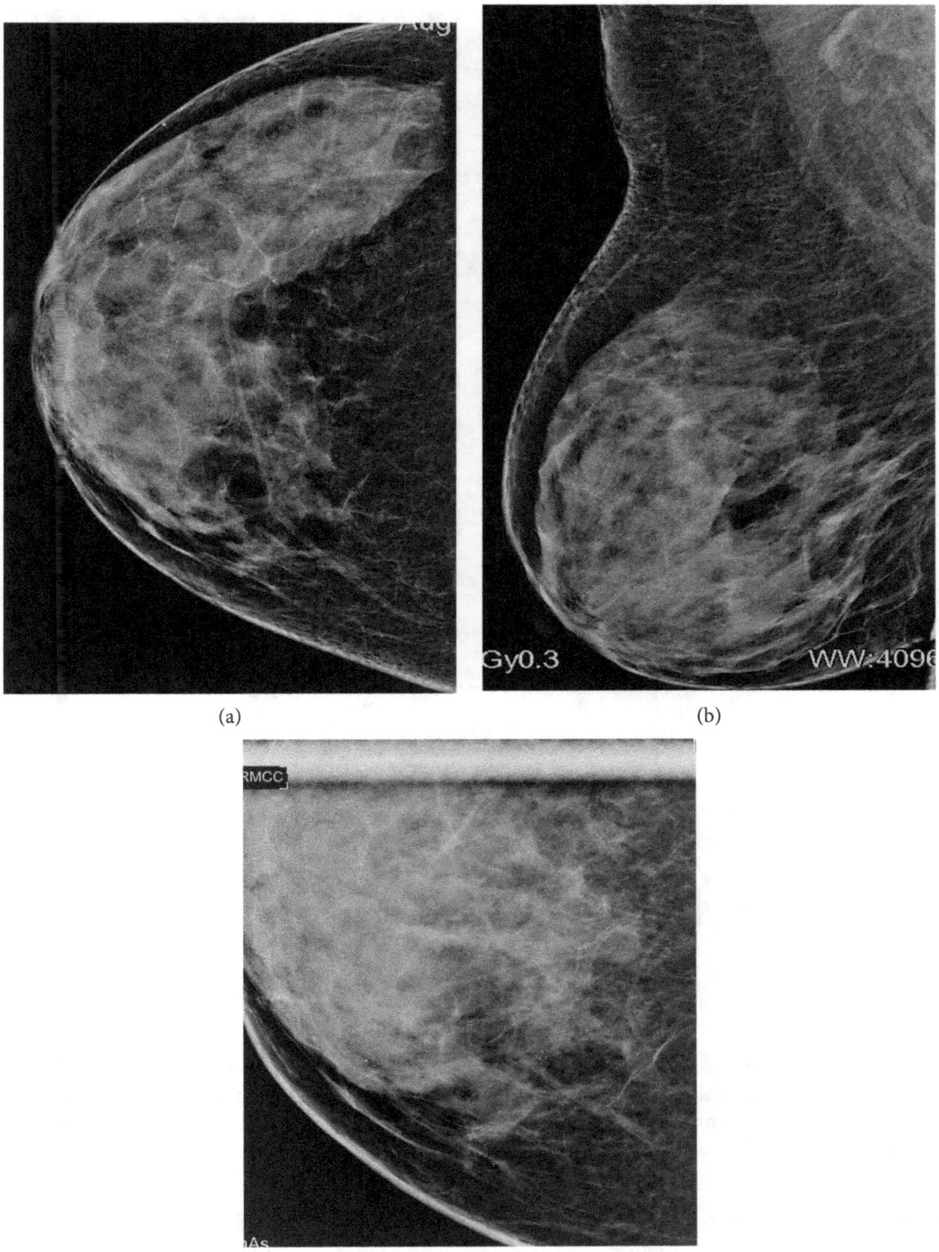

(a) (b) (c)

FIGURE 4: CC, MLO, and magnified CC view of right breast. (a) Biopsy-proven infiltrating ductal carcinoma Her-2 neu enrich tumor. (b) There are suspicious microcalcifications in the lower-outer quadrant which lead us to do a magnified CC view which shows clustered microcalcifications. (c) No definite mass was identified on mammogram as well as on ultrasound. Sono-mammometry score = 0.

discussed imaging features of two cancer molecular subtypes, i.e., HER-2 positive and triple-negative, with the help of radiomics [26]. Although radiomics is an evolving methodology which has shown to provide insightful results in quantitatively and objectively elucidating tumor biology, there are issues of standardization and lack of reporting guidelines. Furthermore, in economically developing and resource-constrained environment, these advanced engineering techniques are still seemed to be far-fetched and human readers with manual interpretation of images take precedence.

Our results should be comprehended after taking into account the limitations. First, it is a retrospective study with a small number of patients. Prospective studies with larger numbers of patients are needed to validate these results. Sono-mammometry score should be applied in a prospective population reassessment to see how predictive the model obtained is. Another is that breast density was not taken into

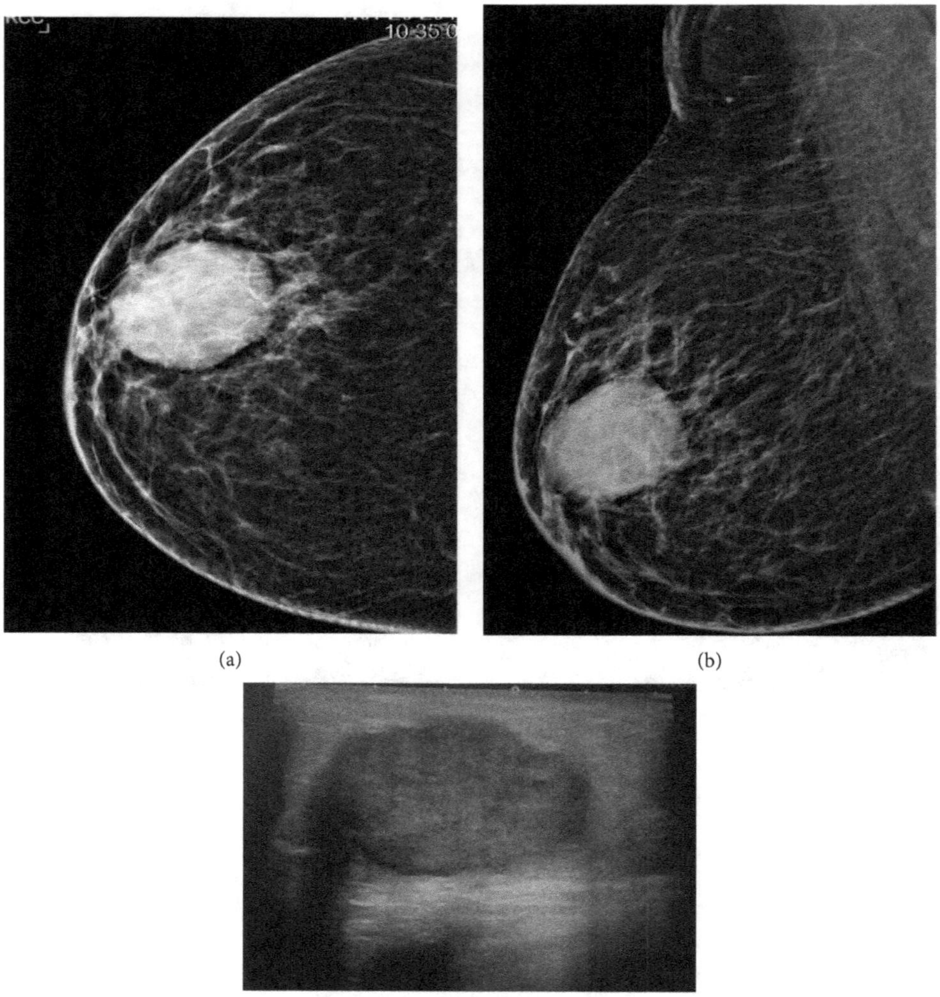

(a) (b) (c)

FIGURE 5: CC and MLO views of right breast. (a) Biopsy-proven metaplastic carcinoma triple-negative (grade III). There is an oval-shaped high-density mass in retroareolar region. Well-defined margins are seen. (b) Peripheral lucent halo is also seen. No microcalcifications are identified. (c) Ultrasound of the same patient shows a hypoechoic mass with microlobulated margins. Posterior acoustic enhancement is seen. Abrupt boundary with antiparallel orientation is also noticed. Sono-mammometry score = 9.

account. Moreover, our analysis was carried out on selected images rather than images acquired during real-time scanning and operator-dependent nature of ultrasound can give rise to biases.

5. Conclusion

Breast cancer exhibits different imaging features according to molecular type. Although imaging characteristics are helpful in the prediction of molecular classification, the prognostication of these features is still weak. There is considerable variation in the imaging features of TNBC as some of its imaging features overlap with those of typical benign tumors, which warrants vigilance towards improved diagnostic performance for early suspicion and recognition of malignancy. To help better understand these features, our sono-mammometry score can serve as a relatively inexpensive and straightforward test which assumes to be functional and productive in resource-limited settings. Our next step would be to apply this score in prospective study to assess its predictive value.

Acknowledgments

The authors would like to express their gratitude towards Dr. Abbas and Dr. Farina from Sindh Institute of Urology and Transplantation for their special consultation regarding the statistical analysis.

References

[1] L. Fan, P. E. Goss, and K. Strasser-Weippl, “Current status and future projections of breast cancer in asia,” *Breast Care*, vol. 10, no. 6, pp. 372–378, 2015.

[2] J. Kim, M. Jang, S. M. Kim et al., "Clinicopathological and imaging features of breast cancer in Korean women under 40 years of age," *Journal of the Korean Society of Radiology*, vol. 76, no. 6, pp. 375–385, 2017.

[3] I. Lee, S. M. Le Blanc, J. David et al., "Molecular classification of infiltrating breast cancer: toward personalized therapy," *Radio Graphics*, vol. 34, no. 5, pp. 1178–1195, 2014.

[4] N. Cho, "Molecular subtypes and imaging phenotypes of breast cancer," *Ultrasonography*, vol. 35, no. 4, pp. 281–288, 2016.

[5] S. Rashmi, S. Kamala, S. S. Murthy, S. Kotha, Y. S. Rao, and K. V. Chaudhary, "Predicting the molecular subtype of breast cancer based on mammography and ultrasound findings," *Indian Journal of Radiology and Imaging*, vol. 28, no. 3, pp. 354–361, 2018.

[6] L. Zhang, J. Li, Y. Xiao et al., "Identifying ultrasound and clinical features of breast cancer molecular subtypes by ensemble decision," *Scientific Reports*, vol. 5, no. 1, p. 11085, 2015.

[7] *American College of Radiology, ACR Practice Parameter for the Performance of a Breast Ultrasound Examination*, https://www.acr.org/-/media/ACR/Files/Practice-Parameters/US-Breast, 2016.

[8] *American College of Radiology, ACR Practice Parameter for the Performance of Screening and Diagnostic Mammography*, https://www.acr.org/-/media/ACR/Files/Practice-Parameters/screen-diag-mammo, 2018.

[9] F. Çelebi, K. N. Pilanci, C. Ordu et al., "The role of ultrasonographic findings to predict molecular subtype, histologic grade, and hormone receptor status of breast cancer," *Diagnostic and Interventional Radiology*, vol. 21, no. 6, pp. 448–453, 2015.

[10] S. Wojcinski, A. A. Soliman, J. Schmidt, L. Makowski, F. Degenhardt, and P. Hillemanns, "Sonographic features of triple-negative and non-triple-negative breast cancer," *Journal of Ultrasound in Medicine*, vol. 31, no. 10, pp. 1531–1541, 2012.

[11] S. Lui, X.-D. Wu, W.-J. Xu, Q. Lin, X.-J. Liu, and Y. Li, "Is there a correlation between the presence of a spiculated mass on mammogram and luminal A subtype breast cancer?" *Korean Journal of Radiology*, vol. 17, no. 6, pp. 846–852, 2016.

[12] J. Lin, K. Zhang, Z. Ting Shi et al., "Triple-negative invasive breast carcinoma: the association between the sonographic appearances with clinicopathological feature," *Scientific Reports*, vol. 8, p. 9040, 2018.

[13] S. G. Elias, A. Adams, D. J. Wisner et al., "Imaging features of HER-2 overexpression in breast cancer: a systematic review and meta-analysis," *Cancer Epidemiology, Biomarkers & Prevention*, vol. 23, no. 8, pp. 1464–1483, 2014.

[14] M. B. Lacroix, G. M. Grogan, M. Debled et al., "Radiological features of triple negative breast cancers (about 73 cases)," *Diagnostic and Interventional Imaging*, vol. 93, no. 3, pp. 183–190, 2012.

[15] D. Cen, L. Xu, N. Li et al., "BI-RADS 3-5 microcalcifications can preoperatively predict breast cancer HER-2 and Luminal a molecular subtype," *Oncotarget*, vol. 8, no. 8, pp. 13855–13862, 2017.

[16] S. H. Lee, J. M. Chang, S. U. Shin et al., "Imaging features of breast cancers on digital breast tomosynthesis according to molecular subtype: association with breast cancer detection," *The British Journal of Radiology*, vol. 90, no. 1080, p. 20170470, 2017.

[17] Q. I. Yang, H. Y. Liu, D. Liu, and Y. Q. Song, "Ultrasonographic features of triple-negative breast cancer: a comparison with other breast cancer subtypes," *Asian Pacific Journal of Cancer Prevention: APJCP*, vol. 16, no. 8, pp. 3229–3232, 2015.

[18] B. E. Dogan and L. W. Turnbull, "Imaging of triple-negative breast cancer," *Annals of Oncology*, vol. 23, pp. vi23–vi29, 2012.

[19] G. Dilorenzo, M. Telegrafo, D. La Forgia, A. A. Stabile Ianora, and M. Moschetta, "Breast MRI background parenchymal enhancement as an imaging bridge to molecular cancer subtype," *European Journal of Radiology*, vol. 113, pp. 148–152, 2019.

[20] A. Stabile Ianora, M. Bernini, D. La Forgia et al., "Six-year prospective evaluation of second-look US with volume navigation for MRI-detected additional breast lesions," *European Radiology*, vol. 29, no. 4, pp. 1799–1808, 2019.

[21] L. Fanizzi, A. Fanizzi, T. M. A. Basile et al., "Radiomics analysis on contrast-enhanced spectral mammography images for breast cancer diagnosis: a pilot study," *Entropy*, vol. 21, no. 11, p. 1110, 2019.

[22] A. Fanizzi, T. M. Basile, L. Losurdo et al., "Ensemble discrete wavelet transform and gray-level co-occurrence matrix for microcalcification cluster classification in digital mammography," *Applied Sciences*, vol. 9, no. 24, p. 5388, 2019.

[23] A. Fanizzi, T. M. A. Basile, L. Losurdo et al., "Machine learning approach on multiscale texture analysis for breast microcalcification diagnosis," *BMC Bioinformatics*, vol. 21, no. Suppl 2, 2020.

[24] L. Losurdol, A. Fanizzi, T. M. A. Basile et al., *A Combined Approach of Multiscale Texture Analysis and Interest Point/ Corner Detectors for Microcalcifications Diagnosis*, pp. 302–313, Springer International Publishing, NY, USA, 2018.

[25] A. Fanizzi, T. M. A. Basile, L. Losurdo et al., "Hough transform for clustered microcalcifications detection in full-field digital mammograms," in *Applications of Digital Image Processing XL*, A. G. Tescher, Ed., vol. 10396, p. 41, SPIE, Bellingham, Washington, USA, 2017.

[26] D. L. Forgia, A. Fanizzi, and F. Campobasso, "Radiomic analysis in contrast-enhanced spectral mammography for predicting breast cancer histological outcome," *Diagnostics*, vol. 10, no. 9, p. 708, 2020.

25

A Review of Doses for Dental Imaging in 2010–2020 and Development of a Web Dose Calculator

Hawon Lee[1,2] **and Andreu Badal**[2]

[1]*Montgomery Blair High School, Silver Spring, MD, USA*
[2]*Division of Imaging, Diagnostics and Software Reliability, OSEL, CDRH, Food and Drug Administration, Silver Spring, MD, USA*

Correspondence should be addressed to Hawon Lee; gracehawonlee@gmail.com

Academic Editor: André Luiz Ferreira Costa

Dental imaging is one of the most common types of diagnostic radiological procedures in modern medicine. We introduce a comprehensive table of organ doses received by patients in dental imaging procedures extracted from literature and a new web application to visualize the summarized dose information. We analyzed articles, published after 2010, from PubMed on organ and effective doses delivered by dental imaging procedures, including intraoral radiography, panoramic radiography, and cone-beam computed tomography (CBCT), and summarized doses by dosimetry method, machine model, patient age, and technical parameters. Mean effective doses delivered by intraoral, 1.32 (0.60–2.56) μSv, and panoramic, 17.93 (3.47–75.00) μSv, procedures were found to be about1% and 15% of that delivered by CBCT, 121.09 (17.10–392.20) μSv, respectively. In CBCT imaging, child phantoms received about 29% more effective dose than the adult phantoms received. The effective dose of a large field of view (FOV) (>150 cm^2) was about 1.6 times greater than that of a small FOV (<50 cm^2). The maximum CBCT effective dose with a large FOV for children, 392.2 μSv, was about 13% of theeffective dose that a person receives on average every year from natural radiation, 3110 μSv. Monte Carlo simulations of representative cases of the three dental imaging procedures were then conducted to estimate and visualize the dose distribution within the head. The user-friendly interactive web application (available at http://dentaldose.org) receives user input, such as the number of intraoral radiographs taken, and displays total organ and effective doses, dose distribution maps, and a comparison with other medical and natural sources of radiation. The web dose calculator provides a practical resource for patients interested in understanding the radiation doses delivered by dental imaging procedures.

1. Introduction

Dental imaging is one of the most common types of diagnostic radiological procedures taken by the average person. Popular dental imaging procedures include intraoral radiography, which has the longest history of use, followed by panoramic radiography, and more recently, cone-beam computed tomography (CBCT) [1]. Intraoral radiography, a simple two-dimensional (2D) projection imaging, is often used to detect periodontal disease and cavities at regular dental check-ups. Panoramic radiography, a more comprehensive 2D image that combines a series of narrow 2D images, has been widely used to provide a wide range of information about the dentition and jaws. Introduced in the late 1990s, three-dimensional (3D) imaging technology, CBCT, offers a comprehensive set of cross-sectional images, the ability of vertical scanning, and real-time intraoperative assessment. All three procedures expose different portions of the head, from small parts of the teeth to the whole lower head, to ionizing radiation. There are concerns about the increasing use of imaging procedures as well as the resulting radiation dose, especially for pediatric patients [2, 3].

Absorbed dose is defined as the energy deposited to a given volume divided by the mass (measured in gray, Gy, in the International System of Units) [4]. Equivalent dose (measured in sieverts, Sv) is derived from the absorbed dose multiplied by the radiation weighting factor, which represents the effectiveness of the biological damage to the exposed tissue. Effective dose (measured in sieverts, Sv) is then derived by adding all equivalent doses multiplied by tissue weighting factors and provides a relative measure of the risk of stochastic effects that might result from irradiation. The most fundamental dose quantity, organ dose, of dental imaging can be obtained through two methods: measurement and computer simulation. First, organ doses can be physically measured with dosimeters placed within anatomy models, called physical human phantoms, that are exposed to dental radiation. Second, organ doses can be calculated through computer simulations where the simulation model of an imaging device is combined with digital anatomy models, called computational human phantoms [5]. Different types of pediatric and adult computational human phantoms are available for dose calculations. Many studies report organ doses from dental imaging procedures estimated by measurement or simulation. However, there are few resources that summarize a variety of data and present the radiation dose with a user-friendly interface.

The current study was intended to provide a practical resource for patients interested in understanding the radiation doses delivered by dental imaging procedures for the period of 2010–2020 and comparison with other radiation sources that are commonly faced in daily life. We established a comprehensive table of organ doses for dental imaging procedures by extracting data from literature and developed a user-friendly web application to present the summarized information.

2. Materials and Methods

We obtained articles from PubMed, published after 2010, on organ and effective doses delivered by dental imaging procedures including intraoral radiography, panoramic radiography, and CBCT, and summarized doses by dosimetry method, machine model, patient age, and technical parameters. Monte Carlo simulations of representative cases of the three dental imaging procedures were conducted to estimate and visualize the dose distribution within the head. Finally, we developed an interactive web-based dose calculator to provide easy access to the dental doses and to compare them with other radiation sources commonly faced in daily life.

2.1. Literature Search. We searched for articles on organ and effective doses delivered by dental imaging in PubMed (https://pubmed.ncbi.nlm.nih.gov, National Library of Medicine, National Center for Biotechnology Information) available on October 1, 2020, using the following keywords:

(i) "dental intraoral organ dose" (for intraoral)
(ii) "dental panoramic organ dose" (for panoramic)
(iii) "dental cone beam CT organ dose" (for CBCT)

These keywords brought up 41, 49, and 54 papers (144 in total) for intraoral, panoramic, and CBCT procedures, respectively. We selected papers published after 2010:a total of 81 papers (14, 20, and 47 papers for intraoral, panoramic, and CBCT, respectively) out of 144 papers. The papers that were not written in English (except for non-English articles with dose tables in English) or did not include the dose to bone marrow, brain, salivary glands, and thyroid and effective doses were excluded from the review process. After the exclusion, we finally used 3, 9, and 11 papers providing organ and effective doses for intraoral, panoramic, and CBCT procedures, respectively.

2.2. Data Collection. The following data were extracted from the papers:

(i) Dosimetry methods: simulation or measurement
(ii) Imaging machine model
(iii) Age represented by physical (measurement) or computational (simulation) phantoms: we denoted the age of 35 as the minimum age for all adult phantoms, which is the International Commission on Radiological Protection (ICRP) reference age of adults [6]
(iv) Dose calculation program for simulation studies or dosimeter type for measurement studies
(v) Beam rotation angle (only for CBCT)
(vi) Imaging protocol
(vii) Dose area product (DAP) (mGy-cm^2) (for intraoral and CBCT)
(viii) Tube potential (kVp)
(ix) The width and height of field of view (FOV) (cm) (for intraoral and CBCT)
(x) Effective dose (E) (μSv)
(xi) Doses to the bone marrow, brain, salivary glands, and thyroid (μGy)

When a single paper provided multiple dose data in multiple categories, the dose in each category was considered a separate dose set. Simulation and measurement data were analyzed separately when both were reported in a single paper. When an effective dose was missing but organ doses were reported, an effective dose was derived from the organ doses using tissue weighting factors from ICRP Publication 103 [4]: 0.12 (bone marrow), 0.01 (brain), 0.01 (salivary glands), and 0.04 (thyroid). We assumed zero doses for other organs outside the head region in the calculation of the effective dose. The extracted data were tabulated in three detailed tables for intraoral, panoramic, and CBCT, respectively.

To efficiently analyze the doses, we averaged the organ and effective doses over different data sources. As for CBCT, which had more available data for different phantom ages and FOVthan intraoral and panoramic, we further arranged organ and effective doses by phantom age group (children and adults) and/or the area (height *x* width) of FOV (small $<50\,cm^2$, medium $50–150\,cm^2$, and large $>150\,cm^2$).

2.3. Monte Carlo Simulation of Dental Imaging Procedures. We conducted Monte Carlo simulations of intraoral, panoramic, and CBCT imaging procedures by using a computational human head phantom and multimodal imaging-based detailed anatomical (MIDA) [7]combined with a Monte Carlo radiation transport code, MC-GPU [8]. The voxel resolution of the head phantom was $0.5 \times 0.5 \times 0.5\,mm^3$. Key technical parameters for Monte Carlo simulations that were collected from literature are summarized in Table 1. In the case of panoramic imaging, a simplified image acquisition was modeled by concatenating 9,153 simulations with a 1-pixel-wide field of view of $10 \times 0.05\,cm^2$ instead of the realistic field of view of $10 \times 0.2\,cm^2$ since the image overlap in real machines could not be reliably simulated. Our simulations had two purposes: to evaluate the proportion of the dose distribution among different tissues during the three imaging modalities and to visualize dose distribution across the head anatomy in the web program.

2.4. Development of a Web-Based Dose Calculator. After the summary dose tables were established, we developed a web-based dose calculation program to allow for convenient access to the organ and effective doses and comparison of the dental doses with doses from other radiation sources.

The web program was designed to allow an input from the user for the following parameters: type of imaging modalities, number of image sets, patient age group (child or adult), and size of imaging region, which is the area of the FOV (small $<50\,cm^2$, medium $50–150\,cm^2$, and large $>150\,cm^2$). The last two parameters were only used for CBCT dose as the dose data for intraoral and panoramic imaging were not enough to be stratified by age and FOV. The user has the option of "I do not know" for the patient age group and FOV, in which case the average dose of the age groups and/or the size of FOV were presented.

Based on the input data from a user, the web application presents the following information:

(i) Dose delivered to the bone marrow, brain, salivary glands, and thyroid and effective dose; the doses are calculated by multiplying the dose per imaging by the number of image sets inputted by a user. Limited pediatric data points were available for intraoral and panoramic, andonly a total of 22 pediatric data points were extracted for CBCT. Since the data points were not enough to derive age dependency of dose for finer age resolution, we combined the 22 data points for CBCT into the pediatric age group. In the case of CBCT, when the user selects both age group and FOV, age and FOV dependent doses are displayed. FOV-averaged doses are displayed when a user selects "I do not know" for FOV. Age-averaged dose is displayed when a user selects "I do not know" for age.

(ii) 2D and 3D dose distribution for the selected imaging procedures and the fraction of dose delivered to different tissues

(iii) Comparison of the total effective dose (effective dose multiplied by the number of image sets) with that from other radiation sources: 37 μSv (London-to-New York flight), 100 μSv (chest X-ray) and 3110 μSv (annual natural background) [9]

The web dose calculator was developed using the commercial cross-platform language, Xojo (Xojo, Inc., Austin, TX). The Xojo development tool provides a graphical user interface-based programming environment to develop multiplatform apps for macOS, Windows, Linux, and Web. We used the web application platform to develop our web-based dose calculator. We created two versions of the web interface for web browsers on a personal computer and a smart phone to account for differences in screen size. The web application was deployed through Xojo Cloud hosting, which was connected to the domain name http://dentaldose.org. Figure 1 shows the workflow of the web program, where the user input data and output data are described.

3. Results

We tabulated technical parameters and doses for a total of 4, 18, and 51 dose sets for intraoral (Table 2), panoramic (Table 3), and CBCT (Table 4) procedures, respectively.

3.1. Technical Parameters and Methods Used in Dosimetry Studies. About 56% ($n = 57$) of the dose sets were from measurements, and the remaining 44% ($n = 44$) were from simulation studies. In the measurement studies, different types of dosimeters were used: the thermoluminescent dosimeter (TLD) (86%), the optically stimulated luminescent dosimeter (OSLD) (7%), the Gafchromic film (5%), and the metal-oxide-silicon field-effect transistor (MOSFET) (2%). The physical head phantoms used for measurements included the Alderson Radiation Therapy (ART) phantom (Radiology Support Devices Inc., Long Beach, CA) (70%), the ATOM adult and child phantoms (CIRS, Norfolk, VA) (20%), and CDP-R1 (Chengdu Fangtuo Simulation Technology Company Limited, China) (10%). In the simulation studies, the EGS program [27] produced about 60% of all dose sets followed by MCNP [28] (22%) and PCXMC [29] (STUK, Helsinki, Finland) (18%). A variety of computational head phantoms were used for the simulation studies: in-house head phantoms developed from patient CT images (44%), the Zubal head phantom [30] (22%), the Oak Ridge National Laboratory (ORNL)-stylized phantoms (18%), and the ICRP adult phantoms [31] (16%). The tube potential for intraoral imaging ranged from 60 to 70 kVp. The panoramic and CBCT scans used 62–73 kVp and 70–120 kVp, respectively. In the case of CBCT, the width and height of the FOV ranged from about 4 to 26 cm and the area (width × height) ranged from about 15 [11] to 600 [24] cm^2. The beam rotation angle for CBCT was between 180° and 360°. The DAP for CBCT ranged from 91 to 1080 $mGy\text{-}cm^2$.

3.2. Organ and Effective Doses. The organ and effective doses reported in the literature are summarized in Table 5. Mean effective doses delivered by intraoral, 1.32 (0.60–2.56) μSv,

TABLE 1: Technical parameters for intraoral, panoramic, and cone-beam computed tomography collected from literature, which were used for Monte Carlo simulations conducted using MC-GPU to estimate dose distribution within the head.

Parameters	Intraoral	Panoramic	Cone-beam computed tomography
X-ray energy (kVp)	60	73	90
Filtration (mm Al)	3.5	2.5	2.8
FOV (cm^2)	4×3	10×0.2	10×10
SRD[1] (cm)	75	35	50
Rotation angle per view (degree)	0[2]	240	360
Number of views per acquisition	1	9153	360
Number of X-rays per simulated view	10^{11}	5×10^7	5×10^9
Total simulation time (min)[3]	33	143	760

[1]Source-to-rotation axis distance. [2]The rectangular field was rotated 30° cranially. [3]Simulation run in an NVIDIA GeForce GTX 1080 GPU.

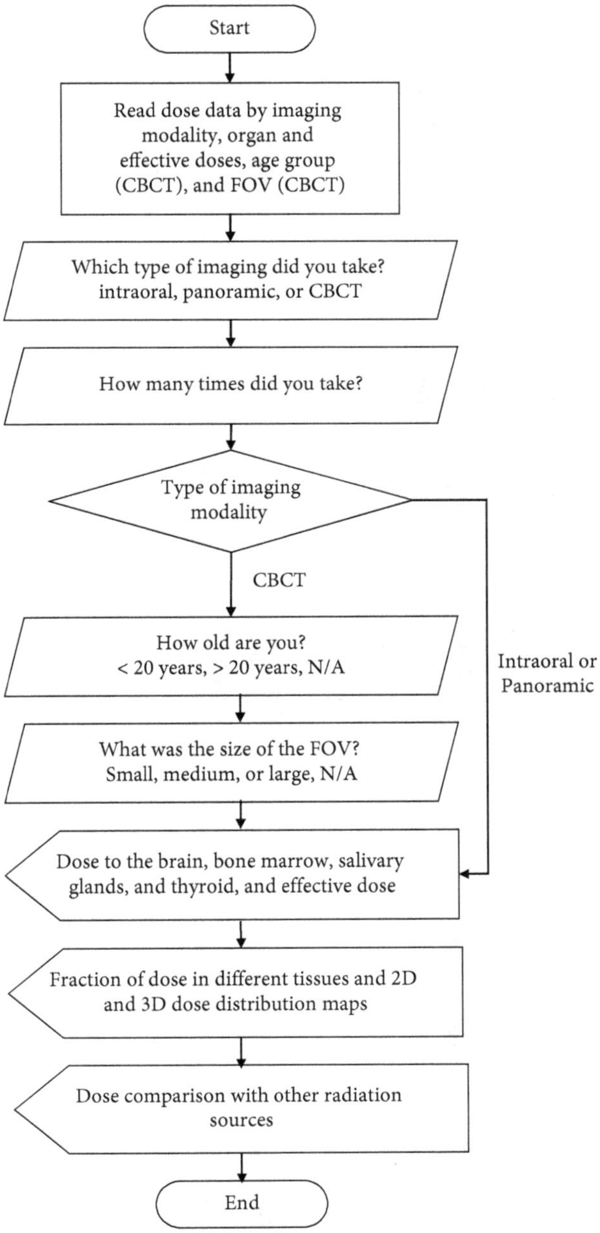

FIGURE 1: Flowchart of the web application for dental radiation dose calculations and dose display.

Table 2: Dosimetry method, machine model, phantom age, technical parameters, and effective and organ (bone marrow, brain, salivary gland, and thyroid) doses for intraoral imaging procedures. No simulation-based doses are reported.

Method	Machine model	Age	Dosimeter	Phantom	Imaging protocols	DAP (mGy × cm^2)	kVp	FOV width (cm)	FOV height (cm)	Effective dose (uSv)	Organ dose (uGy)				Reference
											Bone marrow	Brain	Salivary gland	Thyroid	
Measurement	Gendex Oralix DC	35	TLD	ART	Bitewing single image		60	3.5	4.5	0.85	0.50	0.00	27.00	2.00	Granlund et al. 2015 [10]
Measurement	Gendex Oralix DC	35	TLD	ART	Full-mouth single image		60	3.5	4.5	0.83	0.33	0.00	25.11	2.94	Granlund et al. 2015 [10]
Measurement	Prostyle	10	Gafchromic film	ATOM 706C	Periapical lateral	7.42	66	4.5	5.5	0.60	1.20	0.30	5.50	0.00	Kadesjo et al. 2018 [11]
Measurement	Prostyle	10	Gafchromic film	ATOM 706C	Periapical central	7.42	66	4.5	5.5	0.70	0.00	0.00	0.01	0.00	Kadesjo et al. 2018 [11]
Measurement	Focus	35	TLD	CDP-R1	Maxillary premolar left		70	4.5	3.5	2.56	0.55	6.12	45.25	24.47	Li et al. 2020 [12]
Measurement	Focus	35	TLD	CDP-R1	Maxillary premolar left		70	4.5	3.5	2.39	1.19	7.76	33.88	18.38	Li et al. 2020 [12]

DAP, dose area product; FOV, field of view.

TABLE 3: Dosimetry methods, machine model, phantom age, technical parameters, and effective and organ (bone marrow, brain, salivary gland, and thyroid) doses for panoramic imaging procedures.

Method	Machine model	Age (year)	Dosimeter/MC code	Phantom	Imaging protocols	kVp	Effective dose (uSv)	Organ dose (uGy)				Reference
								Bone marrow	Brain	Salivary gland	Thyroid	
Measurement	AZ3000	35	TLD	RANDO	Temporomandibular	70	11.00	3.30	29.50	549.90	29.80	Matsuo et al. 2011 [13]
Measurement	OP-200	35	TLD	ART		66	10.73	9.94	10.03	311.78	27.89	Han et al. 2013 [14]
Measurement	ORTHOPHOS CD	35	TLD	ART		71	14.33	10.74	9.41	419.17	67.87	Han et al. 2013 [14]
Measurement	ORTHOPHOS XG Plus	35	TLD	ART		69	19.06	15.99	18.41	604.05	54.60	Han et al. 2013 [14]
Measurement	ProMax	35	TLD	ART		66	26.26	14.53	15.12	939.55	54.95	Han et al. 2013 [14]
Measurement	Cranex Tome Ceph	35	TLD	ART	Jaw	66	19.00	11.00	26.00	1028.00	40.00	Granlund et al. 2015 [10]
Measurement	Cranex Tome Ceph	35	TLD	ART	Dental	66	22.00	10.00	10.00	1182.00	48.00	Granlund et al. 2015 [10]
Measurement	Veraviewepocs	35	TLD	ART	Jaw	66	23.00	13.00	10.00	869.00	53.00	Granlund et al. 2015 [10]
Measurement	Veraviewepocs	35	TLD	ART	Dental	66	30.00	18.00	5.00	939.00	52.00	Granlund et al. 2015 [10]
Measurement	Scanora	35	TLD	ART	Jaw	66	75.00	54.00	18.00	2887.00	126.00	Granlund et al. 2015 [10]
Measurement	Scanora	35	TLD	ART	Dental	66	49.00	38.00	19.00	2428.00	111.00	Granlund et al. 2015 [10]
Measurement	OP-200	5	TLD	ATOM 705	Long collimator P1	66	11.40	1.90	43.00	94.00	37.00	Davis 2015 [15]
Measurement	OP-200	5	TLD	ATOM 705	Short collimator P2	66	7.70	1.50	19.00	103.00	30.00	Davis et al. 2015 [15]
Measurement	OP-100	35	TLD	RANDO		73	7.15	5.00	72.00	109.00	24.00	Lee et al. 2016 [16]
Simulation	OP-100	35	PCXMC	ORNL		73	9.39	10.00	9.00	299.00	20.00	Lee et al. 2016 [16]
Measurement	ProMax 2D	10	Gafchromic film	ATOM 706C		62	4.10	1.80	0.00	160.00	17.00	Kadesjo et al. 2018 [11]
Measurement	ORTHOPHOSXG/ Cep	35	TLD	RANDO		64	13.00	24.00	37.00	622.00	256.00	Qiang et al. 2019 [17]
Measurement	OP-100	5	TLD	ATOM 705-D		66	3.85	38.33	55.64	54.40	35.85	Lee et al. 2019 [18]
Simulation	OP-100	5	PCXMC	ORNL		66	3.47	10.51	20.00	4.32	13.29	Lee et al. 2019 [18]
Measurement	PP1	35	TLD	CDP-R1	Maxillofacial	73	8.15	8.08	33.10	113.30	54.31	Li et al. 2020 [12]
Measurement	PP1	35	TLD	CDP-R1	Maxillofacial	73	8.99	8.34	29.59	148.55	63.90	Li et al. 2020 [12]

Table 4: Dosimetry methods, machine model, phantom age, technical parameters, and effective and organ (bone marrow, brain, salivary gland, and thyroid) doses for cone-beam computed tomography procedures.

Method	Machine model	Age	Dosimeter/ MC code	Phantom	Rotation (degree)	Imaging protocols	DAP (mGy × cm^2)	kVp	FOV width (cm)	FOV height (cm)	Effective dose (uSv)	Organ dose (uGy)				Reference
												Bone marrow	Brain	Salivary gland	Thyroid	
Measurement	Galileos	35	TLD	ART		Maxillofacial		85	15	15	84.00	82.00	124.00	2104.00	380.00	Pauwels et al. 2012 [19]
Measurement	i-CAT	35	TLD	ART		Maxillofacial		120	16	13	83.00	116.00	375.00	1830.00	355.00	Pauwels et al. 2012 [19]
Measurement	Iluma Elite	35	TLD	ART		Maxillofacial		120	21	14	368.00	660.00	3415.00	7225.00	1230.00	Pauwels et al. 2012 [19]
Measurement	Kodak 9500	35	TLD	ART		Maxillofacial		90	20	18	136.00	206.00	1205.00	2676.00	585.00	Pauwels et al. 2012 [19]
Measurement	NewTom VG	35	TLD	ART		Maxillofacial		110	15	10	83.00	115.00	251.00	1690.00	354.00	Pauwels et al. 2012 [19]
Measurement	NewTom VGi	35	TLD	ART		Maxillofacial		110	15	15	194.00	186.00	605.00	2855.00	2045.00	Pauwels et al. 2012 [19]
Measurement	Scanora 3D	35	TLD	ART		Maxillofacial		85	14.5	13.5	68.00	86.00	255.00	1568.00	296.00	Pauwels et al. 2012 [19]
Measurement	SkyView	35	TLD	ART		Maxillofacial		90	17	17	87.00	134.00	719.00	1582.00	474.00	Pauwels et al. 2012 [19]
Measurement	3D Accuitomo 170	35	TLD	ART		Maxilla		90	10	5	54.00	112.00	189.00	2138.00	148.00	Pauwels et al. 2012 [19]
Measurement	i-CAT NG	35	TLD	ART		Mandible		120	16	6	45.00	33.00	46.00	973.00	251.00	Pauwels et al. 2012 [19]
Measurement	Kodak 9500	35	TLD	ART		Dentoalveolar		90	15	8	92.00	85.00	91.00	2166.00	541.00	Pauwels et al. 2012 [19]
Measurement	NewTom VGi	35	TLD	ART		Dentoalveolar		110	12	8	265.00	294.00	431.00	6372.00	1293.00	Pauwels et al. 2012 [19]
Measurement	Picasso trio	35	TLD	ART		Dentoalveolar		85	12	7	123.00	126.00	134.00	2982.00	551.00	Pauwels et al. 2012 [19]

TABLE 4: Continued.

Method	Machine model	Age	Dosimeter/ MC code	Phantom	Rotation (degree)	Imaging protocols	DAP (mGy × cm^2)	kVp	FOV width (cm)	FOV height (cm)	Effective dose (uSv)	Organ dose (uGy)				Reference
												Bone marrow	Brain	Salivary gland	Thyroid	
Measurement	Picasso trio	35	TLD	ART		Dentoalveolar		85	12	7	81.00	62.00	39.00	1837.00	583.00	Pauwels et al. 2012 [19]
Measurement	ProMax 3D	35	TLD	ART		Dentoalveolar		84	8	8	122.00	88.00	53.00	2576.00	1021.00	Pauwels et al. 2012 [19]
Measurement	ProMax 3D	35	TLD	ART		Dentoalveolar		84	8	8	28.00	27.00	28.00	596.00	202.00	Pauwels et al. 2012 [19]
Measurement	Scanora 3D	35	TLD	ART		Dentoalveolar		85	10	7.5	46.00	42.00	45.00	1285.00	148.00	Pauwels et al. 2012 [19]
Measurement	Scanora 3D	35	TLD	ART		Mandible		85	10	7.5	47.00	34.00	25.00	1052.00	352.00	Pauwels et al. 2012 [19]
Measurement	Scanora 3D	35	TLD	ART		Maxilla		85	10	7.5	45.00	37.00	31.00	1117.00	240.00	Pauwels et al. 2012 [19]
Measurement	Veraviewepocs 3D	35	TLD	ART		Dentoalveolar		70	8	8	73.00	55.00	40.00	1956.00	330.00	Pauwels et al. 2012 [19]
Measurement	3D Accuitomo 170	35	TLD	ART		Lower jaw, molar region		90	4	4	43.00	37.00	37.00	2120.00	195.00	Pauwels et al. 2012 [19]
Measurement	Kodak 9000 3D	35	TLD	ART		Upper jaw, front region		70	5	3.7	19.00	21.00	18.00	523.00	30.00	Pauwels et al. 2012 [19]
Measurement	Kodak 9000 3D	35	TLD	ART		Lower jaw, molar region		70	5	3.7	40.00	78.00	290.00	709.00	251.00	Pauwels et al. 2012 [19]
Measurement	Pax-Uni3D	35	TLD	ART		Upper jaw, front region		85	5	5	44.00	47.00	28.00	1073.00	209.00	Pauwels et al. 2012 [19]
Measurement	ProMax 3D	35	MOSFET	RANDO RAN102	200		574		8	8	153.00	25.00	4.30	32.00	32.00	Koivisto et al. 2012 [20]
Simulation	ProMax 3D	35	PCXMC	ORNL Phantom	200		574		8	8	131.00	6.90	2.80	41.00	8.40	Koivisto et al. 2012 [20]

Table 4: Continued.

Method	Machine model	Age	Dosimeter/ MC code	Phantom	Rotation (degree)	Imaging protocols	DAP (mGy × cm^2)	kVp	FOV width (cm)	FOV height (cm)	Effective dose (uSv)	Organ dose (uGy) Bone marrow	Brain	Salivary gland	Thyroid	Reference
Simulation	i-CAT	35	EGS4	ICRP ADULT	360		556		16	13	66.00	50.00	590.00	1270.00	80.00	Morant et al. 2013 [21]
Simulation	i-CAT	35	EGS4	ICRP ADULT	360		476		16	11	58.00	40.00	310.00	1230.00	80.00	Morant et al. 2013 [21]
Simulation	i-CAT	35	EGS4	ICRP ADULT	360		415		16	10	53.00	30.00	190.00	1150.00	70.00	Morant et al. 2013 [21]
Simulation	Accuitomo 170	5	EGSnrc	In-house	360	Standard resolution		90	6	6	172.26	1052.00	89.00	2965.00	387.00	Stratis et al. 2016 [22]
Simulation	Accuitomo 170	5	EGSnrc	In-house	360	Standard resolution		90	8	8	297.97	1478.00	181.00	4204.00	1919.00	Stratis et al. 2016 [22]
Simulation	Accuitomo 170	8	EGSnrc	In-house	360	Standard resolution		90	6	6	119.35	518.00	92.00	2623.00	751.00	Stratis et al. 2016 [22]
Simulation	Accuitomo 170	8	EGSnrc	In-house	360	Standard resolution		90	8	8	228.32	986.00	181.00	3831.00	1747.00	Stratis et al. 2016 [22]
Simulation	Accuitomo 170	12	EGSnrc	In-house	360	Standard resolution		90	6	6	111.76	607.00	42.00	1862.00	497.00	Stratis et al. 2016 [22]
Simulation	Accuitomo 170	12	EGSnrc	In-house	360	Standard resolution		90	8	8	250.95	913.00	90.00	2961.00	2772.00	Stratis et al. 2016 [22]
Simulation	Accuitomo 170	35	EGSnrc	ICRP AF	360	Standard resolution		90	6	6	81.54	376.00	112.00	2830.00	175.00	Stratis et al. 2016 [22]
Simulation	Accuitomo 170	35	EGSnrc	ICRP AF	360	Standard resolution		90	8	8	126.68	565.00	224.00	4308.00	339.00	Stratis et al. 2016 [22]
Simulation	i-CAT	35	PCXMC	ORNL Phantom	360			120	16	13	30.99	42.90	269.58	738.29	46.97	Yeh and Chen 2018 [23]
Simulation	ProMax 3D	5	EGSnrc	In-house		Canine XS/ND		96	4.2	5.5	134.90	200.00	152.00	3558.00	214.00	Marcu et al. 2018 [24]

Table 4: Continued.

Method	Machine model	Age	Dosimeter/ MC code	Phantom	Rotation (degree)	Imaging protocols	DAP (mGy × cm^2)	kVp	FOV width (cm)	FOV height (cm)	Effective dose (uSv)	Organ dose (uGy)				Reference
												Bone marrow	Brain	Salivary gland	Thyroid	
Simulation	ProMax 3D	5	EGSnrc	In-house		Molars XS/ND		96	4.2	5.5	155.90	222.00	170.00	4352.00	256.00	Marcu et al. 2018 [24]
Simulation	ProMax 3D	5	EGSnrc	In-house		Molars XS/ND		96	5	5.5	220.20	23.80	15.80	336.30	67.90	Marcu et al. 2018 [24]
Simulation	ProMax 3D	5	EGSnrc	In-house		Molars XS/ND		96	10	9	68.60	77.70	62.70	1400.60	315.30	Marcu et al. 2018 [24]
Simulation	ProMax 3D	5	EGSnrc	In-house		Molars XS/ND		96	10	5.5	55.70	45.00	28.60	1211.00	308.80	Marcu et al. 2018 [24]
Simulation	ProMax 3D	5	EGSnrc	In-house		Molars XS/ND		96	13	16	75.60	149.60	948.20	1453.60	206.60	Marcu et al. 2018 [24]
Simulation	ProMax 3D	5	EGSnrc	In-house		S/ND		96	23	26	178.40	614.00	4324.00	1596.00	2677.00	Marcu et al. 2018 [24]
Simulation	ProMax 3D	8	EGSnrc	In-house		Canine XS/ND		96	4.2	5.5	124.60	85.00	126.00	3080.00	157.00	Marcu et al. 2018 [24]
Simulation	ProMax 3D	8	EGSnrc	In-house		Molars XS/ND		96	4.2	5.5	128.60	93.00	141.00	3458.00	187.00	Marcu et al. 2018 [24]
Simulation	ProMax 3D	8	EGSnrc	In-house		Molars XS/ND		96	5	5.5	17.10	15.20	14.40	419.00	38.60	Marcu et al. 2018 [24]
Simulation	ProMax 3D	8	EGSnrc	In-house		Molars XS/ND		96	10	9	60.80	54.30	48.70	1389.00	290.90	Marcu et al. 2018 [24]
Simulation	ProMax 3D	8	EGSnrc	In-house		Molars XS/ND		96	10	5.5	47.90	31.70	219.00	1028.00	270.60	Marcu et al. 2018 [24]
Simulation	ProMax 3D	8	EGSnrc	In-house		Molars XS/ND		96	13	16	64.70	104.70	772.20	1319.00	202.60	Marcu et al. 2018 [24]
Simulation	ProMax 3D	8	EGSnrc	In-house		S/ND		96	23	26	392.20	518.00	4247.00	4007.00	2908.00	Marcu et al. 2018 [24]

Table 4: Continued.

Method	Machine model	Age	Dosimeter/ MC code	Phantom	Rotation (degree)	Imaging protocols	DAP (mGy × cm^2)	kVp	FOV width (cm)	FOV height (cm)	Effective dose (uSv)	Organ dose (uGy)				Reference
												Bone marrow	Brain	Salivary gland	Thyroid	
Simulation	ProMax 3D	35	EGSnrc	ICRP AM				96	23	26	256.10	362.80	4653.00	4378.00	294.00	Marcu et al. 2018 [24]
Simulation	Cranex3Dx	35	MCNP6.1	ZUBAL Head	180	Maxillary first molar/SR	168	90	5	5	40.00	375.00	105.00	1154.00	139.00	Kralik et al. 2018 [25]
Simulation	Cranex3Dx	35	MCNP6.1	ZUBAL Head	180	Mandibular dental arch/SR	280	90	6.1	7.8	75.00	370.00	55.00	1278.00	1252.00	Kralik et al. 2018 [25]
Simulation	Cranex3Dx	35	MCNP6.1	ZUBAL Head	180	Both dental arches	338	90	7.8	7.8	74.00	578.00	1155.00	2045.00	535.00	Kralik et al. 2018 [25]
Simulation	Cranex3Dx	35	MCNP6.1	ZUBAL Head	180	Mandible/SR	528	90	7.8	15	142.00	564.00	96.00	2275.00	2465.00	Kralik et al. 2018 [25]
Simulation	Cranex3Dx	35	MCNP6.1	ZUBAL Head	180	Viscerocranium/ SR	755	90	13	15	170.00	1034.00	552.00	2847.00	2370.00	Kralik et al. 2018 [25]
Simulation	Cranex3Dx	35	MCNP6.1	ZUBAL Head	360	Maxillary first molar/SR	168	90	5	5	37.00	335.00	78.00	592.00	104.00	Kralik et al. 2018 [25]
Simulation	Cranex3Dx	35	MCNP6.1	ZUBAL Head	360	Mandibular dental arch/SR	280	90	6.1	7.8	105.00	400.00	49.00	1161.00	789.00	Kralik et al. 2018 [25]
Simulation	Cranex3Dx	35	MCNP6.1	ZUBAL Head	360	Both dental arches	338	90	7.8	7.8	92.00	621.00	153.00	1559.00	789.00	Kralik et al. 2018 [25]
Simulation	Cranex3Dx	35	MCNP6.1	ZUBAL Head	360	Mandible/SR	528	90	7.8	15	184.00	607.00	87.00	2035.00	3533.00	Kralik et al. 2018 [25]
Simulation	Cranex3Dx	35	MCNP6.1	ZUBAL Head	360	Viscerocranium/ SR	755	90	13	15	214.00	1005.00	523.00	2371.00	3384.00	Kralik et al. 2018 [25]
Measurement	ProMax 3D	10	TLD	ATOM 706C	360		510	90	4	5	88.00	130.00	510.00	1800.00	200.00	Kadesjo et al. 2018 [11]
Measurement	NewTom5G	10	TLD	ATOM 706C	360		1080	110	6	6	172.00	270.00	760.00	3800.00	340.00	Kadesjo et al. 2018 [11]

Table 4: Continued.

Method	Machine model	Age	Dosimeter/ MC code	Phantom	Rotation (degree)	Imaging protocols	DAP (mGy × cm^2)	kVp	FOV width (cm)	FOV height (cm)	Effective dose (uSv)	Organ dose (uGy) Bone marrow	Brain	Salivary gland	Thyroid	Reference
Measurement	Galileos	35	TLD	RANDO		Maxillofacial		85	15	15	203.00	278.00	636.00	7775.00	8727.00	Qiang et al. 2019 [17]
Simulation	CS9300	35	PCXMC	ORNL Phantom	360	Facial	251	90	17	13.5	160.90	180.00	460.00	4570.00	450.00	Lee et al. 2020 [26]
Simulation	CS9300	35	PCXMC	ORNL Phantom	360	Dual jaw	91	90	10	10	94.40	100.00	230.00	1950.00	580.00	Lee et al. 2020 [26]
Simulation	RAYSCAN	35	PCXMC	ORNL Phantom	360	Large jaw	177	80	16	10	198.00	200.00	220.00	5360.00	320.00	Lee et al. 2020 [26]
Simulation	RAYSCAN	35	PCXMC	ORNL Phantom	360	Jaw	91	80	10	10	195.20	190.00	280.00	4700.00	410.00	Lee et al. 2020 [26]
Measurement	CS9300	35	OSLD	ATOM 702C	360	Facial	251	90	17	13.5	181.40	20.00	1020.00	3160.00	1210.00	Lee et al. 2020 [26]
Measurement	CS9300	35	OSLD	ATOM 702C	360	Dual jaw	91	90	10	10	90.70	10.00	230.00	1950.00	580.00	Lee et al. 2020 [26]
Measurement	RAYSCAN	35	OSLD	ATOM 702C	360	Large jaw	177	80	16	10	228.50	10.00	380.00	4540.00	1680.00	Lee et al. 2020 [26]
Measurement	RAYSCAN	35	OSLD	ATOM 702C	360	Jaw	91	80	10	10	213.80	10.00	570.00	3930.00	1500.00	Lee et al. 2020 [26]
Measurement	KaVo 3D eXami	35	TLD	CDP-R1		Maxillofacial		120	14.5	8.5	56.63	15.22	427.82	1177.24	476.04	Li et al. RPD 2020 [12]
Measurement	KaVo 3D eXami	35	TLD	CDP-R1		Maxillofacial		120	14.5	8.5	55.18	11.63	494.50	1314.85	452.68	Li et al. RPD 2020 [12]

DAP, dose area product; FOV, field of view.

Table 5: Minimum, mean, and maximum values of effective and organ (bone marrow, brain, salivary gland, and thyroid) doses from intraoral, panoramic, and cone-beam computed tomography procedures reported in the selected publications.

Procedures		Effective dose (μSv)	Organ dose (μGy)			
			Bone marrow	Brain	Salivary gland	Thyroid
Intraoral ($n = 6$)	Mean	1.32	0.63	2.36	22.79	7.97
	Min	0.60	0.00	0.00	0.01	0.00
	Max	2.56	1.20	7.76	45.25	24.47
Panoramic ($n = 21$)	Mean	17.93	14.66	23.28	660.24	57.93
	Min	3.47	1.50	0.00	4.32	13.29
	Max	75.00	54.00	72.00	2887.00	256.00
Cone-beam computed tomography ($n = 76$)	Mean	121.09	254.78	471.65	2333.95	811.16
	Min	17.10	6.90	2.80	32.00	8.40
	Max	392.20	1478.00	4653.00	7775.00	8727.00

and panoramic, 17.93 (3.47–75.00) μSv, procedures are about 1% and 15% of that delivered by CBCT, 121.09 (17.10–392.20) μSv. Among the three imaging modalities, the salivary glands received the greatest dose: 22.79 μGy (intraoral), 660.24 μGy (panoramic), and 2333.95 μGy (CBCT). Among the four organs of interest, the smallest dose was delivered to the bone marrow, except for intraoral where the brain received the smallest dose.

In CBCT imaging, the child phantoms tended to receive greater doses compared with the adult phantoms, except for the salivary glands and thyroid doses (Table 6). The child phantoms received about 29% greater effective dose than the adult phantoms. The bone marrow dose of the child phantoms was about 80% greater than that of the adult phantom.

The effective dose for the larger FOV in CBCT is greater than that for the smaller FOV (Table 7). The effective dose for the large FOV (greater than 150 cm^2) is about 1.6 times greater than that for the small FOV (less than 50 cm^2). The brain dose for the large FOV is about eight times greater than that for the small FOV.

Table 8 shows the age- and FOV size-dependent organ and effective doses. A similar trend by age group shown in Table 6 (child's dose is greater than adult's dose) and by FOV size shown in Table 7 (large FOV gives greater dose than small FOV) is also observed.

3.3. Monte Carlo Dose Distribution. 2D dose distribution at the level of the center of the lower teeth for intraoral, panoramic, and CBCT calculated by MC-GPU simulations are presented in Figure 2. The angles of radiation incidence to the head phantom used in the simulations (Table 1) are visible on the head anatomy: 30° from the patient's front for intraoral; 240° rotation behind the patient's head for panoramic; and 360° rotation for CBCT. Movie clips presenting a rotating 3D dose distribution for panoramic and CBCT were created and included in the web dose calculator.

The fraction of dose in different tissues (brain, muscle, bone, skin, soft tissue, cerebrospinal, blood, and eye lens) out of the total dose for intraoral, panoramic, and CBCT is shown in Figure 3. A larger portion of the radiation dose is delivered to the bone (55%) in intraoral imaging compared with panoramic and CBCT, each of which contributes about 35% of the total radiation dose to the bone. The dose delivered to the brain is nearly zero in intraoral but slightly increased to 1% in panoramic and 2% in CBCT. The dose delivered to skin and soft tissue remarkably increases from 12% (soft tissue) and 10% (skin) in intraoral to 26% (soft tissue) and 12% (skin) in panoramic and 22% (soft tissue) and 11% (skin) in CBCT.

3.4. Web Dose Calculator. A user-friendly interactive web program was developed for a user to input the following: the type of imaging procedure, the number of image sets, age group, and FOV size (Figure 4(a)). The web interface displays organ and effective doses (Figure 4(b)), dose fraction in tissues and 2D and 3D dose distributions in the head (Figure 4(c)), and dose comparison with other radiation sources (Figure 4(d)).

4. Discussion

Dental imaging is one of the most common radiological imaging procedures. Although the dose level is known to be relatively low, it is still important to monitor the trend of dental dose in different dental imaging modalities. We evaluated the radiation dose received from dental imaging practices by extracting data from literature published after 2010. To efficiently present the results of the study, an interactive web-based dose calculator was created.

We compared our results from intraoral imaging with those published by Fontana et al. [32], which report the dose to the brain, salivary gland, and thyroid delivered by imaging conducted from 1940 to 2009, with the increment of ten years. To simplify the comparison, we averaged their doses in three time periods: 1940–1969, 1970–1989, and 1990–2009. The period 2010–2020 adopted in our study follows the end of their study period. A clear dose reduction was observed in the brain dose by period. Compared with the organ doses reported for the earliest period (1940–1969), the doses to the brain, salivary gland, and thyroid resulted from our study were smaller by 77%, 93%, and 93%, respectively. Compared with the latest period, 1990–2009, in Fontana et al., our organ doses were smaller by 7%, 64%, and 62% for the brain, salivary gland, and thyroid, respectively. The dose reduction may be due to the change in technical parameters and the

Table 6: Minimum, mean, and maximum values of effective and organ (bone marrow, brain, salivary gland, and thyroid) doses from cone-beam computed tomography procedures by age group (children and adults) reported in the selected publications.

Age group		Effective dose (μSv)	Organ dose (μGy)			
			Bone marrow	Brain	Salivary gland	Thyroid
Children ($n = 22$)	Mean	143.9	372.2	600.7	2393.3	759.7
	Min	17.1	15.2	14.4	336.3	38.6
	Max	392.2	1478.0	4324.0	4352.0	2908.0
Adults ($n = 54$)	Mean	111.8	207.0	419.1	2309.7	832.1
	Min	19.0	6.9	2.8	32.0	8.4
	Max	368.0	1034.0	4653.0	7775.0	8727.0

Table 7: Minimum, mean, and maximum values of effective and organ (bone marrow, brain, salivary gland, and thyroid) doses from cone-beam computed tomography procedures by field-of-view area (FOV width × height, cm^2) reported in the selected publications.

FOV area (cm^2)		Effective dose (μSv)	Organ dose (μGy)			
			Bone marrow	Brain	Salivary gland	Thyroid
Small (<50) ($n = 20$)	Mean	96.5	262.8	144.2	1984.7	312.0
	Min	17.1	15.2	14.4	336.3	38.6
	Max	220.2	1052.0	760.0	4352.0	1252.0
Medium (50–150) ($n = 32$)	Mean	113.7	246.4	184.9	2137.2	780.7
	Min	28.0	6.9	2.8	32.0	8.4
	Max	298.0	1478.0	1155.0	4700.0	3533.0
Large (>150) ($n = 24$)	Mean	151.4	259.3	1126.8	2887.3	1267.7
	Min	31.0	10.0	124.0	738.3	47.0
	Max	392.2	1034.0	4653.0	7775.0	8727.0

Table 8: Minimum, mean, and maximum values of effective and organ (bone marrow, brain, salivary gland, and thyroid) doses from cone-beam computed tomography procedures by age group (children and adults) and field-of-view area (FOV width × height, cm^2) reported in the selected publications.

FOV area (cm^2) age group			Effective dose (μSv)	Organ dose (μGy)			
				Bone marrow	Brain	Salivary gland	Thyroid
Small (<50)	Children ($n = 11$)	Mean	131.3	292.4	192.0	2568.5	281.4
		Min	17.1	15.2	14.4	336.3	38.6
		Max	220.2	1052.0	760.0	4352.0	751.0
	Adults ($n = 9$)	Mean	53.8	226.6	85.8	1271.1	349.3
		Min	19.0	21.0	18.0	523.0	30.0
		Max	105.0	400.0	290.0	2830.0	1252.0
Medium (50–150)	Children ($n = 7$)	Mean	144.3	512.2	115.9	2289.2	1089.1
		Min	47.9	31.7	28.6	1028.0	270.6
		Max	298.0	1478.0	219.0	4204.0	2772.0
	Adults ($n = 25$)	Mean	105.2	172.0	204.3	2094.7	694.4
		Min	28.0	6.9	2.8	32.0	8.4
		Max	265.0	621.0	1155.0	6372.0	3533.0
Large (>150)	Children ($n = 4$)	Mean	177.7	346.6	2572.9	2093.9	1498.6
		Min	64.7	104.7	772.2	1319.0	202.6
		Max	392.2	614.0	4324.0	4007.0	2908.0
	Adults ($n = 20$)	Mean	146.1	241.9	837.6	3046.0	1221.5
		Min	31.0	10.0	124.0	738.3	47.0
		Max	368.0	1034.0	4653.0	7775.0	8727.0

improvement in imaging quality with the same amount of radiation.

The average effective dose from CBCT, delivering the greatest dose compared with intraoral and panoramic, was more than 92 times greater than that from intraoral and seven times greater than that from panoramic (Table 4). However, the maximum CBCT effective dose, with a large FOV, for children, 392.2 μSv [5], is about 13% of the dose from the natural radiation that a person receives on average every year, 3110 μSv [9], disregarding the radiation received from occupations and medical procedures.

We are aware of the following limitations in the current study. First, without dose calibration using measurements from clinical machines, absolute doses could not be

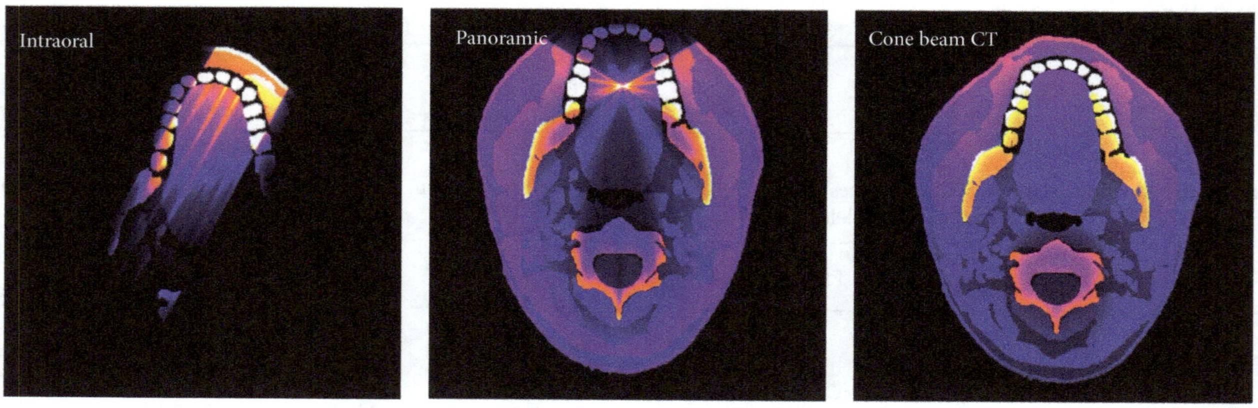

(a) (b) (c)

FIGURE 2: Dose distribution at the level of the lower teeth generated by MC-GPU simulations for (a) intraoral radiography, (b) panoramic radiography, and (c) cone-beam computed tomography.

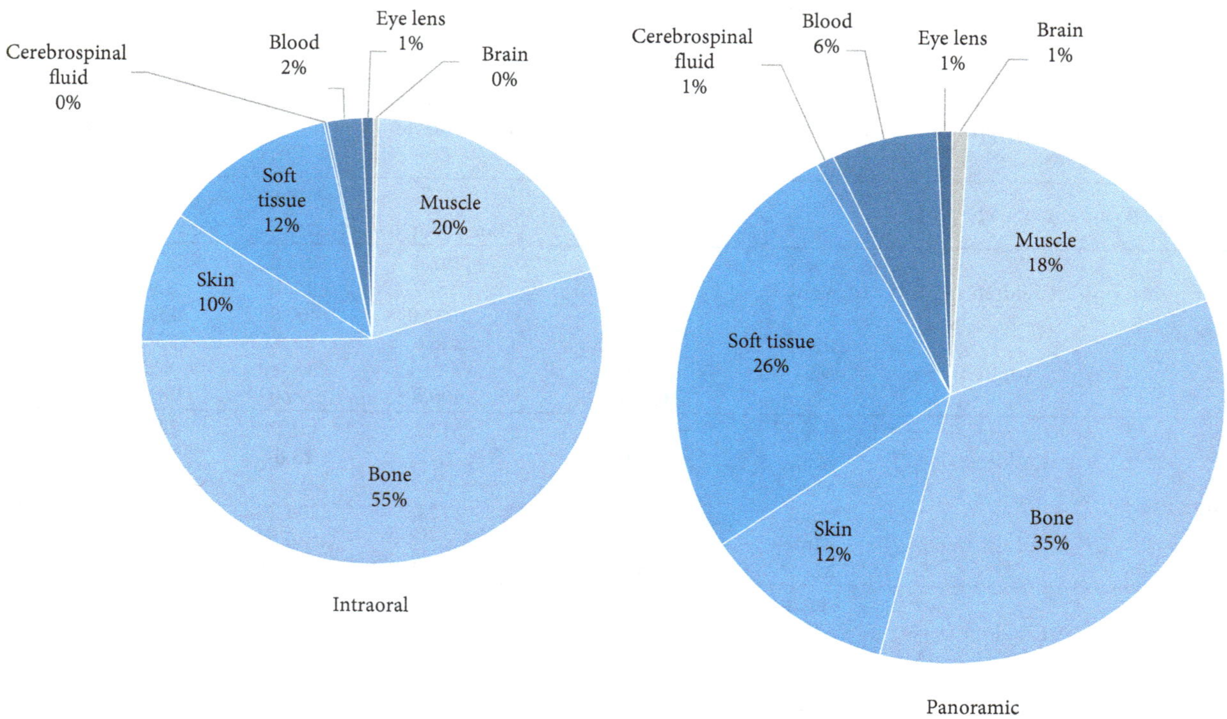

(a) (b)

FIGURE 3: Continued.

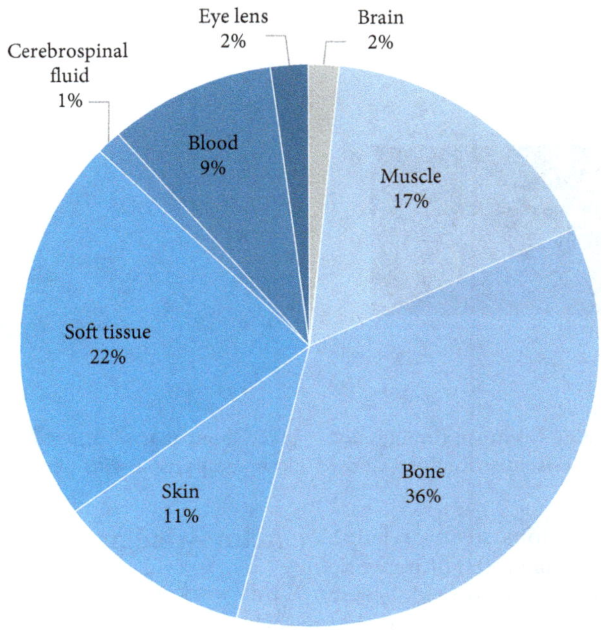

CBCT

(c)

FIGURE 3: Percent fraction of radiation dose for the different tissues in the head derived from the MC-GPU simulation of the human head phantom exposed to (a) intraoral radiography, (b) panoramic radiography, and (c) cone-beam computed tomography.

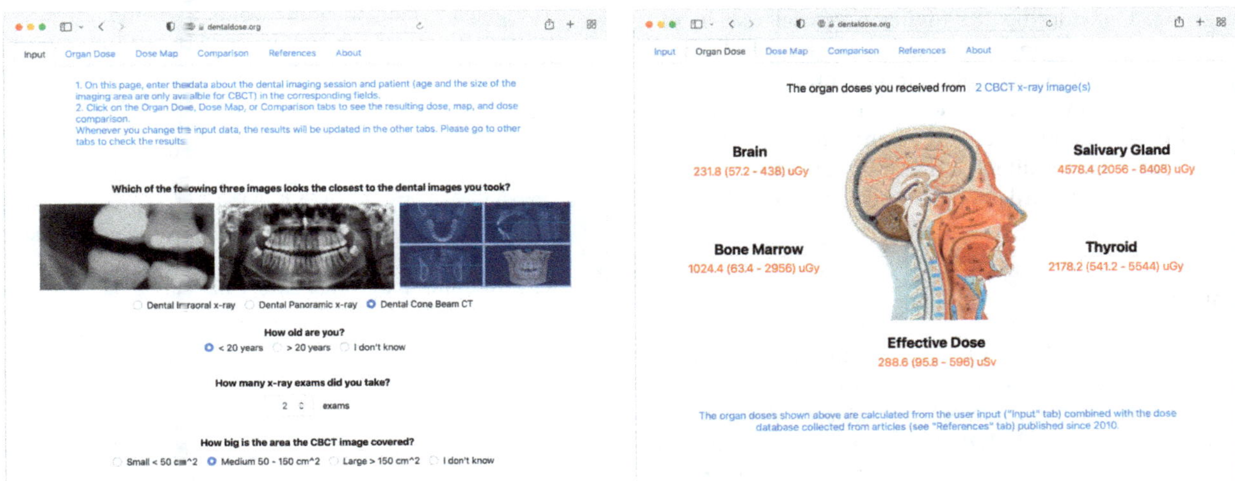

(a)

(b)

FIGURE 4: Continued.

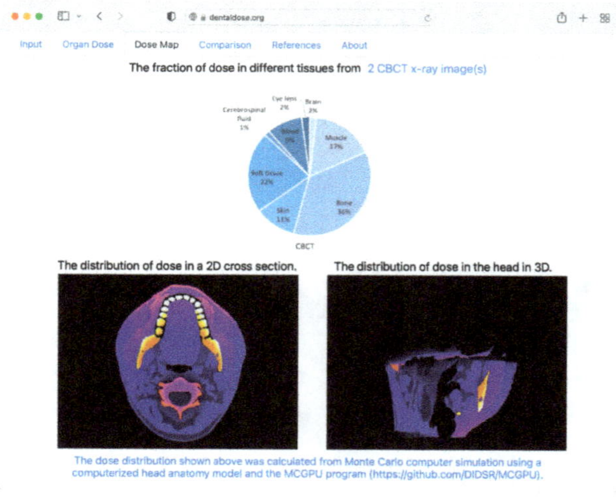

(c)

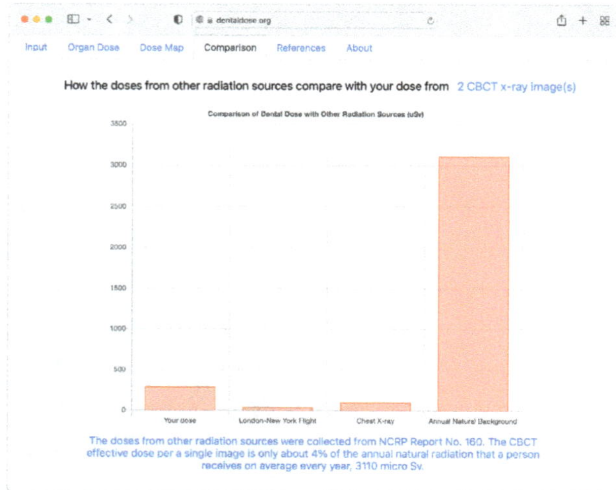
Input Organ Dose Dose Map Comparison References About
How the doses from other radiation sources compare with your dose from 2 CBCT x-ray image(s)
The doses from other radiation sources were collected from NCRP Report No. 160. The CBCT effective dose per a single image is only about 4% of the annual natural radiation that a person receives on average every year, 3110 micro Sv.

(d)

FIGURE 4: Web interfaces for (a) user input, (b) organ (brain, salivary gland, bone marrow, thyroid) and effective doses, (c) the fraction of dose in different tissues and 2D and 3D dose distributions, and (d) dose comparison with other radiation sources.

estimated with our Monte Carlo simulations, so only relative dose distributions were obtained and analyzed. Future work may involve accurate dose measurements to provide absolute doses for a comprehensive library of technical parameters for panoramic and CBCT procedures. Second, we found that pediatric dose data were relatively limited in literature compared with those of adults, so we grouped age-dependent dose data into pediatric (age <20) and adult (age ≥ 20) for CBCT only,for which a total of 22 pediatric data points were available. Since a clear age dependency for those limited data points was not observed, possibly due to large variability, we categorized the pediatric ages into a single group. Considering the higher potential risk in pediatric patients, due to increased radiosensitivity and longer expected life span after the irradiation event, it is important to more accurately evaluate the doses delivered to them once additional dose data are available in the future. Lastly, our literature search was limited to one bibliographic database, PubMed, to the keywords we defined, and to the papers written in English.

5. Conclusion

A comprehensive table of the organ and effectives doses delivered by intraoral, panoramic, and CBCT dental imaging procedures was established from previously published articles collected from PubMed. We found that organ and effective doses from intraoral and panoramic radiography are substantially smaller than those from CBCT, and the maximum CBCT effective dose is about 13% of the dose from annual natural radiation. Our dose summary should be useful for comparison among doses from different dental imaging methods as well as comparison with doses from other radiation sources. The user-friendly, interactive web application (http://dentaldose.org) allows for receiving user input and displaying doses, dose distribution maps, and dose comparison with other radiation sources.

Acknowledgments

This work was funded by the 2020 Oak Ridge Institute for Science and Education (ORISE) Research Fellowship Program at the US Food and Drug Administration.

References

[1] Ö Özalp, H. A. Tezerişener, B. Kocabalkan et al., "Comparing the precision of panoramic radiography and cone-beam computed tomography in avoiding anatomical structures critical to dental implant surgery: a retrospective study," *Imaging Science in Dentistry*, vol. 48, pp. 269–275, 2018.

[2] A. Stratis, G. Zhang, R. Jacobs, R. Bogaerts, and H. Bosmans, "The growing concern of radiation dose in paediatric dental and maxillofacial CBCT: an easy guide for daily practice," *European Radiology*, vol. 29, no. 12, pp. 7009–7018, 2019.

[3] E. Pakbaznejad Esmaeili, M. Ekholm, J. Haukka, M. Evälahti, and J. Waltimo-Sirén, "Are children's dental panoramic tomographs and lateral cephalometric radiographs sufficiently optimized?" *The European Journal of Orthodontics*, vol. 38, no. 1, pp. 103–110, 2016.

[4] ICRP, *The 2007 Recommendations of the International Commission on Radiological Protection*, ICRP Publication 103, Ann, ICRP 37, 2007.

[5] X. G. Xu, "An exponential growth of computational phantom research in radiation protection, imaging, and radiotherapy: a review of the fifty-year history," *Physics in Medicine and Biology*, vol. 59, no. 18, pp. R233–R302, 2014.

[6] ICRP, *Basic Anatomical and Physiological Data for Use in Radiological Protection Reference Values*, ICRP Publication 89, Ann, ICRP 32, 2002.

[7] M. I. Iacono, E. Neufeld, E. Akinnagbe et al., "MIDA: a multimodal imaging-based detailed anatomical model of the human head and neck," *PLoS One*, vol. 10, no. 4, p. e0124126, 2015.

[8] A. Badal and A. Badano, "Accelerating Monte Carlo simulations of photon transport in a voxelized geometry using a massively parallel graphics processing unit," *Medical Physics*, vol. 36, no. 11, pp. 4878–4880, 2009.
[9] N. C. RP. Ionizing, *Radiation Exposure of the Population of the United States*, National Council on Radiation Protection and Measurement, Bethesda, MD, USA, 2009.
[10] C. Granlund, A. Thilander-Klang, B. Ylhan, S. Lofthag-Hansen, and A. Ekestubbe, "Absorbed organ and effective doses from digital intra-oral and panoramic radiography applying the ICRP 103 recommendations for effective dose estimations," *The British Journal of Radiology*, vol. 89, no. 1066, p. 20151052, 2016.
[11] N. Kadesjö, R. Lynds, M. Nilsson, and X. Q. Shi, "Radiation dose from X-ray examinations of impacted canines: cone beam CT vs two-dimensional imaging," *Dento Maxillo Facial Radiology*, vol. 47, p. 20170305, 2018.
[12] Y. Li, B. Huang, J. Cao et al., "Estimating radiation dose to major organs IN dental X-ray examinations: a phantom study," *Radiation Protection Dosimetry*, vol. 192, no. 3, pp. 328–334, 2020.
[13] A. Matsuo, T. Okano, K. Gotoh et al., "The absorbed dose and the effective dose of panoramic temporo mandibular joint radiography," *Japanese Journal of Radiological Technology*, vol. 67, no. 10, pp. 1275–1283, 2011.
[14] G.-S. Han, J.-G. Cheng, G. Li, and X.-C. Ma, "Shielding effect of thyroid collar for digital panoramic radiography," *Dentomaxillofacial Radiology*, vol. 42, no. 9, p. 20130265, 2013.
[15] A. T. Davis, H. Safi and S. M. Maddison, "The reduction of dose in paediatric panoramic radiography: the impact of collimator height and programme selection," *Dentomaxillofacial Radiology*, vol. 44, no. 2, p. 20140223, 2015.
[16] C. Lee, S.-S. Lee, J.-E. Kim et al., "Comparison of dosimetry methods for panoramic radiography: thermoluminescent dosimeter measurement versus personal computer-based Monte Carlo method calculation," *Oral Surgery, Oral Medicine, Oral Pathology and Oral Radiology*, vol. 121, no. 3, pp. 322–329, 2016.
[17] W. Qiang, F. Qiang, and L. Lin, "Estimation of effective dose OF dental X-ray devices," *Radiation Protection Dosimetry*, vol. 183, pp. 417–421, 2019.
[18] C. Lee, B. Park, S.-S. Lee et al., "Efficacy of the Monte Carlo method and dose reduction strategies in paediatric panoramic radiography," *Scientific Reports*, vol. 9, no. 1, p. 9691, 2019.
[19] R. Pauwels, J. Beinsberger, B. Collaert et al., "Effective dose range for dental cone beam computed tomography scanners," *European Journal of Radiology*, vol. 81, no. 2, pp. 267–271, 2012.
[20] J. Koivisto, T. Kiljunen, M. Tapiovaara, J. Wolff, and M. Kortesniemi, "Assessment of radiation exposure in dental cone-beam computerized tomography with the use of metal-oxide semiconductor field-effect transistor (MOSFET) dosimeters and Monte Carlo simulations," *Oral Surgery, Oral Medicine, Oral Pathology and Oral Radiology*, vol. 114, no. 3, pp. 393–400, 2012.
[21] J. Morant, M. Salvadó, I. Hernández-Girón, R. Casanovas, R. Ortega, and A. Calzado, "Dosimetry of a cone beam CT device for oral and maxillofacial radiology using Monte Carlo techniques and ICRP adult reference computational phantoms," *Dentomaxillofacial Radiology*, vol. 42, no. 3, p. 92555893, 2013.
[22] A. Stratis, G. Zhang, R. Jacobs, R. Bogaerts, and H. Bosmans, "Rotating and translating anthropomorphic head voxel models to establish an horizontal Frankfort plane for dental CBCT Monte Carlo simulations: a dose comparison study," *Physics in Medicine and Biology*, vol. 61, no. 24, pp. N681–N696, 2016.
[23] J.-K. Yeh and C.-H. Chen, "Estimated radiation risk of cancer from dental cone-beam computed tomography imaging in orthodontics patients," *BMC Oral Health*, vol. 18, no. 1, p. 131, 2018.
[24] M. Marcu, M. Hedesiu, B. Salmon et al., "Estimation of the radiation dose for pediatric CBCT indications: a prospective study on ProMax3D," *International Journal of Paediatric Dentistry*, vol. 28, no. 3, pp. 300–309, 2018.
[25] I. Kralik, D. Faj, T. Lauc, M. Škarica, J. Popić, and H. Brkic, "Dose area product in estimation of effective dose of the patients undergoing dental cone beam computed tomography examinations," *Journal of Radiological Protection*, vol. 38, no. 4, pp. 1412–1427, 2018.
[26] C. Lee, J. Yoon, S.-S. Han et al., "Dose assessment in dental cone-beam computed tomography: comparison of optically stimulated luminescence dosimetry with Monte Carlo method," *PLoS One*, vol. 15, no. 3, p. e0219103, 2020.
[27] I. Kawrakow and D. W. O. Rogers, *The EGSnrc Code System: Monte Carlo Simulation of Electron and Photon Transport*, National Research Council of Canada, Ottawa, Canada, 2003.
[28] J. F. Briesmeister, *MCNP - A General Monte Carlo N-Particle Transport Code*, Los Alamos National Laboratory, Los Alamos, NM, USA, 1997.
[29] M. Tapiovaara, M. Lakkisto, and A. Servomaa, *PCXMC-A PC-Based Monte Carlo Program for Calculating Patient Doses in Medical X-Ray Examinations*, Radiation and Nuclear Safety Authority (STUK), Helsinki, Finland, 2nd edition, 2008.
[30] I. G. Zubal, C. R. Harrell, E. O. Smith, Z. Rattner, G. Gindi, and P. B. Hoffer, "Computerized three-dimensional segmented human anatomy," *Medical Physics*, vol. 21, no. 2, pp. 299–302, 1994.
[31] ICRP, "Adult reference computational phantoms. ICRP publication 110," ICRP Publication, ICRP 39, 2, 2009.
[32] R. C. Fontana, E. Pasqual, D. L. Miller, S. L. Simon, E. Cardis, and I. Thierry-Chef, "Trends in estimated thyroid, salivary gland, brain, and eye lens doses from intraoral dental radiography over seven decades (1940 TO 2009)," *Health Physics*, vol. 118, no. 2, pp. 136–148, 2020.

26

Preoperative Portal Vein Embolization in Hepatic Surgery: A Review about the Embolic Materials and Their Effects on Liver Regeneration and Outcome

Jose Hugo M. Luz,[1,2] Filipe V. Gomes,[1,2] Elia Coimbra,[1] Nuno V. Costa,[1,2] and Tiago Bilhim[1,2]

[1]*Interventional Radiology Unit, Curry Cabral Hospital CHULC, Rua Beneficencia 8, Zip Code 1069-166, Lisbon, Portugal*
[2]*Nova Medical School, Faculdade de Ciências Médicas, Universidade Nova de Lisboa, Lisbon, Portugal*

Correspondence should be addressed to Jose Hugo M. Luz; jhugoluz@gmail.com

Academic Editor: Paul Sijens

Liver volume and function after hepatectomies are directly correlated to postoperative complications and mortality. Consequently contemporary liver surgery has focused on reaching an adequate future liver remnant so as to diminish postoperative morbidity and mortality. Portal vein embolization has evolved and is the standard of care as a liver regenerative strategy in many surgery departments worldwide before major liver resections. Different embolic materials have been used for portal vein embolization including gelfoam, ethanol, polyvinyl-alcohol particles, calibrated microspheres, central vascular plugs, coils, n-butyl-cyanoacrylate glue, fibrin glue, polidocanol-foam, alcoholic prolamin solution, and ethylene vinyl alcohol copolymer, as sole occluders or in varied combinations. While to date there has been no prospective controlled trial comparing the efficacy of different embolic materials in portal vein embolization, retrospective data insinuates that the use of n-butyl-cyanoacrylate and absolute ethanol produces higher contralateral liver hypertrophies. In this review, we evaluated publications up to August 2019 to assess the technical and regenerative results of portal vein embolization accomplished with different embolic materials. Special attention was given to specific aspects, advantages, and drawbacks of each embolic agent used for portal vein embolization, its liver regenerative performance, and its influence on patient outcome.

1. Introduction

Liver unique regenerative ability has been known for a long time, as suggested by the ancient Greek tale of Prometheus, in which an eagle feeds daily on his exposed liver [1]. However, it was not until 1920 that a report correlated portal vein flow interruption to liver parenchymal atrophy in the obstructed side and liver regeneration in the contralateral one [2]. Likewise, modern liver surgery has focused on regenerative strategies to obtain adequate volumes and function for the future liver remnant (FLR) in order to reduce postoperative complications and mortality [3, 4]. Furthermore, the FLR volume and function after surgery are directly associated with rates of complications and mortality after liver resections [5, 6]. The very first reports of the percutaneous approach to portal vein branches occlusion, known as preoperative portal vein embolization (PVE), came with Makuuchi et al. in 1982 [7] and Kinoshita et al. [8] in 1986. Since then, PVE has gained relevant support worldwide, and presently many hepatobiliary and oncological surgery units implement this approach before major liver resections.

Concerning the different embolic materials adopted for PVE to date, there is considerable heterogeneity among groups. Miscellaneous embolic materials were embraced and reported in the PVE literature such as gelatin sponge, absolute ethanol, polyvinyl-alcohol (PVA) particles, calibrated tris-acryl microspheres, vascular plugs, coils, n-butyl-cyanoacrylate (NBCA) glue, fibrin glue, polidocanol-foam, alcoholic prolamin solution (Ethibloc), and DMSO-based agents as sole occluders or in varied combinations [9]. Randomized controlled trials evaluating the efficacy of different embolic materials in head-to-head comparisons are lacking, although reported data suggests that the use of NBCA and ethanol produces higher FLR hypertrophies [10, 11]. We assessed publications up to August 2019 to review the results of each embolic agent and mixtures used for PVE, focusing on their handling, safety profiles, and liver hypertrophy regenerative results and exemplified clinical cases from our own experience.

2. Indications for PVE and Liver Assessment

Some aspects have to be addressed in order to more precisely determine the results of PVE. First, the percentage of the FLR must be calculated and currently there are two frequently adopted measurement methods. One is derived from the patient's total body surface through the calculation of the standardized liver volume (the formula to obtain the volume for the standardized liver is $-794 + 1267 \times$ body surface area) [12]. The other one is obtained from direct computed tomography volumetric measurements [13]. The FLR percentage or FLR ratio is its direct proportion to the total functional liver volume (TFLV) and provides a clear-cut analysis of the FLR relation to the entire tumor-free liver parenchyma. This parameter has historically influenced PVE application, and thus PVE is commonly indicated if the FLR represents less than 25% in healthy and 40% in diseased livers. Patients with chronic liver disease, cholestatic liver tumors, high-dose chemotherapy burden, or significant NASH compromise are those who will need a greater FLR [14, 15].

Nonetheless there are other assessment tests that can and should be used. The indocyanine green test is a clearance test available worldwide due to its simplicity and low cost [16, 17]. It is currently used to assess liver functional reserve before, during, and after hepatic resection [18]. During liver transplantation it is used for serial evaluations of the hepatic function throughout the several stages of this complex surgery [19]. However in some particular situations (i.e., hyperbilirubinemia state) its interpretation can be misleading. Generally an indocyanine green retention ratio above 10% in 15 minutes precludes extended hepatectomies [19]. Nuclear medicine functional studies have come a long way also to play a role in liver assessment. While CT is the established method for volume measurements before and after PVE, liver function evaluation might be more vital and its assessment may shorten the interval between PVE and resection [20, 21]. The liver function cutoff to direct patients to preoperative PVE before liver surgery was established at $2.7\%/\text{min}/\text{m}^2$ as accessed by mebrofenin hepatobiliary scintigraphy [22].

3. PVE Technical Aspects: The Percutaneous Access

3.1. Ipsilateral Access. In this approach portal vein access is obtained through liver that will be removed in the near future surgery and has the clear advantaged of not crossing or puncturing the FLR. If segment IV embolization is planned, this approach might offer a more straightforward rout to those branches. The anterior segment of the right portal vein should preferably be elected since there is evidence of more complications when puncturing the posterior branch [23]. Disadvantages of the ipsilateral approach are the need to use longer, 180° reverse-curve catheters (e.g., Simons catheters), which might be troublesome. Other disadvantages include the risk of puncture through tumor tissue, which might lead to tumor seeding, and embolic material dislodgment when crossing back and forward though an already embolized branch [24].

3.2. Contralateral Access. In the contralateral access the puncture is performed in the FLR, usually a segment III branch, or if portal branches are too thin, puncture of the Rex recess can be adopted [24]. Rex recess is defined as the space between segments 3 and 4 under the liver bridge and similarly refers to the point where the portal vein bifurcates to supply those segments [25]. Some authors advise to avoid the Rex recess puncture due to the thick and fibrotic tissue around the periportal area [26]. One immediate advantage of the contralateral access is the use of shorter catheters (e.g., 30 cm to 40 cm long), which are easier to handle and might prevent the use of an introducer and microcatheter. Furthermore the inside volume capacity of shorter catheters ("dead space") is considerably less than the longer, curved catheters used for ipsilateral approach. This reduced volume is advantageous when adopting liquids for embolization, decreasing the entrapment of embolic material inside the catheters. Other advantages include having the catheters always pointed in the targeted branches flow direction, making this approach technically simpler and quicker. Embolization of segment IV might be troublesome especially if central portal access is obtained [27]. A clear contralateral access disadvantage is FLR puncture and catheterization through its portal branches. Complications involving the FLR might make the planned surgical resection impossible. Overall, the option regarding the contralateral or ipsilateral approach should be made bearing in mind the liver tumor burden, the embolic material used, and local expertise, Figures 1 and 2.

4. The Embolic Materials

The optimal embolization material for PVE would combine greatest and fastest hypertrophy induction with minimal adverse events while being easy to handle, elected by well designed, controlled, prospective comparative studies [28].

4.1. Gelatin Foam. Gelatin sponge or foam (Gelfoam; Pfizer Inc., New York, USA) is a biologic substance prepared from filtered skin gelatin. Although it is very inexpensive and has been used for more than 30 years, its temporary occlusion feature is detrimental in the PVE scenario. In fact, early reports with gelatin foam described recurrent recanalization [7, 29] and less liver hypertrophy than with more definitive,

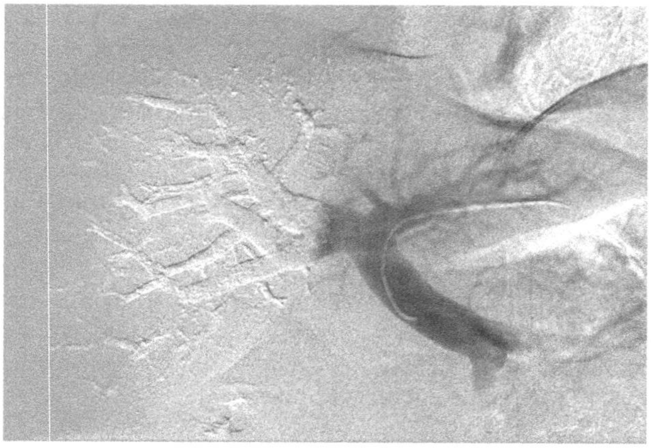

Figure 1: Final portography aspect after portal vein embolization with NBCA accomplished through a contralateral portal vein access.

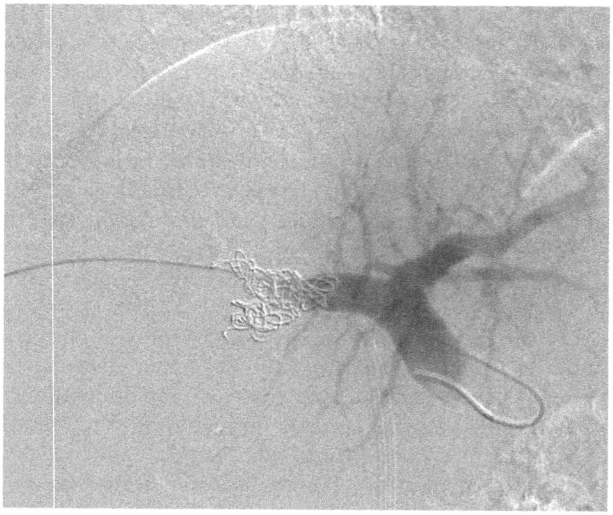

Figure 2: Final portography aspect after portal vein embolization with PVA plus coils accomplished through an ipsilateral portal vein access.

non-temporary embolic material [30]. Studies adopting gelatin foam for PVE have reported degrees of FLR hypertrophy from 18 to 38%. Some groups have mixed gelatin foam with other embolic materials such as iodized oil (Lipiodol; Andre Guerbet, Aulnay-sous-Bois, France) [31]. One possible advantage of using gelatin foam for PVE is the apparent lack of an inflammatory reaction or histological changes after embolization, although this might translate into less hypertrophy since liver regeneration triggering may be related to the periportal inflammation [32]. More recently gelatin foam has been less reported due to the superiority of the other available embolic agents used for PVE.

4.2. Ethibloc/Lipiodol Mixture. Ethibloc (Ethicon, Ethnor Laboratories, Germany) is a mixture that induces thrombosis and is composed of an alcoholic solution of zein and other compounds [33, 34]. After being exposed to any liquid medium, it condenses instantaneously acquiring a more thicken and chomping texture. This mixture has been scarcely reported with results coming mainly from few groups [35, 36]. Although they reported solid hypertrophy results with this embolic material (61% and 25% in the aforementioned studies), disadvantages such as the suspension behavior (not emulsion), higher price, and anecdotal reports of fatal Ethibloc emboli to the brain have limited their widespread usage [37].

4.3. Polyvinyl-Alcohol (PVA) Particles and Microspheres. PVA particles were one of the first materials available for embolization, being offered since 1974. PVA particles are obtained from a piece of dehydrated foam and cut in varied sizes [38, 39], extending from approximately 50 μm to 1200 μm. Nonspherical PVA particles have differences from calibrated microspheres (e.g., Embosphere Trisacryl Microspheres, Biosphere Medical, MA, USA), and the latter is known to be more regular in size and spherical and have a more predictable behavior during transcatheter embolization [40, 41]. Covey et al. adopting PVE with PVA particles, reported a FLR hypertrophy of 31.9% and a FLR ratio increase of 10% in 58 consecutive patients with nondiseased liver [42]. van den Esschert et al. reported an increase in FLR ratio of 8.7% in a metastatic cohort of patients [43] and Leung et al. reported a FLR ratio increase of 9% and a FLR hypertrophy of 29% in a mixed cohort of primary and secondary liver malignancies [44].

4.4. PVA Particles and Microspheres Plus Coils or Vascular Plugs. PVE accomplished with PVA particles plus central vascular plug or coils (CP/C) is currently one of the preferred embolic approaches, principally in the United States. The enhancement effect of deploying CP/C after first utilizing PVA particles or microspheres for distal embolization seems reasonable since it will promote a more proximal and definitive occlusion. Also embolization of segment I might be achieved by central occlusion. Substantial increases in FLR hypertrophy have been published such as the study by Geisel et al. [45]. In their cohort, PVE with PVA particles plus a central vascular plug showed a statistically higher regeneration result, reaching 53% of FLR growth, when compared to patients submitted to PVE with PVA particles alone. Likewise publications from other groups encountered similar results when adopting PVE with PVA particles with the increment of central coils [46]. Remarkably in this latter report one patient developed main and left portal vein thrombosis diagnosed in the routine follow-up CT, a rare complication after PVE. Nevertheless the authors were able to obtain recanalization of the portal vein, and the patient was successfully submitted to the planned liver surgery. Albeit the credible benefit in liver regeneration with the addition of coils in PVA PVE, recanalization with this technique has been reported [47].

Spherical microspheres were also elected for PVE with the intention of promoting a more distal, homogeneous, and regular embolization compared to irregular PVA particles [48]. Madoff et al. published an interesting study about the

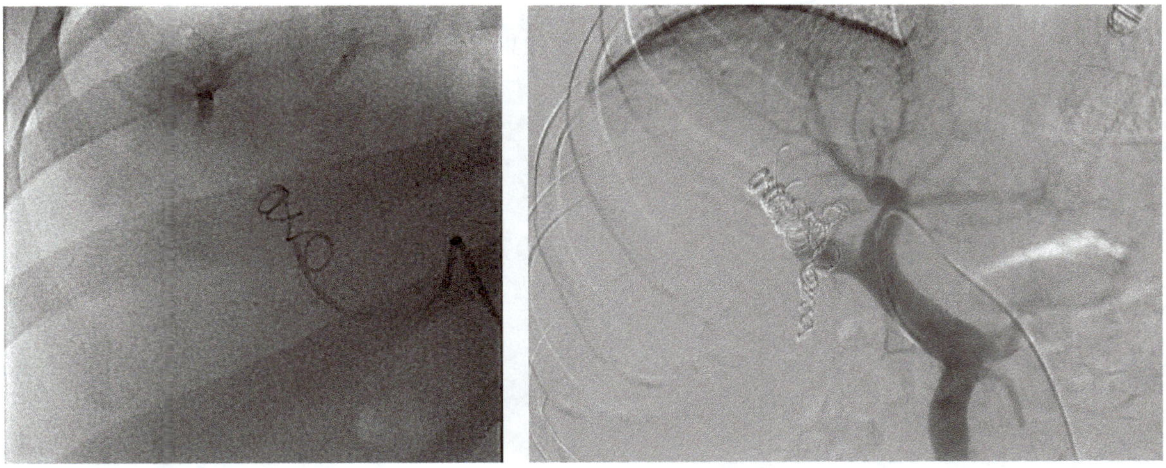

(a) (b)

FIGURE 3: Portal vein embolization accomplished with PVA plus coils. Fluoroscopy image shows the first coil (a) and the last coil (b) deployed in a right portal vein embolization.

use of microspheres in PVE. Besides the liver regenerative benefit obtained in the group of patients submitted to PVE with microspheres plus coils; they also could demonstrate better resection rates in this population. It is important to note that the entire cohort consisted of patients who underwent right hepatectomy plus segment four [48], Figures 3(a) and 3(b).

4.5. N-Butyl-cyanoacrylate. N-butyl-cyanoacrylate (NBCA) is a liquid, uncolored embolic agent, supplied in 0.5 up to 1.0 ml vials. It polymerizes when in contact with ionic mediums forming a strong bound to the adjacent tissue [49]. Lipiodol (Lipiodol Ultra-Fluid, Aulnay-sous-Bois, France) is added to NBCA to provide radiographic opacification and to act as a polymerization regulator. Varying the Lipiodol-NBCA ratio will alter polymerization rate and influence the solution's behavior during embolization. Different lipiodol-NBCA ratios are used and its selection will depend on the portal vein flow, the vein diameter, the level of distal embolization desired, the use of short or long catheters to deliver NBCA, and the operator experience. Catheters must always be flushed with nonionic liquids such as dextrose to avoid NBCA polymerization inside their lumen. Plastic polypropylene syringes are recommended because the NBCA-lipiodol mixture frequently dissolves polycarbonate [50]. Specifically for portal vein embolization, small aliquots of the NBCA-lipiodol mixture (i.e., 0.5 to 0.3 ml) should be injected each time and thoroughly flushed with D5W to prevent any attachment inside the catheter. The contralateral approach to the portal system is advocated by some groups due to the advantage of using short-length catheters [24, 30]. Nonetheless groups have reported entire series adopting the ipsilateral approach to accomplish NBCA PVE [51].

Different groups have reported robust liver regenerative results when adopting glue for PVE, which might be related and explained by the fact that NBCA distinguished intense inflammatory effect in endothelial cells [49, 52]. Nonetheless

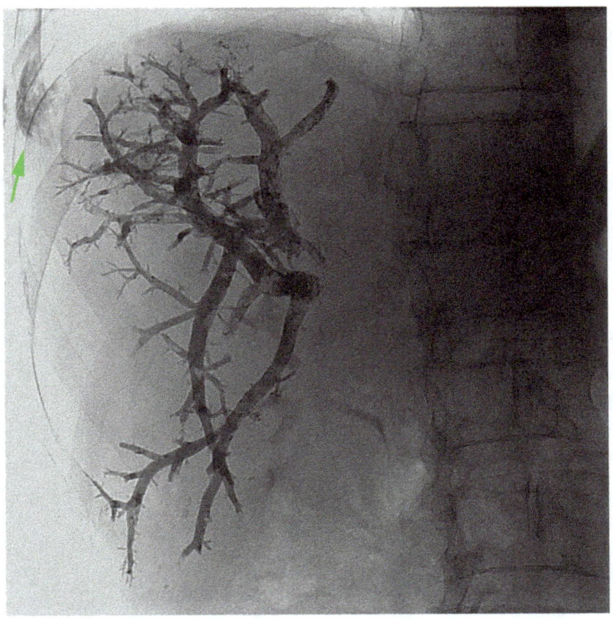

FIGURE 4: Portal vein embolization accomplished with NBCA and lipiodol with a 1:5 ratio. The green arrow shows the liver tract embolization from the ipsilateral approach.

the use of this liquid embolic material requires a steeper learning curve. Reflux to nonintended locations may occur, and although scarcely reported, catheters can become entrapped in the occluded vessel [53]. In a recent systematic review the authors identified thirteen eligible published studies and concluded that NBCA PVE is safe and has a low complication rate. In addition, FLR hypertrophy rates were noticeably high, in some studies reaching 74% 30 days after PVE. Besides a high regeneration yield, other advantages from adopting NBCA PVE have been consistently reported such as significantly less amount of contrast and less fluoroscopy time per procedure [10, 28]. Guiu et al. reported average contrast volume of 264 ml and 162 ml, for microparticles plus coils

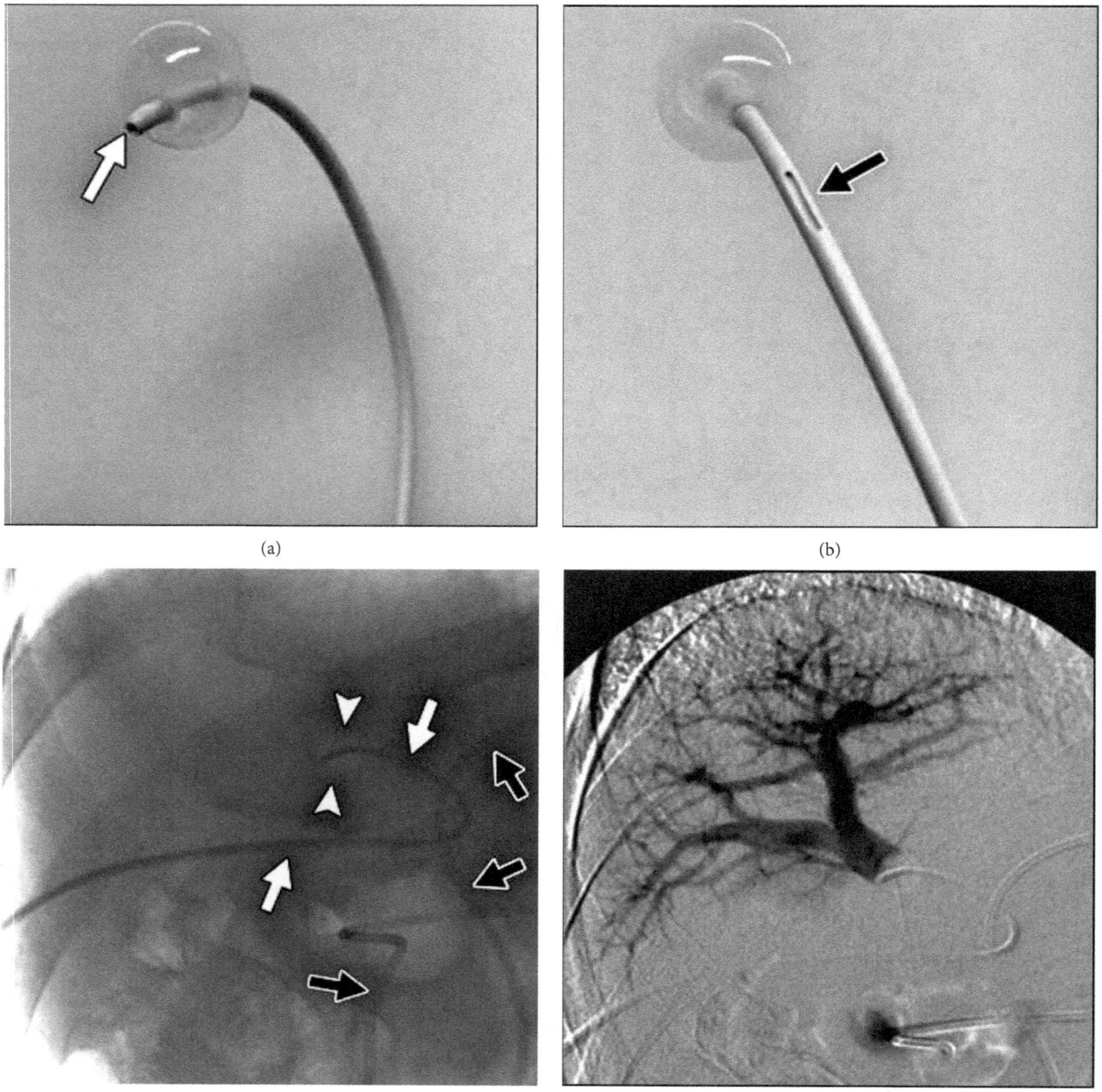

(a) (b) (c) (d)

Figure 5: (a and b). Catheter used for portal vein embolization with absolute alcohol. This 5 French catheter has an end hole for ethanol administration, a side hole for contrast flushing, and an in-between balloon to prevent alcohol reflux (reprinted with permission from the American Journal of Roentgenology). (c). The triple lumen catheter (white arrow heads) with the balloon inflated is placed in the right portal vein. The black arrows refer to a nasobiliary drain. (d). Portography with the balloon inflated shows the anterior sectorial branch, which was embolized with absolute alcohol through the end hole (reprinted with permission from the *American Journal of Roentgenology*).

PVE and NBCA PVE, respectively. Jaberi et al. reported a median fluoroscopy time of 11 minutes for NBCA PVE and 23 minutes for PVA plus coils PVE, Figure 4.

4.6. Absolute Alcohol. This liquid embolic material has an aggressive profile in tissues and blood vessels, with reports of protein denaturation leading to immediate thrombus formation inside blood vessels [50]. For PVE it is frequently used with antireflux strategies such as administration distal to inflated balloons or from a surgically ligated portal vein to prevent any reflux [54]. Many reports, mainly from the Japanese experience, have demonstrated robust hypertrophy results. The regenerative performance of ethanol has been shown as a FLR absolute growth of 35% up to 46% and a degree of hypertrophy ranging from 10% to 12%, even in the cirrhotic population [55–57]. Recently a retrospective analysis demonstrated higher FLR ratio increments after PVE adopting absolute ethanol

Table 1: Embolization Materials reported for portal vein embolization.

PVE material	No. of studies	No. of patients	DH	FLR absolute growth
Gelatin sponge	9*1	355	8.5% up to 11%	17% up to 37%
PVA	4	325	9.6% up to 10%	24% up to 45%
PVA/microspheres plus coils/VP	13*2	869	8.6% up to 11%	27% up to 57%*3
Ethanol	3	382	10.8% up to 12%	33.6% up to 40%
Fibrin glue	3	161	10%	27% up to 31%
NBCA	19*4	583	9% up to 13%	27% up to 74%
EVOH	2	40	10% up to 14%	53%
Ethibloc	2	34	10% up to 11%	25% up to 61%
Aethoxysklerol/air-foam	2	30	7.4% up to 8.5%	NR

PVE: portal vein embolization; PVA: polyvinyl-alcohol particles; DH: degree of hypertrophy; VP: vascular plug; NR: not reported; NBCA: n-butyl-cyanoacrylate; EVOH: ethylene vinyl alcohol; *1One publication reported gelatin sponge associated with other embolic material. *2Two publications reported also other materials for PVE in the same study. *3One publication reported 69% hypertrophy, but it was in patients submitted to right PVE plus segment IV. *4One study mixed NBCA with gelatin sponge and two studies used a vascular plug for central occlusion.

Table 2: Embolic materials used for PVE: advantages and drawbacks.

Material	Main advantages	Drawbacks	Occlusion	Pain
Gelatin sponge	Easy handling Low inflammation	Recanalization	Transient	Mild
PVA/MS plus coils/VP	Distal and proximal occlusion	Time consuming; more contrast and fluoroscopy time	Definitive*2	Mild
Fibrin glue	Robust hypertrophy	Very expensive*1; fatal emboli to the brain reported	Definitive	NR
NBCA-lipiodol	Best hypertrophy? Cheap	Steeper learning curve	Definitive	Moderate to severe
Ethanol	Robust hypertrophy Cheap	Occlusion balloon usually adopted	Definitive	Moderate to severe
Foam	Cheap	Recanalization; occlusion balloon adopted	Definitive	Mild
EVOH	Controlled administration	Many vials needed; very expensive; time consuming	Definitive	Moderate to severe

PVA: polyvinyl-alcohol particles; MS: microspheres; VP: vascular plug; NBCA: n-butyl-cyanoacrylate; EVOH: ethylene vinyl alcohol; NR: not reported; *1Some groups reported interruption of its use due to its elevated cost. *2There are reports of recanalization.

versus NBCA [11]. Interestingly also in the later report, FLR growth after PVE did not differ significantly between groups, and grade 3 and 4 toxicity were seen more commonly in the absolute ethanol cohort. Technical disadvantages of absolute alcohol embolization include the need of antireflux apparatus, significant pain during the procedure, and rapid dilution by vascular inflow. Changes in serum liver enzyme levels are commonly seen and may increase dramatically, up to tenfold, on the first day after PVE [56].

4.7. Ethylene Vinyl Alcohol (EVOH) Copolymer. This liquid material is a DMSO- (dimethyl sulfoxide, a strong solvent) based embolic agent. It is composed by a plastic polymer conjugated with tantalum powder for radiopacity [58]. Its fluidity and liquid form is maintained while in contact with DMSO and solidifies when blood separates it from its solvent. Unlike other liquid embolic materials such as NBCA, this plastic polymer does not have adhesive properties as it only fills the vascular lumen [58]. Very few groups have reported the use of EVOH for PVE. Biggemann et al. compared right PVE with PVA, PVE with EVOH, and portal vein ligation. Interestingly the authors in this study opted to occlude the right portal vein with a vascular plug to prevent EVOH reflux [59]. In this study PVE with EVOH delivered a higher FLR hypertrophy than embolization with PVA and portal ligation although the use of proximal mechanical embolization with vascular plug prevented the EVOH individual hypertrophy evaluation. Né et al. reported 6 cases of PVE using different concentrations of EVOH. As in the rationale for PVA and microspheres embolization, the authors in this work accomplished more distal embolization with lesser viscous preparation of EVOH for deeper penetration and more proximal embolization with viscous formulations. An interesting and may be promising application of EVOH PVE was described recently. The authors used this cohesive liquid embolic material in more challenging portal branches, such as segment IV [59]. All targeted portal branches were successfully embolized without any occurrence of nontarget embolization. An evident drawback of using EVOH is the elevated price of this product and the necessity of large amount of vials with a mean of 12.3 vials per procedure [60], Tables 1 and 2.

5. Discussion

There are a limited number of reports comparing embolic materials for PVE, and none in the prospective, randomized form. Besides, their head-to-head comparisons are problematic. Different FLR measurement models, different timing between PVE and volumetric and functional

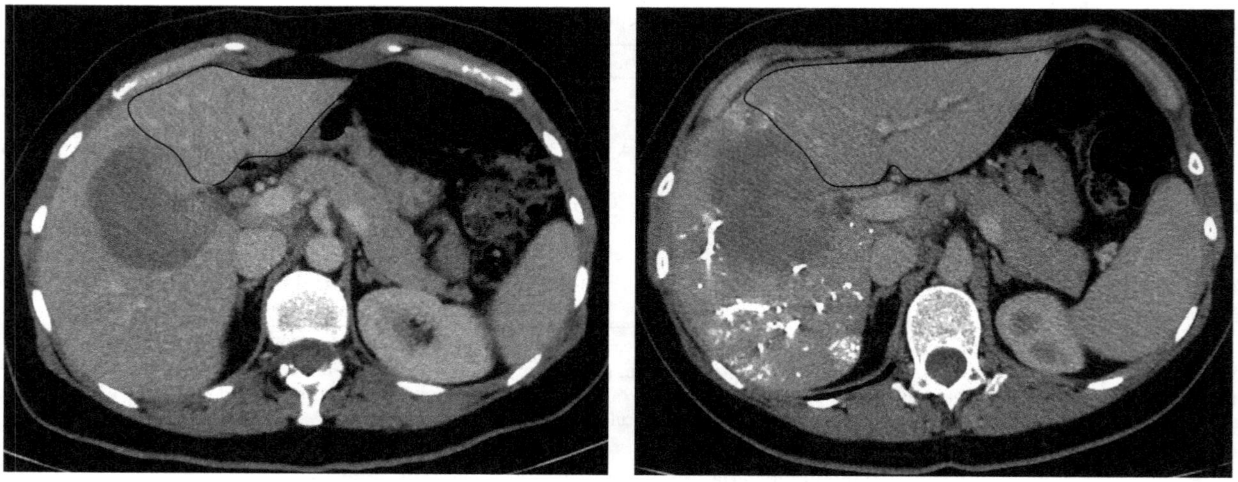

(a) (b)

Figure 6: (a) Computed tomography in the portal venous phase acquired before portal vein embolization shows a small left liver (future liver remnant circled in black line). (b) Computed tomography in the portal venous phase shows a significant increase in the left liver (future liver remnant circled in black line) 28 days after portal vein embolization with NBCA.

evaluation (diverging from 2 up to 8 weeks), differences in normal and diseased liver regeneration rates, all influence the hypertrophy results and prevent fair comparisons among publications [14, 15]. Two publications with animal models compared different materials for PVE. Larger hepatic lobules were found in the regenerated animal's livers submitted to PVE with NBCA one week after the procedure [9]. The histology analysis showed more fibrosis in the embolized liver submitted to PVE with NBCA and 50–150 μm PVA, suggesting the causative role of inflammation in liver regeneration [9]. The other animal study demonstrated higher liver regenerative increments in CT volumetry 14 and 28 after PVE for the group in which NBCA was elected as the embolic material. Geisel et al. have compared PVA PVE to PVA plus coils/vascular plug PVE. The analysis of their retrospective cohort of 70 patients showed that the addition of proximal coils or a vascular plug yielded superior FLR hypertrophy results [45]. Madoff et al. compared right plus segment IV PVE accomplished with PVA plus coils versus PVE with microspheres plus coils in a retrospective cohort. There was a significant increment in liver hypertrophy and better resection rates after PVE with microspheres and coils [48]. In a colorectal liver metastases cohort different embolic agents were tested for PVE. Patients were submitted to PVE with either one of three embolic regimens: PVA plus coils, PVA plus NBCA and coils (combination group), and NBCA. The NBCA PVE group presented significantly higher regeneration results, followed by the combination group and lastly by the PVA plus coils group [61].

Jaberi et al. compared liver hypertrophy results in 45 patients submitted to PVE with NBCA plus a vascular plug versus 40 patients submitted to PVE with PVA plus coils. FLR regeneration results were more robust in the NBCA group (degree of hypertrophy of 16.2% versus 12.3% and kinetic growth rate of 3.5% versus 2.6%). Interestingly it was also shown that fluoroscopy time and contrast volumes used were significantly lower in the NBCA group [28]. Guiu et al. compared a cohort of 14 successive patients submitted to right PVE accomplished with spherical microparticles plus coils with 20 other consecutive patients submitted to right PVE with NBCA. In spite of the few number of patients, they reported a noteworthy disparity in FLR regenerative capacity between groups, with differences as high as 74% for the NBCA group and 23% for the microspheres plus coils group. It was also shown that the amount of contrast is significantly less when adopting NBCA to perform PVE. Complications rates and toxicity were not different among the two studied groups [10]. van Lienden et al. published a comprehensive review, which addressed many aspects of PVE. They compared the FLR volume increase achieved with different embolic agents, of which NBCA had the most powerful effect [62], Figures 5(a) and 5(b).

6. Conclusion

Permanent embolic materials, such as ethanol, NBCA, microparticles, coils, and plugs, seem to yield superior liver regeneration. NBCA and absolute ethanol PVE might deliver more robust FLR hypertrophy results, although no prospective randomized study is currently available.

Acknowledgments

The authors would like to express their great gratitude to Prof. Dr. Paula Mendes Luz and Prof. Dr. Beatriz Vaz de Melo Mendes for their support and insights.

References

[1] T. S. Chen and P. S. Chen, "The myth of Prometheus and the liver," *Journal of the Royal Society of Medicine*, vol. 87, no. 12, pp. 754-755, 1994.

[2] P. Rous and L. D. Larimore, "Relation of the portal blood to liver maintenance: a demonstration of liver atrophy conditional on compensation," *The Journal of Experimental Medicine*, vol. 31, no. 5, pp. 609–632, 1920.

[3] M. J. Schindl, D. N. Redhead, K. C. Fearon, O. J. Garden, and S. J. Wigmore, "The value of residual liver volume as a predictor of hepatic dysfunction and infection after major liver resection," *Gut* vol. 54, no. 2, pp. 289–296, 2005.

[4] V. Pamecha, G. Glantzounis, N. Davies, G. Fusai, D. Sharma, and B. Davidson, "Long-term survival and disease recurrence following portal vein embolisation prior to major hepatectomy for colorectal metastases," *Annals of Surgical Oncology*, vol. 16, no. 5, pp. 1202–1207, 2009.

[5] E. K. Abdalla, C. C. Barnett, D. Doherty, S. A. Curley, and J. N. Vauthey, "Extended hepatectomy in patients with hepatobiliary malignancies with and without preoperative portal vein embolization," *Archives of Surgery*, vol. 137, no. 6, pp. 675–680, 2002.

[6] K. Shirabe, M. Shimada, T. Gion et al., "Postoperative liver failure after major hepatic resection for hepatocellular carcinoma in the modern era with special reference to remnant liver volume," *Journal of the American College of Surgeons*, vol. 188, no. 3, pp. 304–309, 1999.

[7] M. Makuuchi, B. L Thai, K. Takayasu et al., "Preoperative portal embolization to increase safety of major hepatectomy for hilar bile duct carcinoma: a preliminary report," *Surgery*, vol. 107, no. 5, pp. 521–527, 1990.

[8] H. Kinoshita, K. Sakai, K. Hirohashi, S. Igawa, O. Yamasaki, and S. Kubo, "Preoperative portal vein embolization for hepatocellular carcinoma," *World Journal of Surgery*, vol. 10, no. 5, pp. 803–808, 1986.

[9] T. de Baere, A. Denys, and V. Paradis, "Comparison of four embolic materials for portal vein embolization: experimental study in pigs," *European Radiology*, vol. 19, no. 6, pp. 1435–1442, 2009.

[10] B. Guiu, P. Bize, D. Gunthern, N. Demartines, N. Halkic, and A. Denys, "Portal vein embolization before right hepatectomy: improved results using n-butyl-cyanoacrylate compared to microparticles plus coils," *Cardiovascular and Interventional Radiology*, vol. 36, no. 5, pp. 1306–1312, 2013.

[11] S. Sugawara, Y. Arai, M. Sone et al., "Retrospective comparative study of absolute ethanol with N-butyl-2-cyanoacrylate in percutaneous portal vein embolization," *Journal of Vascular and Interventional Radiology*, vol. 30, no. 8, pp. 1215–1222, 2019.

[12] J. Vauthey, E. K. Abdalla, D. A. Doherty et al., "Body surface area and body weight predict total liver volume in Western adults," *Liver Transplantation*, vol. 8, no. 3, pp. 233–240, 2002.

[13] T. M. Lodewick, C. W. K. P. Arnoldussen, M. J. Lahaye et al., "Fast and accurate liver volumetry prior to hepatectomy," *HPB*, vol. 18, no. 9 pp. 764–772, 2016.

[14] K. Kubota, M. Makuuchi, K. Kusaka et al., "Measurement of liver volume and hepatic functional reserve as a guide to decision-making in resectional surgery for hepatic tumors," *Hepatology*, vol. 26 no. 5, pp. 1176–1181, 1997.

[15] D. Azoulay, D. Castaing, J. Krissat et al., "Percutaneous portal vein embolization increases the feasibility and safety of major liver resection for hepatocellular carcinoma in injured liver," *Annals of Surgery*, vol. 232, no. 5, pp. 665–672, 2000.

[16] T. Mizuguchi, M. Kawamoto, M. Meguro, T. T. Hui, and K. Hirata, "Preoperative liver function assessments to estimate the prognosis and safety of liver resections," *Surgery Today*, vol. 44, no. 1, pp. 1–10, 2014.

[17] J. J. Vos, J. K. G. Wietasch, A. R. Absalom, H. G. D. Hendriks, and T. W. L. Scheeren, "Green light for liver function monitoring using indocyanine green? An overview of current clinical applications," *Anaesthesia*, vol. 69, no. 12, pp. 1364–1376, 2014.

[18] Y. Seyama and N. Kokudo, "Assessment of liver function for safe hepatic resection," *Hepatology Research*, vol. 39, no. 2, pp. 107–116, 2009.

[19] A. D. Gasperi, E. Mazza, and M. Prosperi, "Indocyanine green kinetics to assess liver function: ready for a clinical dynamic assessment in major liver surgery?" *World Journal of Hepatology*, vol. 8, no. 7, pp. 355–367, 2016.

[20] T. Beppu, H. Hayashi, H. Okabe et al., "Liver functional volumetry for portal vein embolization using a newly developed 99mTc-galactosyl human serum albumin scintigraphy SPECT-computed tomography fusion system," *Journal of Gastroenterology*, vol. 46, no. 7, pp. 938–943, 2011.

[21] W. de Graaf, K. P. van Lienden, J. W. van den Esschert, R. J. Bennink, and T. M. van Gulik, "Increase in future remnant liver function after preoperative portal vein embolization," *British Journal of Surgery*, vol. 98, no. 6, pp. 825–834, 2011.

[22] W. de Graaf, K. P. van Lienden, S. Dinant et al., "Assessment of future remnant liver function using hepatobiliary scintigraphy in patients undergoing major liver resection," *Journal of Gastrointestinal Surgery*, vol. 14, no. 2, pp. 369–378, 2010.

[23] Y. Kodama, T. Shimizu, H. Endo, N. Miyamoto, and K. Miyasaka, "Complications of percutaneous transhepatic portal vein embolization," *Journal of Vascular and Interventional Radiology*, vol. 13, no. 12, pp. 1233–1237, 2002.

[24] D. R. Di Stefano, T. de Baere, A. Denys et al., "Preoperative percutaneous portal vein embolization: evaluation of adverse events in 188 patients," *Radiology*, vol. 234, no. 2, pp. 625–630, 2005.

[25] S. T. Orcutt, K. Kobayashi, M. Sultenfuss et al., "Portal vein embolization as an oncosurgical strategy prior to major hepatic resection: anatomic, surgical, and technical considerations," *Frontiers in Surgery*, vol. 3, no. 1, p. 14, 2016.

[26] N. Narula and T. A. Aloia, "Portal vein embolization in extended liver resection," *Langenbeck's Archives of Surgery*, vol. 402, no. 5, pp. 727–735, 2017.

[27] R. Avritscher, T. de Baere, R. Murthy, F. Deschamps, and D. Madoff, "Percutaneous transhepatic portal vein embolization: rationale, technique, and outcomes," *Seminars in Interventional Radiology*, vol. 25, no. 2, pp. 132–145, 2008.

[28] A. Jaberi, S. S. Toor, D. K. Rajan et al., "Comparison of clinical outcomes following glue versus polyvinyl alcohol portal vein embolization for hypertrophy of the future liver remnant prior to right hepatectomy," *Journal of Vascular and Interventional Radiology*, vol. 27, no. 12, pp. 1897–1905, 2016.

[29] J. H. Shin, H.-K. Yoon, J. Kwon et al., "Volumetric analysis of the liver after right portal vein embolization: mid-term follow-up based on embolization score," *Clinical Radiology*, vol. 65, no. 4, pp. 288–296, 2010.

[30] T. Debaere, A. Roche, D. Elias, P. Lasser, C. Lagrange, and V. Bousson, "Preoperative portal vein embolization for extension of hepatectomy indications," *Hepatology*, vol. 24, no. 6, pp. 1386–1391, 1996.

[31] H. Kakizawa, N. Toyota, K. Arihiro et al., "Preoperative portal vein embolization with a mixture of gelatin sponge and

iodized oil: efficacy and safety," *Acta Radiologica*, vol. 47, no. 10, pp. 1022–1028, 2006.

[32] A. Denys, J. Prior, P. Bize et al., "Portal vein embolization: what do we know?" *Cardiovascular and Interventional Radiology*, vol. 35, no. 5, pp. 999–1008, 2012.

[33] C. Adamsbaum, H. Leclet, and G. Kalifa, "Intralesional ethibloc injections in bone cysts," *Seminars in Musculoskeletal Radiology*, vol. 1, no. 2, pp. 301–304, 1997.

[34] M. A. Emran, J. Dubois, L. Laberge, A. Al-Jazaeri, A. Bütter, and S. Yazbeck, "Alcoholic solution of zein (Ethibloc) sclerotherapy for treatment of lymphangiomas in children," *Journal of Pediatric Surgery*, vol. 41, no. 5, pp. 975–979, 2006.

[35] R. Ladurner, G. Brandacher, C. Riedl-Huter et al., "Percutaneous portal vein embolisation in preparation for extended hepatic resection of primary nonresectable liver tumours," *Digestive and Liver Disease*, vol. 35, no. 10, pp. 716–721, 2003.

[36] B. Radeleff, S. Schawo, K. Hoffmann et al., "Efficacy and safety of percutaneous transhepatic portal embolization before right liver resection using an ethibloc/lipiodol mixture: a single-center experience," *Digestive Surgery*, vol. 25, no. 1, pp. 52–59, 2008.

[37] A. Peraud, J. M. Drake, D. Armstrong, D. Hedden, P. Babyn, and G. Wilson, "Fatal ethibloc embolization of vertebrobasilar system following percutaneous injection into aneurysmal bone cyst of the second cervical vertebra," *AJNR: American Journal of Neuroradiology*, vol. 25, no. 6, pp. 1116–1120, 2004.

[38] M. Herrera, J. Rysavy, F. Kotula, B. Rusnak, W. R. Castaneda-Zuniga, and K. Amplatz, "Ivalon shavings: technical considerations of a new embolic agent," *Radiology*, vol. 144, no. 3, pp. 638–640, 1982.

[39] S. M. Tadavarthy, J. H. Moller, and K. Amplatz, "Polyvinyl alcohol (Ivalon)—a new embolic material," *American Journal of Roentgenology*, vol. 125, no. 3, pp. 609–616, 1975.

[40] C. P. Derdeyn, V. B. Graves, M. S. Salamat, and A. Rappe, "Collagen-coated acrylic microspheres for embolotherapy: in vivo and in vitro characteristics," *AJNR. American Journal of Neuroradiology*, vol. 18, no. 4, pp. 647–653, 1997.

[41] A. Laurent, "Microspheres and nonspherical particles for embolization," *Techniques in Vascular and Interventional Radiology*, vol. 10, no. 4, pp. 248–256, 2007.

[42] A. M. Covey, S. Tuorto, L. A. Brody et al., "Safety and efficacy of preoperative portal vein embolization with polyvinyl alcohol in 58 patients with liver metastases," *American Journal of Roentgenology*, vol. 185, no. 6, pp. 1620–1626, 2005.

[43] J. W. van den Esschert, W. de Graaf, K. P. van Lienden et al., "Volumetric and functional recovery of the remnant liver after major liver resection with prior portal vein embolization : recovery after PVE and liver resection," *Journal of Gastrointestinal Surgery*, vol. 13, no. 8, pp. 1464–1469, 2009.

[44] U. Leung, A. L. Simpson, R. L. C. Araujo et al., "Remnant growth rate after portal vein embolization is a good early predictor of post-hepatectomy liver failure," *Journal of the American College of Surgeons*, vol. 219, no. 4, pp. 620–630, 2014.

[45] D. Geisel, M. Malinowski, M.-J. Powerski et al., "Improved hypertrophy of future remnant liver after portal vein embolization with plugs, coils and particles," *Cardiovascular and Interventional Radiology*, vol. 37, no. 5, pp. 1251–1258, 2014.

[46] D. C. Madoff, M. E. Hicks, E. K. Abdalla, J. S. Morris, and J.-N. Vauthey, "Portal vein embolization with polyvinyl alcohol particles and coils in preparation for major liver resection for hepatobiliary malignancy: safety and effectiveness—study in 26 patients," *Radiology*, vol. 227, no. 1, pp. 251–260, 2003.

[47] M. Malinowski, D. Geisel, V. Stary et al., "Portal vein embolization with plug/coils improves hepatectomy outcome," *Journal of Surgical Research*, vol. 194, no. 1, pp. 202–211, 2015.

[48] D. C. Madoff, E. K. Abdalla, S. Gupta et al., "Transhepatic ipsilateral right portal vein embolization extended to segment IV: improving hypertrophy and resection outcomes with spherical particles and coils," *Journal of Vascular and Interventional Radiology*, vol. 16, no. 2, pp. 215–225, 2005.

[49] J. S. Pollak and R. I. White, "The use of cyanoacrylate adhesives in peripheral embolization," *Journal of Vascular and Interventional Radiology*, vol. 12, no. 8, pp. 907–913, 2001.

[50] S. Vaidya, K. Tozer, and J. Chen, "An overview of embolic agents," *Seminars in Interventional Radiology*, vol. 25, no. 3, pp. 204–215, 2008.

[51] J. H. M. Luz, P. M. Luz, T. Bilhim et al., "Portal vein embolization with n-butyl-cyanoacrylate through an ipsilateral approach before major hepatectomy: single center analysis of 50 consecutive patients," *Cancer Imaging*, vol. 17, no. 1, p. 25, 2017.

[52] O. Levrier, C. Mekkaoui, P. H. Rolland et al., "Efficacy and low vascular toxicity of embolization with radical versus anionic polymerization of n-butyl-2-cyanoacrylate (NBCA). An experimental study in the swine," *Journal of Neuroradiology*, vol. 30, no. 2, pp. 95–102, 2003.

[53] J. M. Mathis, A. J. Evans, A. J. DeNardo et al., "Hydrophilic coatings diminish adhesion of glue to catheter: an in vitro simulation of NBCA embolization," *AJNR American Journal of Neuroradiology*, vol. 18, no. 6, pp. 1087–1091, 1997.

[54] G.-Q. Zhang, Z.-W. Zhang, W.-Y. Lau, and X.-P. Chen, "Associating liver partition and portal vein ligation for staged hepatectomy (ALPPS): a new strategy to increase resectability in liver surgery," *International Journal of Surgery*, vol. 12, no. 5, pp. 437–441, 2014.

[55] Y. Sakuhara, D. Abo, Y. Hasegawa et al., "Preoperative percutaneous transhepatic portal vein embolization with ethanol injection," *American Journal of Roentgenology*, vol. 198, no. 4, pp. 914–922, 2012.

[56] K. Sofue, Y. Arai, K. Shimada et al., "Right portal vein embolization with absolute ethanol in major hepatic resection for hepatobiliary malignancy," *British Journal of Surgery*, vol. 101, no. 9, pp. 1122–1128, 2014.

[57] G.-Y. Ko, K.-B. Sung, H.-K. Yoon, J.-H. Kim, Y. C. Weon, and H.-Y. Song, "Preoperative portal vein embolization with a new liquid embolic agent," *Radiology*, vol. 227, no. 2, pp. 407–413, 2003.

[58] M. Saeed Kilani, J. Izaaryene, F. Cohen et al., "Ethylene vinyl alcohol copolymer (Onyx®) in peripheral interventional radiology: indications, advantages and limitations," *Diagnostic and Interventional Imaging*, vol. 96, no. 4, pp. 319–326, 2015.

[59] R. Breguet, S. Boudabbous, L. F. Pupulim et al., "Ethylene vinyl alcohol copolymer for occlusion of specific portal branches during preoperative portal vein embolisation with n-butyl-cyanoacrylate," *European Radiology*, vol. 28, no. 11, pp. 4810–4817, 2018.

[60] R. Né, O. Chevallier, N. Falvo et al., "Embolization with ethylene vinyl alcohol copolymer (Onyx) for peripheral hemostatic and non-hemostatic applications: a feasibility and safety study," *Quantitative Imaging in Medicine and Surgery*, vol. 8, no. 3, pp. 280–290, 2018.

[61] S. K. Dhaliwal, G. Annamalai, N. Gafoor, R. Pugash, C. Dey, and E. N. David, "Portal vein embolization: correlation of future liver remnant hypertrophy to type of embolic agent used," *Canadian Association of Radiologists Journal*, vol. 69, no. 3, pp. 316–321, 2018.

[62] K. P. van Lienden, J. W. van den Esschert, W. de Graaf et al., "Portal vein embolization before liver resection: a systematic review," *Cardiovascular and Interventional Radiology*, vol. 36, no. 1, pp. 25–34, 2013.

27

An Experimental Intervention Study Assessing the Impact of a Thin Silicone Gel Surface Overlay on Interface Pressure

Seth Kwadjo Angmorterh[1] **Andrew England,**[2] **Sonia Aboagye,**[3] **Eric Kwasi Ofori,**[1] **and Peter Hogg**[4]

[1]*Department of Medical Imaging, School of Allied Health Sciences, University of Health and Allied Sciences (UHAS), Ho, Ghana*
[2]*School of Allied Health Professions, Keele University, Staffordshire, Newcastle, UK*
[3]*Department of Speech, Language & Hearing Sciences, School of Allied Health Sciences, University of Health and Allied Sciences (UHAS), Ho, Ghana*
[4]*Directorate of Radiography, School of Healthcare Sciences, Allerton Building, University of Salford, Salford—Greater Manchester, UK*

Correspondence should be addressed to Seth Kwadjo Angmorterh; sangmorterh@uhas.edu.gh

Academic Editor: Daniele La Forgia

Introduction. The incidence of pressure ulcers (PUs) presents a substantial threat to patients, especially geriatric patients, those with restricted mobility, and patients suffering from chronic diseases such as cancer. PUs creates a huge financial burden on healthcare authorities and patients, costing billions to treat and manage. Radiography and radiotherapy patients may experience medical device related (MDR) PUs and studies have shown that high interface pressure (IP) values exist for the head when placed on an X-ray table without a mattress. These high IP values pose a PU risk to patients, especially those accessing prolonged radiography/radiology and radiotherapy procedures. The current study assessed the impact on IP values for the head from using a thin silicone gel surface overlay during radiographic procedures and identified whether this reduced the risk of PUs. *Materials and Methods.* A calibrated XSENSOR pressure mat was used to measure IP for the head on an X-ray table with and without a thin silicone gel surface overlay. Prior to pressure mapping, the silicone gel surface overlay was assessed for its impact on radiation attenuation and image quality. *Results.* Study participants were 14 males (70%) and six females (30%), with an age range of 25–53 years (mean $= 34.4 \pm 7.0$). Paired-samples t-test results indicated that there was a statistically significant decrease in the mean IP for the head on the X-ray table without the silicone gel surface overlay (mean $= 83.9 \pm 8.2$ in mmHg) and the X-ray table with the gel surface overlay (mean $= 62.4 \pm 6.1$ in mmHg), $p \leq 0.001$. Paired-samples t-test results indicated that there was a statistically significant decrease in the mean peak pressure index (PPI) for the head on the X-ray table without the silicone gel surface overlay (mean $= 205.1 \pm 28.2$ in mmHg) and the X-ray table with the gel surface overlay (mean $= 159.8 \pm 26.8$ in mmHg), $p \leq 0.001$. *Conclusions.* The use of a thin silicone gel surface overlay could reduce IP risk for the head by approximately 25%. The reduction in IP risk could have a significant impact in reducing the risk of developing a PU. To ensure maximum benefit, the silicone gel surface overlay should be evaluated to address the specific needs within radiography and radiotherapy planning and treatment settings.

1. Introduction

Pressure ulcers (PUs) are wounds to the skin and underlying tissue caused by sustained pressure on the skin. They can develop within a short space of time or over days. Geriatric patients, those with restricted mobility, and patients suffering from chronic diseases such as cancer are at greater risk of developing a PU [1, 2]. PUs are a common problem in healthcare and significant effort and international attention has been directed towards reducing their incidence. However, rates continue to rise, resulting in increasing numbers of PU sufferers worldwide [3, 4]. Prevalence of PUs across hospital settings and nursing homes in the United Kingdom (UK), Canada, and the United States of America (USA) is

4.7%, 36.8%, and 12.3%, respectively, [5–7]. PUs place a huge financial burden on healthcare authorities, costing billions to treat and manage [8–10]. They also lead to negative physical and psychological effects on patients, thereby reducing their quality of life [11, 12]. Due to the harmful effects of PUs, the National Institute for Health and Care Excellence (NICE) of the United Kingdom (UK) has recommended that rigorous scientific research should be conducted into the aetiology and prevention of PUs to help prevent or minimise their incidence [13].

In radiography and radiotherapy, patients are likely to be exposed to medical device related (MDR) PUs. These are localised injuries to the skin and/or underlying tissue because of sustained pressure from a medical or therapeutic device [14]. MDRs usually appear visually on the superficial layer of the skin and take the shape of the device [15, 16]. In radiography, because of the need to minimise error and produce diagnostically acceptable images, patients are usually transferred onto medical imaging surfaces prior to a procedure [17]. These hard surfaces often have a thin radiolucent mattress on their surface, to aid patient comfort. During radiographic procedures, a pillow may be used, which has valuable consequences for PU minimisation. However not all cases permit a pillow to be used. Furthermore, in some countries such as Portugal and Ghana, diagnostic radiography procedures are typically conducted on hard carbon fibre X-ray tables. By contrast, in radiotherapy, it is important to maintain reproducibility of patient position during planning and treatment, so patients are usually positioned on hard couch surfaces again with no mattress [18]. It is essential that the daily radiotherapy treatment position is the same as that in planning to ensure accuracy of the radiotherapy procedure [19]. Lying on hard imaging and radiotherapy treatment surfaces with no mattress could be harmful to at-risk populations such as elderly patients and those suffering from cancer because of their fragile skin [20]. Confounding this is the fact that some of these procedures take a very long time to complete. For example, cranial stereotactic radiotherapy takes between 40 and 60 minutes depending on the clinical history of the patient [21]. Cervical vertebroplasty, an interventional radiography procedure, takes over an hour to complete and sometimes longer when several cervical fractures are present [22]. Another confounding factor is that patients are intentionally immobilised to minimise image artefacts during the procedure. Immobilisation is harsher in radiotherapy because patient positioning during treatment needs to be assured. For example, the use of immobilisation devices such as full head masks helps to reduce positioning errors but limits patient motion. These are necessary to minimise misdirection of prescribed radiation doses [19]. All these factors could contribute to high interface pressure (IP) between the head and the radiography/radiotherapy surface.

Interface pressure (IP), defined as the pressure between the human body and a supporting surface, plays a crucial role in skin damage [23, 24]. Seminal works have shown that IP greater than 47 mmHg sustained for a period longer between 30 minutes is most likely to compromise blood circulation and may cause tissue ischaemia, which may lead to PUs [25–29]. PUs are prone to occurring at the head (occiput), sacrum, and heels, due to the prominent bony features found at these anatomical sites [30, 31]. A study conducted by Justham et al. [32] indicated that there is the potential of high IP on medical imaging and radiotherapy surfaces. Angmorterh et al. [33] followed up on this study and more recently confirmed that high IP values do exist on X-ray tables without mattresses. The high IP values pose a PU risk to patients and could increase the risk of developing PUs in patients accessing prolonged radiography/radiology and radiotherapy procedures. High IP risk could have a more severe negative impact among geriatric patients and those suffering from chronic diseases such as cancer due to the poor collagen and elastin content in their skin and the presence of comorbidities among these patient populations [34]. The study by Angmorterh et al. [33] also found that lying on an X-ray table without a mattress can be very uncomfortable and, in some cases, patients may experience pain centred in the head region. Such discomfort could have negative implications on patient management as research has highlighted a link between patient comfort and the accuracy of radiotherapy procedures [35].

It is common for patients not to be given pillows during radiographic and/or radiotherapy procedures as the pillow could induce diagnostic and radiotherapy planning and treatment errors. In some countries, for example, Ghana, fluoroscopic X-ray machines do not use mattresses. Patients undergoing fluoroscopic procedures such as cervical vertebroplasty are required to lie on hard rigid fluoroscopic X-ray surfaces for the duration of the procedure. It must be stated that patients' heads are not supported on pillows during cervical vertebroplasty due to the possibility that the pillow might elevate the head above the level of the cervical spine, thereby putting pressure on the already distressed cervical spine. These may both increase the pain in the cervical spine, as well as cement leaks within the vertebrae [36]. Additionally, the proximity of the cervical vertebrae to the head demands that the head is not supported on pillows because the use of pillows could produce artefacts, which might affect the diagnostic quality of the fluoroscopic image. It is a common practice in radiography and radiotherapy that any anatomical area which to be irradiated and its immediate surroundings are kept free of foreign materials [17]. However, the absence of a pillow or any form of cushioning at the head, combined with rigid immobilisation, could induce tissue damage because the head will be in direct contact with a rigid fluoroscopic surface for prolonged period of time. It is therefore important to explore ways of minimising the high IP risks identified for the head when using X-ray tables without mattresses. This empirical intervention study aimed to assess the results of using a thin silicone gel surface overlay as an intervention to minimise the high IP risk for the head. The outcome of this study may help inform measures to reduce the incidence of PUs among patients accessing prolonged radiography and radiotherapy planning and treatment procedures.

2. Materials and Methods

2.1. Study Design, Setting, and Ethical Considerations. This was a quantitative experimental study, conducted at the medical imaging facility of the University of Salford (UoS) in Manchester, UK. The study was approved by the UoS College of Health and Social Care Ethics Committee (HSCR 15–141).

2.2. Pressure Redistributing Surface Overlays. Pressure redistributing surface overlays are characterised by design, by materials in the finished product, and as dynamic (alternating) or static (constant). The primary aim of pressure redistributing support surfaces such as mattresses, surface overlays, and cushions is to relieve IP so as to provide some level of cushioning to high risk parts of the body and distribute the IP more evenly. The two main types of pressure redistributing surface overlays—alternating and static—provide different functions [37]. Alternating pressure redistribution surface overlays cause periodic high and low movement. However, they cannot be applied in radiography or radiotherapy planning and treatment procedures because of the risk of errors and subsequent negative impact on patient management. For the purposes of this intervention study, a range of static pressure surface overlays were scrutinized for selection. Foams and air-filled surface overlays are not applicable in radiotherapy planning and treatment procedures because they have the tendency to squeeze and sometimes collapse under patient weight. This can induce movement during procedures; hence, they were not used in this study. Following extensive searching and contact with clinicians, tissue viability nurses, occupational therapists, manufacturers, and distributors of pressure redistribution surface overlays, five static pressure redistribution surface overlays were identified and procured. The physical characteristics of the surface overlays are detailed in Table 1.

2.3. Radiation Tests. Radiation tests were conducted on the five pressure redistribution surface overlays listed in Table 1. The main aim of these tests was to determine the one with the least impact on radiation dose attenuation and image quality and apply it during interventional radiography and radiotherapy planning and treatment procedures. The radiation tests were conducted in three stages. Firstly, a dosimetry test was conducted to assess the impact of each surface on radiation attenuation. Secondly, an assessment was made of the impact of each surface overlay on image quality. Thirdly, computed tomography (CT) scanning of each surface overlay was conducted to provide a detailed internal three-dimensional visualisation of each surface overlay. The information from the CT images was used to calculate the Hounsfield unit, hence, the linear attenuation coefficient of each surface overlay. The attenuation coefficient is a measure of how easily a surface overlay can be penetrated by an incident X-ray beam and describes the fraction of a beam of X-ray that is absorbed or scattered per unit thickness of the surface overlay.

2.3.1. Dosimetry Test. The X2 R/F dosimeter (RaySafe, UK) is a modern piece of equipment fitted with high sensor technology that ensures accurate measurement of radiation dose. It was used to assess the impact of each surface overlay on radiation dose attenuation. The dosimeter has a dose range of 40–150 kVp and can detect dosages ranging from 1 nGy to 9999 Gy, with an accuracy of ±5% of calibrated values. The X2 R/F dosimeter has the ability to measure dose rate, peak kilovoltage (kVp), half-value layer (HVL), total filtration, exposure time, pulses, pulse rate, and dose/pulse in one exposure.

The method used for the dosimetry test involved placing the X2 R/F dosimeter on an X-ray table. The radiation field was tightly collimated to the edges of the dosimeter. Using a standard 100 cm source to image-receptor distance (SID), three exposures were made at both high kilovoltage (kV) (75 kV, 2 mAs) and low kV (50 kV, 2 mAs) with a fine focal spot. The mean recorded dose for high and low kVs was 37.28 and 10.72 mGy, respectively. These values served as the control. To assess the impact of each surface overlay on radiation dose attenuation, each surface overlay was placed on the dosimeter. Three exposures were made using the same exposure parameters as the control. The mean recorded dose for each surface overlay and the percentage difference from the control at low and high kVs is reported in Table 2.

To objectively determine the amount of radiation incident on the detector when the various pressure redistribution surface overlays were used, the exposure index (EI) and the deviation index (DI) of each of the X-ray images with the hand phantom were assessed. The EI is an international standard that measures the amount of radiation exposure on a digital image receptor [38]. A target exposure index (TI) value is a constant value set by the manufacturer for specific anatomical parts [39]. The TI value for the X-ray machine used for the study was 250 μGy. The deviation index (DI) calculates the difference between a desired TI and the actual exposure [39]. The EI and the DI for the exposures on the surface overlays are indicated in Table 3.

2.3.2. Image Quality Assessment. The second part of the radiation tests involved assessing the impact of each surface overlay on radiographic image quality. Each pressure redistribution surface overlay was placed on a 17 × 14 inch Aero digital radiography (DR) cassette (Konica Minolta, Tokyo, Japan). Following this, they were exposed to radiation at high kV (120 kV, 1.2 mAs) and low kV (60 kV, 1.2 mAs) using fine focus. A 23 cm long adult hand anthropomorphic phantom weighing 0.79 kg was placed in the middle of the surface overlay on the cassette. The radiation field was collimated to an area of 20 × 25 cm to conform with clinical standards. The same exposure factors at both high and low kV were repeated. These exposure parameters are consistent with exposure protocols for the hand in clinical settings. In all, four exposures were taken for each surface overlay-two with the hand phantom placed on the surface overlay at high and low kVs and another two with only the surface overlay placed on the cassette, also at high and low

Table 1: Physical characteristics of the five static surface overlays.

Name	Image	Material	Dimension ($L \times W \times T$ in cm)*	Weight (kg)
Gel table/hip pad	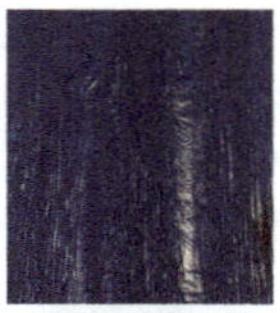	Gel	$45 \times 45 \times 1.4$	3.4
Silicone gel flat pad		Silicone gel	$45 \times 45 \times 0.7$	1.4
Blue hollow overlay	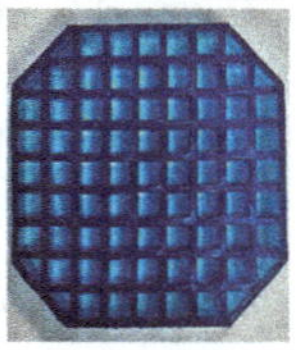	Elastic	$6 \times 6 \times 1.6$	<0.09
Sundance SUN Z3-S	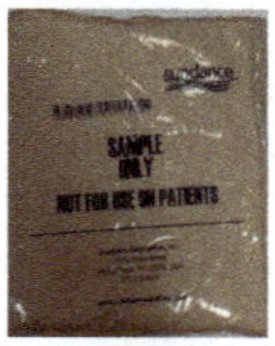	Fluidised	$18 \times 18 \times 1.7$	0.2
Small round gel	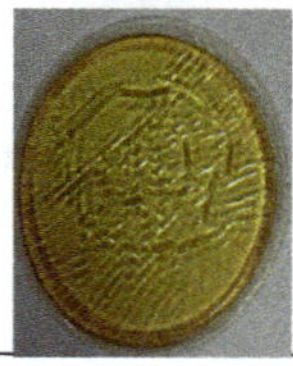	Gel	$8.5 \times 8.5 \times 0.6$	<0.09

*L = length, W = width, and T = thickness.

Table 2: Mean recorded dose at low and high tube potentials with corresponding percentage changes.

Control (no overlay)	Mean dose for high kV (75 kV, 2 mAs)		37.3 mGy	
	Mean dose for low kV (50 kV, 2 mAs)		10.7 mGy	
Surface overlay	**Mean dose at 75 kV, 2 mAs**	**Percentage decrease (%)**	**Mean dose at 50 kV, 2 mAs**	**Percentage decrease (%)**
Gel table/hip pad	32.1 mGy	14.0	8.2 mGy	23.4
Silicone gel flat pad	34.2 mGy	8.3	9.6 mGy	10.3
Blue hollow overlay	35.1 mGy	5.9	10.3 mGy	3.7
Sundance SUN Z3-S	30.0 mGy	19.6	7.8 mGy	27.0
Small round gel	34.3 mGy	8.0	9.6 mGy	10.3

kVs. The images were obtained and processed on AeroDR system (Konica Minolta, Inc.) and its workstation. The acquired radiographic images are presented in Table 4.

2.3.3. Attenuation Coefficient Determination. The third and final stage of the radiation tests involved assessing the density of the various surface overlays to evaluate their Hounsfield unit (HU) measurements and determine the linear attenuation coefficients of the surface overlays. Each surface overlay was scanned using a Toshiba Aquilion 16 slice multidetector CT scanner. To calculate the mean HU of each surface overlay, an area corresponding to a number of pixels was chosen depending on the length and thickness of the surface overlay. For example, when calculating the HU for the silicone gel flat pad (surface 2), 12 areas of 0.2 cm^2 (averaging 40 pixels) were chosen. The HU for each area was calculated and the mean HU for the entire silicone gel surface overlay was also calculated. The procedure was replicated to calculate the HU for the other surface overlays.

Table 3: Exposure and deviation indices for the surface overlays at high and low kVs.

	High kV (120, 1.2 mAs)	Low kV (60, 1.2 mAs)
Control	EI−2940.10 TI−250 DI−10.70	EI224.47 TI−250 DI−−0.46
Gel table/hip pad	EI−2705.38 TI 250 DI−10.34	EI−195.26 TI−250 DI−−1.07
Silicone gel flat pad	EI−2926.91 TI−250 DI−10.68	EI−213.16 TI−250 DI−−0.69
Blue hollow surface	EI−2842.58 TI−250 DI−10.55	EI−207.48 TI−250 DI−−0.80
Sundance SUN Z3-S	EI−2773.14 TI−250 DI−10.45	EI−197.91 TI−250 DI−−1.01
Small round gel	EI−3020.51 TI−250 DI−10.82	EI−222.46 TI−250 DI−−0.50

EI, TI, and DI all in units of microgray (μGy).

The recorded mean HU and standard deviation (SD) of the surface overlays are presented in Table 5.

Based on the findings from the radiation tests, the silicone gel flat pad (surface overlay 2) was chosen as an intervention. It produced no artefact on the resultant radiographic image and had minimal impact on radiation dose attenuation due to a reasonably low linear attenuation coefficient. It also consists of fairly homogenous internal structures making it applicable for radiography and radiotherapy planning and treatment procedures.

2.4. Sampling for Pressure Mapping. A priori power analysis indicated that 20 volunteers would be needed for the research (effect size [0.67], power [0.80], alpha [0.05], and two-tailed repeated measures paired-samples *t*-tests). Effect size, power, and alpha value were determined from the study conducted by Angmorterh et al. [33]. A disproportionate stratified random sampling method was used to recruit 20 students and staff from the UoS. This sampling method was chosen to enable recruitment of volunteers with different characteristics. Inclusion criteria were healthy people aged 18 years and older. Exclusion criterion was volunteers who were >250 kg in weight. These are based on the limitations of the XSENSOR mat. Participation in the study was voluntary.

2.5. Data Collection Instrument. A calibrated XSENSOR PX100.64.160.02 (XSENSOR Technology Corporation, Calgary, Canada) pressure mapping system with its X3 software (v6) was used. The XSENSOR is considered to be the gold standard for pressure mapping and it has previously been used in several studies [33, 40–42]. The XSENSOR mat, fitted with over 10,000 sensing points, had a total area of 68.5 cm × 68.5 cm and a sensing area of 50.8 cm × 50.8 cm, resulting in approximately 200 cells per area [43]. Manufacturer's specification also indicated that the pressure mat had low hysteresis and low creep, an accuracy rate of ±10% of the calibrated values, sampling frame rate of 15.8 per second, and a spatial resolution of 0.51 cm. IP readings were transmitted from the XSENSOR mat to a hand-held monitor. The pressure mapping was conducted on an Arco TN 0055 X-ray table to mimic the imaging surfaces used in radiotherapy. The X-ray table was 240 cm long, 85.3 cm wide, and 2.2 cm thick, made from an industrial grade Rohacell carbon fibre with 0.9 mm aluminium (Al).

2.6. Procedure for Pressure Mapping. The mat was fixed securely to the X-ray table with adhesive tape. To standardise volunteer positioning, a measurement of 2 cm from top (head) of the mat was taken and a tape was placed there to ensure that all volunteers had their heads placed on the same point of the mat. Volunteers were asked to lie on the mat in a supine position with the hands pronated and the hips adjusted to ensure that they were equidistant from the edges of the mat. Following a six-minute settling time [33, 44], the volunteers were asked to remain still for two minutes, whilst pressure mapping data were acquired to serve as control data. At the end of the two minutes, the volunteer was helped off the X-ray table, the silicone gel surface overlay was placed under the pressure mat, and the volunteer was asked to lie again on the pressure mat for the intervention pressure mapping data to be acquired. The same settling and pressure mapping data acquisition times (six and two minutes respectively) were used for the intervention data collection. During pressure mapping, access to the imaging room was restricted to protect volunteers' privacy and also to avoid any distraction. The data acquired were saved onto the hand-held Xsensor device. To ensure high levels of infection control and hygiene, the pressure mat was cleaned in between volunteers using wet wipes as recommended by the manufacturer.

3. Results

3.1. Demographics. The sample comprised 14 males (70%) and six females (30%), with an age range of 25–53 years (mean = 34.4 ± 7.0).

3.2. Normality Testing. The results of normality testing (Kolmogorov–Smirnov tests, $p \geq 0.05$) indicated that the data were normally distributed for all the four variables (mean IP for the head on the X-ray table with and without the silicone gel surface overlay, and the mean peak pressure index (PPI) for the head on the table with and without the gel surface overlay, in mmHg). The mean IP corresponds to the mean of all the cells in the contact area of the head. The mean PPI is defined as the mean of the highest IP within a 10–12 cm^2 area per each frame [42, 45]. In other words, the mean PPI corresponds to the mean of the maximal values within the area under investigation. Studies have shown that this area (10–12 cm^2) is equivalent to a 3 × 3 cell matrix when using the Xsensor pressure mat [42, 45].

Table 4: Radiographic images of the five surfaces at high and low kVs.

Surface overlay	High kV	Low kV	High kV with hand	Low kV with hand	Artefact present
Gel table pad	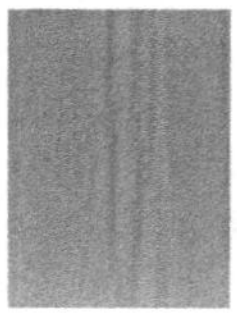		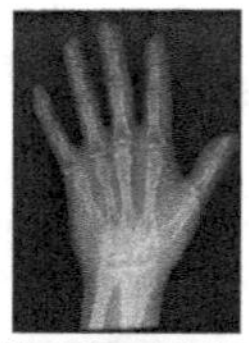	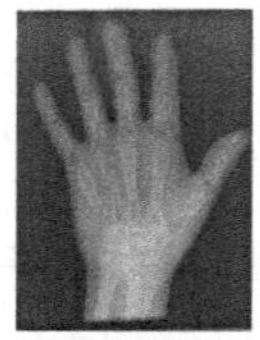	Yes
Silicone gel flat pad			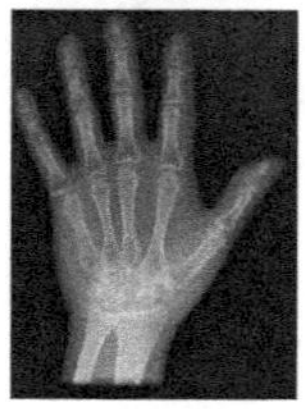	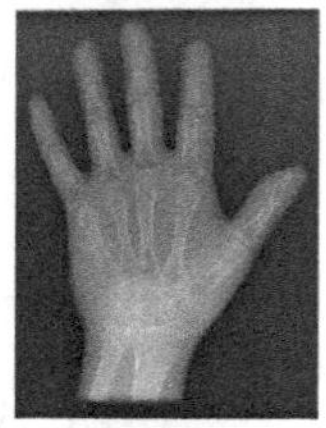	No
Blue hollow gel overlay	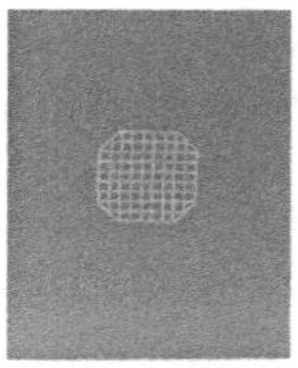		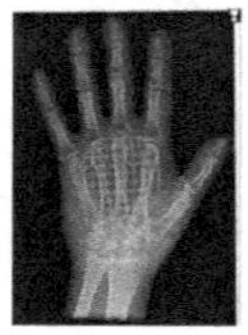	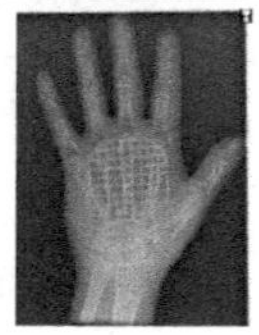	Yes
Sundance SUN Z3-S	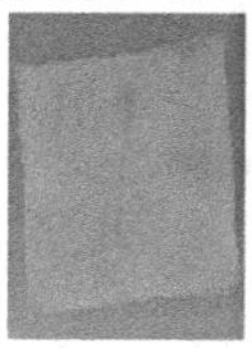		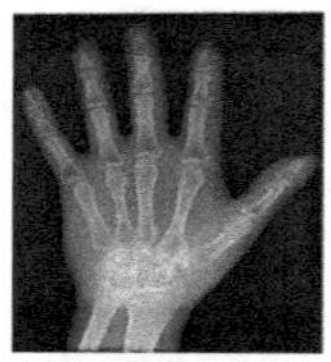	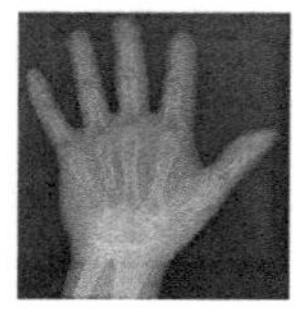	Yes
Small round gel			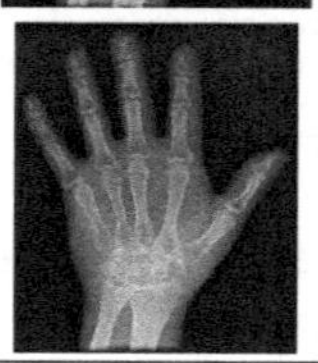	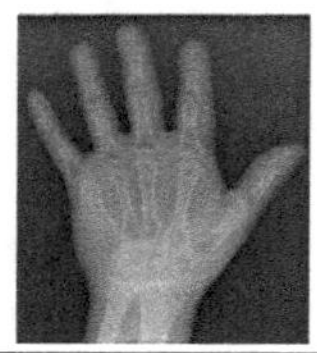	Yes

Table 5: The mean Hounsfield unit (HU) with standard deviation (SD) for the various surface overlays.

Surface no	Surface overlay	Mean HU ± SD
1	Gel table/hip pad	−0.67 ± 22.93
2	Silicone gel flat pad	−12.54 ± 26.80
3	Blue hollow surface	−508.96 ± 37.93
4	Sundance SUN Z3-S	−0.7 ± 15.3
5	Small round gel	−18.17 ± 7.06

3.3. Inferential Statistics. Paired-samples t-test results indicated that there was a statistically significant decrease in the mean IP for the head on the X-ray table without the silicone gel surface overlay (mean = 83.9 ± 8.2 in mmHg) and the X-ray table with the gel surface overlay (mean = 62.4 ± 6.1 in mmHg), $t\ (19) = 14.5$, and $p \leq 0.001$ (two-tailed). The mean decrease in IP was 21.5 mmHg with a 95% confidence interval ranging from 18.4 to 24.6. The eta squared statistic (0.9) indicated a large effect size. The given range of the mean IP values corresponds to the standard deviation of the mean.

Paired-samples t-test results indicated that there was a statistically significant decrease in the mean PPI for the head on the X-ray table without the silicone gel surface overlay (mean = 205.1 ± 28.2 in mmHg) and the X-ray table with the gel surface overlay (mean = 159.8 ± 26.8 in mmHg), $t\ (19) = 5.5$, and $p \leq 0.001$ (two-tailed). The mean decrease in PPI was 45.3 mmHg with a 95% confidence interval ranging from 28.1 to 62.5. The eta squared statistic (0.6) indicated a large effect size. The given range of the mean PPI values corresponds to the standard deviation of the mean. The comparisons of mean IP and PPI on the X-ray table with and without the silicone gel surface overlay are presented graphically in Figure 1.

4. Discussion

This intervention study was conducted to assess the impact on IP values for the head through the use of a thin silicone gel surface overlay during radiographic procedures.

Findings showed that its use resulted in a statistically significant decrease in the mean IP for the head on the X-ray table without the silicone gel surface overlay (mean = 83.9 ± 8.2 in mmHg) and the X-ray table with the gel surface overlay (mean = 62.4 ± 6.1 in mmHg), $p \leq 0.001$. Similarly, the use of the thin silicone gel surface overlay resulted in a statistically

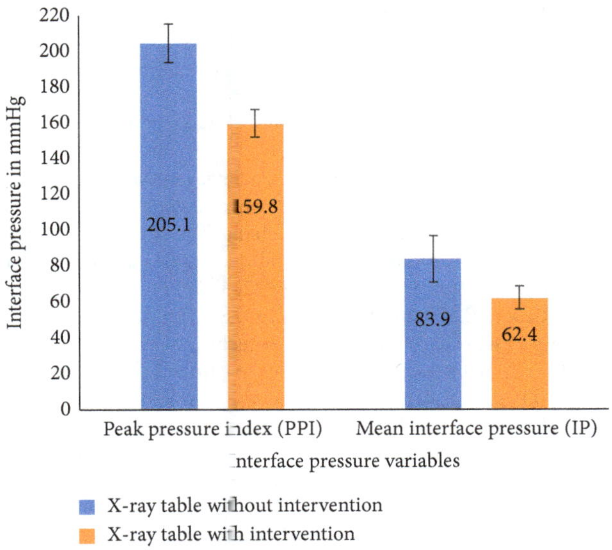

FIGURE 1: Comparison of mean IP and PPI with standard deviation on the X-ray table with and without the intervention.

significant decrease in the mean PPI for the head on the X-ray table without the silicone gel surface overlay (mean = 205.1 ± 28.2 in mmHg) and the X-ray table with the gel surface overlay (mean = 159.8 ± 26.8 in mmHg), $p \leq 0.001$. The findings of this intervention study can be compared to previous studies [46–50] which indicated that gel surface overlays have the ability to significantly reduce interface pressure risk thereby minimising the risk of PUs. It must be stated though that some of these studies were conducted on surfaces and subjects that were different from the conditions and subjects of this study. The silicone gel surface overlay used as an intervention in this study had viscoelastic properties, enabling it to support body weight and shift IP to a larger contact area without bottoming out. The movement of IP to a larger contact area significantly reduces the IP brought to bear on the head. Silicone gel surface overlays also have the ability to resist applied pressure and return to their original state when the applied pressure is removed [49]. These two properties, high viscosity and elasticity, are vital to ensure that the intervention can be applied during radiography and radiotherapy planning and treatment procedures because they minimise movement and errors.

The findings of this intervention study could contribute to efforts to reduce PU risks for the head, particularly among vulnerable patients accessing prolonged radiography and radiotherapy planning and treatment procedures. Patients who are likely to access these procedures are usually older, of poorer health, and mostly suffering from chronic diseases such as cancer [34] Their advanced age comes with a marked reduction in the collagen and elastin content in their skin which makes them highly prone to experiencing skin injuries. Furthermore, the conditions and the specific characteristics of prolonged interventional radiography procedures (e.g., cervical vertebroplasty) and radiotherapy treatment procedures such as cranial stereotactic radiotherapy are likely to expose patients to MDR PUs.

The clinical implication of this study is that patients undergoing prolonged radiography and radiotherapy procedures could be provided with a thin silicone gel surface overlay behind their head. The application of the gel could result in a significant reduction in the interface pressure for the head by approximately 25%. This could have beneficial impact on patient management. However, to ensure that the silicone gel intervention does not have a negative impact on the imaging or therapy procedure, the intervention must be assessed to ensure that it meets the specific conditions within these specialised settings. For example, any silicone gel intervention that would be applied in radiography and radiotherapy planning and treatment must be assessed for its impact on image quality, radiation attenuation, and its ability to prevent patient movement. This is essential because any intervention that produces artefacts will degrade the diagnostic quality of a radiographic image possibly leading to inaccurate diagnosis [17]. As in other cases, this risk should be mitigated against its potential benefit; the benefit in this situation surrounds minimising the risk of developing a PU.

To successfully apply the silicone gel intervention in radiotherapy treatment procedures, it ought to be applied during radiotherapy planning. This is crucial because the radiotherapy planning parameters must be the same as that for treatment [18]. Prior to radiotherapy treatment procedures, patients must undergo a planning scan in a computerised tomography (CT) or a positron emission tomography-computerised tomography (PET-CT) machine. If a gel intervention is to be used during treatment, it has to be applied during the course of the planning to ensure reproducibility of patient position as well as the position of the target tumour, internal organs, and structures. This will help to ensure that the target tumour is not missed during treatment thereby improving the accuracy of the treatment [18].

5. Conclusion

The use of a thin silicone gel surface overlay could reduce IP risk for the head by approximately 25%. The reduction in IP risk could have a significant impact on reducing the risk of developing a PU. To ensure maximum benefit, the silicone gel surface overlay must be assessed to meet the specific needs within radiography and radiotherapy planning and treatment settings.

Acknowledgments

This research paper serves as part of the Ph.D. study of the first author. The Ph.D. work was funded by the Ghana Education Trust Fund (GETFUND).

References

[1] B. Pieper, "Pressure ulcers: impact, etiology, and classification," in *Acute & Chronic Wound. Current Management Concepts*, R. A. Byrant and D. P. Nix, Eds., pp. 123–136, Mosby, Maryland Heights, MO, USA, 2012.

[2] X. Gómez-Batiste, M. Martínez-Muñoz, C. Blay et al., "Prevalence and characteristics of patients with advanced chronic conditions in need of palliative care in the general population: a cross-sectional study," *Palliative Medicine*, vol. 28, no. 4, pp. 302–311, 2014.
[3] M. R. Brennan, D. Laconti, and R. Gilchrist, "Using conformational positioning to reduce hospital-acquired pressure ulcers," *Journal of Nursing Care Quality*, vol. 29, no. 2, pp. 182–187, 2014.
[4] N. A. Stotts, D. S. Brown, N. E. Donaldson, C. Aydin, and M. Fridman, "Eliminating hospital-acquired pressure ulcers," *Advances in Skin & Wound Care*, vol. 26, no. 1, pp. 13–18, 2013.
[5] HSCIC, "NHS safety thermometer: patient harms and harm free care," *Official Statistics*, pp. 1–19, Health and Social Care Information Centre, Leeds, UK, 2014.
[6] C. VanGilder, S. Amlung, P. Harrison, and S. Meyer, "Results of the 2008-2009 international pressure ulcer prevalence survey and a 3-year, acute care, unit-specific analysis," *Ostomy/wound Management*, vol. 55, no. 11, pp. 39–45, 2009.
[7] C. M. Davis and N. G. Caseby, "Prevalence and incidence studies of pressure ulcers in two long-term care facilities in Canada," *Ostomy Wound Manage*, vol. 47, no. 11, pp. 28–34, 2001.
[8] M. Reddy, S. S. Gill, and P. A. Rochon, "Preventing pressure ulcers: a systematic review," *JAMA*, vol. 296, no. 8, pp. 974–984, 2006.
[9] A. Filius, T. H. C. Damen, K. P. Schuijer-Maaskant, S. Polinder, S. E. R. Hovius, and E. T. Walbeehm, "Cost analysis of surgically treated pressure sores stage III and IV," *Journal of Plastic, Reconstructive & Aesthetic Surgery*, vol. 66, no. 11, pp. 1580–1586, 2013.
[10] C. Dealey, J. Posnett, and A. Walker, "The cost of pressure ulcers in the United Kingdom," *Journal of Wound Care*, vol. 21, no. 6, pp. 261–266, 2012.
[11] A. Plaskitt, N. Heywood, and M. Arrowsmith, "Recording pressure ulcer risk assessment and incidence," *Nursing Standard*, vol. 29, no. 46, pp. 54–61, 2015.
[12] P. Kranke, M. H. Bennett, M. Martyn-St James, A. Schnabel, S. E. Debus, and S. Weibel, "Hyperbaric oxygen therapy for chronic wounds," *Cochrane Database of Systematic Reviews*, vol. 2015, no. 6, p. CD004123, 2015.
[13] NICE, "Pressure ulcers: prevention and management of pressure ulcers," National Institute for Health and Care Excellence, London, UK, 2015, https://www.nice.org.uk/guidance/qs89.
[14] J. Pittman, T. Beeson, J. Kitterman, S. Lancaster, and A. Shelly, "Medical device-related hospital-acquired pressure ulcers," *Journal of Wound, Ostomy and Continence Nursing*, vol. 42, no. 2, pp. 151–154, 2015.
[15] M. Visscher and T. Taylor, "Pressure ulcers in the hospitalized neonate: rates and risk factors," *Scientific Reports*, vol. 4, no. 1, pp. 74–79, 2014.
[16] F. Manzano, A. M. Pérez-Pérez, S. Martínez-Ruiz et al., "Hospital-acquired pressure ulcers and risk of hospital mortality in intensive care patients on mechanical ventilation," *Journal of Evaluation in Clinical Practice*, vol. 20, no. 4, pp. 362–368, 2014.
[17] SA. Whitley, C. Charles Sloane, G. Hoadley, AD. Moore, and C. W. Alsop, *Clark's Positioning in Radiography*, Taylor & Francis Publishers., Abingdon, UK, 12th edition, 2005.
[18] A. Barrett, J. Dobbs, and T. Roques, *Practical Radiotherapy Planning*, CRC Press, Boca Raton, FL, USA, 4th edition, 2009.
[19] B. M. Beadle, K. P. Liao, L. S. Elting et al., "Improved survival using intensity-modulated radiation therapy in head and neck cancers: a SEER-Medicare analysis," *Cancer*, vol. 120, no. 5, pp. 702–710, 2014.
[20] O. Stojadinovic, J. Minkiewicz, A. Sawaya et al., "Deep tissue injury in development of pressure ulcers: a decrease of inflammasome activation and changes in human skin morphology in response to aging and mechanical Load," *PLoS One*, vol. 8, no. 8, Article ID e69223, 2013.
[21] J. Rieber, E. Tonndorf-Martini, O. Schramm et al., "Radiosurgery with flattening-filter-free techniques in the treatment of brain metastases," *Strahlentherapie und Onkologie*, vol. 192, no. 11, p. 789, 2016.
[22] C. C. Wong and M. J. McGirt, "Vertebral compression fractures: a review of current management and multimodal therapy," *Journal of Multidisciplinary Healthcare*, vol. 6, pp. 205–214, 2013.
[23] M. N. Pernik, H. H. Seidel, R. E. Blalock et al., "Comparison of tissue-interface pressure in healthy subjects lying on two trauma splinting devices: the vacuum mattress splint and long spine board," *Injury*, vol. 47, no. 8, p. 1801, 2016.
[24] J. Hollington and S. J. Hillman, "Can static interface pressure mapping be used to rank pressure-redistributing cushions for active wheelchair users?" *The Journal of Rehabilitation Research and Development*, vol. 50, no. 1, pp. 53–60, 2013.
[25] E. M. Landis, "Micro-injection studies of capillary blood pressure in human skin," *Heart*, vol. 15, no. 2, pp. 209–228, 1930.
[26] E. M. Landis, "The capillary blood pressure in mammalian mesentery as determined by the micro-injection method," *American Journal of Physiology-Legacy Content*, vol. 93, no. 1, pp. 353–362, 1930.
[27] E. M. Landis, "Micro-injection studies of capillary blood pressure in Raynaud's disease," *Heart-a Journal for the Study of the Circulation*, vol. 15, no. 3, pp. 247–255, 1930.
[28] T. Defloor, "The risk of pressure sores: a conceptual scheme," *Journal of Clinical Nursing*, vol. 8, no. 2, pp. 206–216, 1999.
[29] T. Defloor and M. H. F. Grypdonck, "Sitting posture and prevention of pressure ulcers," *Applied Nursing Research*, vol. 12, no. 3, pp. 136–142, 1999.
[30] J. Casey and L. Gittins, "Use of tilt-in-space in seating systems for adults with physical disabilities," *Physical Therapy Reviews*, vol. 18, no. 4, pp. 285–299, 2013.
[31] L. Clements, M. Moore, T. Tribble, and J. Blake, "Reducing skin breakdown in patients receiving extracorporeal membranous oxygenation," *Nursing Clinics of North America*, vol. 49, no. 1, pp. 61–68, 2014.
[32] D. Justham, C. Michael, and D. Harris, "A healthy volunteer study of skinsurface interface pressure experienced in X-ray departments," *Journal of Tissue Viability*, vol. 6, no. 4, pp. 107–110, 1996.
[33] S. K. Angmorterh, A. England, J. Webb et al., "An investigation of pressure ulcer risk, comfort, and pain in medical imaging," *Journal of Medical Imaging and Radiation Sciences*, vol. 50, no. 1, pp. 43–52, 2019.
[34] C. Forasassi and S. Meaume, "Prise en charge des escarres en soins palliatifs dans les services de gériatrie," *Soins*, vol. 60, no. 792, pp. 35–38, 2015.
[35] F. R. Bartlett, R. M. Colgan, E. M. Donovan et al., "The UK HeartSpare study (Stage IB): randomised comparison of a

voluntary breath-hold technique and prone radiotherapy after breast conserving surgery," *Radiotherapy and Oncology*, vol. 114, no. 1, pp. 66–72, 2015.

[36] R. de la Garza-Ramos, M. Benvenutti-Regato, and E. Caro-Osorio, "Vertebroplasty and kyphoplasty for cervical spine metastases: a systematic review and meta-analysis," *International Journal of Spine Surgery*, vol. 10, pp. 7-8, 2016.

[37] E. McInnes, A. Jammali-Blasi, S. E. Bell-Syer, J. C. Dumville, V. Middleton, and N. Cullum, "Support surfaces for pressure ulcer prevention," *Cochrane Database of Systematic Reviews*, vol. 2015, no. 9, Article ID Cd001735, 2015.

[38] S. J. Shepard, J. Wang, M. Flynn et al., "An exposure indicator for digital radiography: AAPM Task Group 116 (executive summary)," *Medical Physics*, vol. 36, no. 7, pp. 2898–2914, 2009.

[39] M. D. Cohen, M. L. Cooper, K. Piersall, and B. K. Apgar, "Quality assurance: using the exposure index and the deviation index to monitor radiation exposure for portable chest radiographs in neonates," *Pediatric Radiology*, vol. 41, no. 5, pp. 592–601, 2011.

[40] S. K. Angmorterh, A. England, J. Anaman-torgbor et al., "A narrative review on pressure ulcer (PU) studies relevant to medical imaging a narrative review on pressure ulcer (PU) studies relevant to medical imaging," *Pan African Medical Journal*, vol. 36, no. 66, Article ID 19431, 2020.

[41] M. J. Peterson, N. Gravenstein, W. K. Schwab, J. H. van Oostrom and L. J. Caruso, "Patient repositioning and pressure ulcer risk—monitoring interface pressures of at-risk patients," *The Journal of Rehabilitation Research and Development*, vol. 50, no. 4, pp. 477–488, 2013.

[42] B. Hemmes, P. R. G. Brink, and M. Poeze, "Effects of unconsciousness during spinal immobilization on tissue-interface pressures: a randomized controlled trial comparing a standard rigid spineboard with a newly developed soft-layered long spineboard," *Injury*, vol. 45, no. 11, pp. 1741–1746, 2014.

[43] Sumed International, "Products and specifications," 2014, http://www.xsensor.com/files/galleries/XSensor_Automotive_Catalogue_August-2014-0002.pdf.

[44] M. D. Stinson, A. P. Porter-Armstrong, and P. A. Eakin, "Pressure mapping systems: reliability of pressure map interpretation," *Clinical Rehabilitation*, vol. 17, no. 5, pp. 504–511, 2003.

[45] K. Davis and S. Sprigle, *The Science of Interface Pressure Mapping-Updates for Clinical Application*, SAGE Publications, Thousand Oaks, CA, USA, 2010.

[46] S. K. Miller, N. Sharma, L. C. Aberegg, K. N. Blasiole, and J. A. Fulton, "Analysis of the pressure distribution qualities of a silicone border foam dressing," *Journal of Wound, Ostomy and Continence Nursing*, vol. 42, no. 4, pp. 346–351, 2015.

[47] S. L. Groah, M. Schladen, C. G. Pineda, and C.-H. J. Hsieh, "Prevention of pressure ulcers among people with spinal cord injury: a systematic review," *PM&R*, vol. 7, no. 6, pp. 613–636, 2015.

[48] N. S. Walsh, A. W Blanck, L. Smith, M. Cross, L. Andersson, and C. Polito, "Use of a sacral silicone border foam dressing as one component of a pressure ulcer prevention program in an intensive care unit setting," *Journal of Wound, Ostomy and Continence Nursing*, vol. 39, no. 2, pp. 146–149, 2012.

[49] N. Chaiken, "Reduction of sacral pressure ulcers in the intensive care unit using a silicone border foam dressing," *Journal of Wound Ostomy and Continence Nursing*, vol. 39, no. 2, pp. 143–145, 2012.

[50] D. Brienza, S. Kelsey, P. Karg et al., "A randomized clinical trial on preventing pressure ulcers with wheelchair seat cushions," *Journal of the American Geriatrics Society*, vol. 58, no. 12, pp. 2308–2314, 2010.

28

The Association between the Pulmonary Arterial Obstruction Index and Atrial Size in Patients with Acute Pulmonary Embolism

Taraneh Faghihi Langroudi,[1] Maryam Sheikh,[1] Mohammadreza Naderian,[2,3] Morteza Sanei Taheri,[1] Amir Ashraf-ganjouei,[4] and Isa Khaheshi[5]

[1] *Radiology Department, Modarres Hospital, Shahid Beheshti University of Medical Sciences, Tehran, Iran*
[2] *Non-Communicable Diseases Research Center, Endocrinology and Metabolism Population Sciences Institute, Tehran University of Medical Sciences, Tehran, Iran*
[3] *Cardiac Outcome Research and Education (CORE), Universal Scientific Education and Research Network (USERN), Tehran, Iran*
[4] *Students' Scientific Research Center (SSRC), Tehran University of Medical Sciences, Tehran, Iran*
[5] *Cardiovascular Research Center, Shahid Beheshti University of Medical Sciences, Tehran, Iran*

Correspondence should be addressed to Amir Ashraf-ganjouei; A-ganjouei@student.tums.ac.ir and Isa Khaheshi; isa.khaheshi@gmail.com

Academic Editor: Paul Sijens

Purpose. Pulmonary embolism (PE) is a common and potentially fatal form of venous thromboembolism. The aim of this study is to investigate the association between the pulmonary arterial obstruction index and atrial size in patients with acute pulmonary embolism. *Basic Procedure.* The study consisted of 86 patients with clinical symptoms of PE. Out of 86 individuals, 50 patients were diagnosed with PE and considered as the patient group. The others were considered as the control group. All patients were scanned by a multidetector CT scanner. Using the radiology workstation, an expert radiologist calculated the left atrium (LA) and right atrium (RA) areas from planimetric measurements obtained from free-hand delineation of the atrial boarders using an electronic pen. Quantitative volumetric measurements of LA and RA were obtained from original axial images. *Main Findings.* There were 25 males and 25 females with PE, who had a mean age of 58 years. There was not a significant difference in the positive history of diabetes mellitus, hypertension, asthma, chronic obstructive pulmonary diseases, ischemic heart disease, and smoking between patients and control group. There was a significant negative correlation between almost all LA measurements and the PAOI. RA area and volume had the highest area under the curves for recognizing larger clot burden. *Principal Conclusions.* A higher clot load is associated with a smaller LA size and increased RA/LA ratios, measured with CTPA. Atrial measurements are correlated with POAI, and they could be used as sensitive parameters in predicting heart failure in patients with PE.

1. Introduction

Pulmonary embolism (PE) is a common and potentially fatal form of venous thromboembolism that causes 200,000-300,000 deaths annually in the United States, mostly occurring in patients with hemodynamically unstable status [1].

Patients with unrecognized acute PE have an estimated mortality rate of 30% [2]. However, the death rate can be reduced to 2-10% if PE is diagnosed at the right time [3]. Computed tomography pulmonary angiography (CTPA) is currently the modality of choice for the evaluation of acute pulmonary embolism [4]. CTPA has a specificity of 95% for identifying clots within distal pulmonary arteries. Moreover, using CTPA can help physicians in the diagnosis of underlying lung diseases [3]. CTPA can also assess clot burden, using scoring systems such as pulmonary artery obstruction index (PAOI) [5].

Acute PE increases the pressure of the pulmonary arterial system and right ventricle (RV) resulting in right ventricle dysfunction (RVD) [6]. RVD followed by PE may cause death generally within the first hour following admission to hospital [7]. Although echocardiography is currently the modality of choice for RVD diagnosis, CPTA can replace echocardiography, because of its ability to detect PE and RVD simultaneously [8]. Studies show that among patients with PE, the PAOI ratio can recognize patients with or without RVD [6, 9].

Determination of CTPA ability in the early detection of circulatory collapse in patients who have increased risk of acute right heart failure caused by PE is still going [10]. In current study, we have investigated the association between the pulmonary arterial obstruction index and atrial size in patients with acute pulmonary embolism.

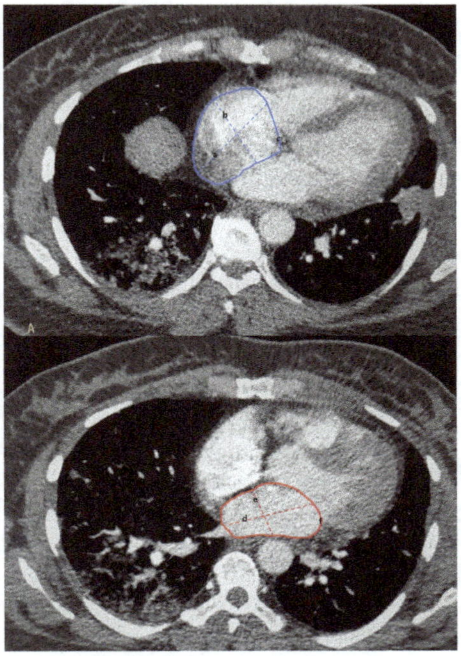

Figure 1: Radiological indices defined in computed tomography pulmonary angiography (CTPA). The figure, depicting a sample of computed tomography pulmonary angiography (CTPA) image and the indices defined for measuring different sizes. a, b, and c imply RA long diameter, short diameter, and area, respectively. d, e, and f imply LA long diameter, short diameter, and area, respectively.

2. Material and Methods

2.1. Study Participants. The study cohort consisted of 86 patients with clinical symptoms of PE who were referred to Shahid Modarres Hospital in Tehran from April 2015 to May 2017. Out of 86 individuals, 50 patients were diagnosed with PE on CTPA and were considered as the patient group. The other 36 patients who did not have any signs of PE on CPTA were considered as the control group. The ethical committee of Shahid Beheshti University of Medical Sciences approved this study and written informed consent was obtained from all participants.

2.2. CT Acquisition and Assessment. All patients were scanned by a multidetector CT scanner (Brilliance 64, Philips medical system, Cleveland, OH, USA). Reconstructed slice thickness was 1.0 mm, with an increment of 0.5 mm. The PE protocol consisted of contrast injections of 50 mL of iodinated contrast material at a concentration of 320 mg iodine/ml (Visipaque, GE healthcare, Ireland, Cork, Ireland). All CT scans were taken at end-of-inspiration during a single breath-hold in a caudal-cranial direction. Using the Radiology workstation (extended brilliance workspace, Philips medical systems Nederlan B.V.), an expert radiologist calculated the left atrium (LA) and right atrium (RA) areas from planimetric measurements obtained from free-hand delineation of the atrial boarders using an electronic pen. Quantitative volumetric measurements of LA and RA were obtained from original axial images, with the protocol used by Aviram et al. [10] (Figure 1). The location of arterial clot presence and the degree of arterial obstruction were scored using the scoring system suggested by Qanadli et al. in this order, the CT obstruction index was described as (n. d) [n, value of the proximal clot location, equal to the number of segmental divisions arising distally; d, extent of obstruction scored as partial obstruction (value of 1) or total obstruction (value of 2)] [5].

2.3. Statistical Analysis. Demographic data were presented as the number of individuals for categorical variables, and as mean with standard deviation (SD) for continuous variables. Student's t-test and Pearson's χ^2 were used to evaluate basic demographic and clinical information in case and control groups. Spearman's rank correlation coefficient was used to assess the correlation between PAOI and LA and RA measurements, as well as LA to RA ratios. Furthermore, to analyze the performance of classification schemes for the different parameters and to compare their ability for identifying higher clot loads, we used a receiver operating characteristic (ROC) curve analysis. Statistical analysis was done using the statistical package SPSS version 22 (IBM Corp., Armonk, N.Y., USA) and *P values* under 0.05 were considered to have statistical significance.

3. Results

There were 25 males and 25 females with PE, who had a mean age of 58 years (SD of 17.93). The control group included 20 males and 16 females, who had a mean age of 55 years (SD of 17.56). The age difference between the two groups was not significant (*P value* of 0.42). The baseline characteristics of the study population are shown in Table 1. There was not a significant difference in the positive history of diabetes mellitus (DM), hypertension (HTN), asthma, chronic obstructive pulmonary diseases (COPD), ischemic heart disease (IHD) and smoking between patients and control group.

Table 2 shows the correlation between the POAI and radiologic parameters of left and right atrium (LA and RA,

TABLE 1: Basic demographic and clinical information in case and control groups.

	Patients (N = 50) Mean (SD), Median (IQR), N (%)	Controls (N = 36) Mean (SD), Median (IQR), N (%)	P value
Male, n	25 (50)	20 (55.6)	0.61
Age, year	58.30 (17.93)	55.14 (17.65)	
Positive History of DM, n	11 (22)	3 (8.3)	0.09
Positive History of HTN, n	18 (36)	9 (25)	0.28
Positive History of Asthma, n	1 (2)	4 (11)	0.07
Positive History of COPD, n	2 (4)	4 (11.1)	0.20
Positive History of IHD, n	6 (12.2)	2 (5.6)	0.30
Positive History of Smoking, n	13 (26.7)	10 (27.8)	0.85
Hospital mortality, n	3 (6)	2 (5.6)	0.93
Reflux Grade, n	2 (1.44)	1.69 (1.49)	0.08
LA Long Diameter, cm	6.39 (1.10)	5.94 (1.16)	0.07
LA Short Diameter, cm	4.06 (0.98)	3.54 (0.87)	**0.01**
LA Height, cm	5.07 (0.99)	5.23 (0.81)	0.42
LA Area, cm^2	20.95 (7.02)	17.75 (7.60)	**0.04**
LA Volume, cm^3	69.28 (36.80)	58.52 (32.36)	0.16
RA Long Diameter, cm	5.13 (1.00)	4.40 (1.01)	**0.01**
RA Short Diameter, cm	5.21 (0.87)	4.87 (0.83)	0.07
RA Height, cm	7.47 (1.62)	7.11 (1.16)	0.25
RA Area, cm^2	21.98 (6.48)	17.35 (6.08)	**<0.01**
RA Volume, cm^3	102.84 (45.60)	78.38 (34.28)	**<0.01**

Abbreviation: DM: diabetes mellitus; HTN: hypertension; IQR: interquartile range; LA: left atrium; RA: right atrium; SD: standard deviation.

TABLE 2: Correlation between PAOI and radiologic parameters in computed tomography (CT) angiography.

	PAOI Spearman's correlation coefficient (ρ)	P Value
LA Long Diameter, cm	-0.205	0.152
LA Short Diameter, cm	-0.380	**0.006**
LA Height, cm	-0.483	**<0.001**
LA Area, cm^2	-0.449	**0.001**
LA Volume, cm^3	-0.472	**0.001**
RA Long Diameter, cm	-00.089	0.538
RA Short Diameter, cm	.334	**0.018**
RA Height, cm	-0.144	0.320
RA Area, cm^2	0.041	0.776
RA Volume, cm^3	-0.015	0.916
RA to LA Long Diameter Ratio	0.05	0.68
RA to LA Short Diameter Ratio	0.50	**<0.01**
RA to LA Height ratio	0.25	0.08
RA to LA Area Ratio	0.44	**<0.01**
RA to LA Volume ratio	0.39	**<0.01**
Reflux Grade, n	-0.033	0.822

Abbreviations: LA: left atrium; PAOI: pulmonary artery obstruction index; RA: right atrium.

TABLE 3: ROC curve analysis of PAOI and different RA and LA measurements.

	AUC	95%	CI	P Value	90% Cut-off	Sensitivity Specificity
LA Long Diameter, cm	0.634	0.512 -	0.756	**0.035**	5.32	75.0
LA Short Diameter, cm	0.665	0.548 -	0.782	**0.009**	2.83	77.8
LA Height, cm	0.426	0.303 -	0.548	0.241	3.95	94.4
LA Area, cm^2	0.675	0.554 -	0.796	**0.006**	13.06	69.4
LA Volume, cm^3	0.609	0.487 -	0.731	0.086	33.09	80.6
RA Long Diameter, cm	0.693	0.577 -	0.809	**0.002**	4.07	55.6
RA Short Diameter, cm	0.624	0.502 -	0.747	**0.050**	4.14	83.3
RA Height, cm	0.550	0.428 -	0.672	0.431	5.75	88.9
RA Area, cm^2	0.724	0.609 -	0.839	**<0.001**	15.61	58.3
RA Volume, cm^3	0.709	0.594 -	0.824	**0.001**	62.83	58.3
RA to LA Long Diameter Ratio	0.610	0.489 -	0.731	0.083	0.60	83.3
RA to LA Short Diameter Ratio	0.432	0.309 -	0.554	0.282	0.98	94.4
RA to LA Height Ratio	0.572	0.451 -	0.693	0.259	1.08	88.9
RA to LA Area Ratio	0.553	0.430 -	0.676	0.406	0.69	88.9
RA to LA Volume Ratio	0.548	0.426 -	00.670	0.446	0.78	100

Abbreviations: AUC: area under the curve; CI: confidence interval; cm: centimeter; LA: left atrium; PAOI: pulmonary artery obstruction index; RA: right atrium.

respectively) on CTPA. There was a significant negative correlation between almost all LA measurements and the PAOI. Regarding RA, only its short diameter was positively correlated with the PAOI. Consequently, RA/LA Short Diameter, RA/LA Area, and RA/LA Volume ratios were positively correlated with the PAOI. It is noteworthy to mention that in the group of patients, the minimum and maximum of PAOI were 1 and 30, respectively, while mean and standard deviation were 10.32 and 8.45, respectively.

Table 3 shows the results of the ROC curve analysis of the PAOI and different RA and LA measurements. We analyzed different cut-offs of the atrial parameters to recognize patients with a large clot burden. RA area and volume had the highest area under the curves. In addition, we had reported cut-offs that achieve 90% sensitivity and the corresponding specificity for these parameters in Table 3.

4. Discussion

The main finding of our study was that a higher clot load is associated with a smaller LA size and increased RA/LA ratios, measured with CTPA. Although RA long diameter, area, and volume were significantly higher in patients in comparison to control group, only an association between a higher clot load and RA short diameter was observed. On the other hand, ROC curve analysis showed that RA area and volume were capable of identifying patients with a large clot burden. Our study suggests that assessing LA and RA dimensions in patients with PE could give the physician some valuable information about the clot load and serve as another prognostic factor for PE.

Pulmonary embolism is one of the fatal conditions of circulatory system. Two series of events may contribute to PE mortality. First, massive PE results in pulmonary arterial hypertension, which subsequently causes pressure overload in right ventricle. This will decrease right heart output, resulting in right ventricular dysfunction and probably right ventricle failure [11]. Consequently, blood flow to left atrium and ventricle would be decreased. On the other hand, increased afterload in the right ventricle would cause dilation in this chamber. The dysfunctional and dilated right ventricle could displace the interventricular septum toward the left ventricle. The leftward shift of the septum impairs the left ventricular preload [7]. All of the mentioned circumstances could decrease cardiac output, resulting in hypotensive shock that could present with catastrophic clinical findings [12]. Studies had shown that even a remarkable proportion of PE patients could present with normal blood pressure while having right ventricular dysfunction [13]. These patients might develop PE-related hemodynamic instability, requiring aggressive therapy. Thus, investigating different variables with CTPA that predicts right and left heart failure could be lifesaving, especially in patients with a higher clot load.

Regarding the degree of vascular obstruction, Qanadli et al. proposed the CT obstruction index that was correlated with the previously described pulmonary angiography index, which could quantify the degree of obstruction [5]. They suggested that a CT obstruction index more than 40% could identify 90% of patients with dilated right ventricle, while an index less than 40% would be unlikely to be observed in a patient who is suffering from acute right ventricular dysfunction [5]. Mastora et al. described that CT severity index could quantitatively assess PE severity, suggesting an applicable scoring system for routine clinical practice [14].

Several studies have investigated pulmonary obstruction indices for their ability to select high-risk PE patients. Van der meer et al. described that both the PAOI and right ventricle (RV) to left ventricle (LV) ratio could be useful in predicting mortality in PE patients that are hemodynamically stable at the presentation [11]. Wu et al. also suggested that quantified

CTPA clot burden analysis could have prominent predictive value on the clinical outcome of patients with PE [15]. On the other hand, Collomb et al., Araoz et al., Pech et al., and Ghaye et al. found that PE clot scores might be poor variables for predicting severe in-hospital morbidity and mortality [3, 16–18]. These contradictory findings could support the hypothesis that both basic cardiopulmonary state and PE clot size contribute to patients' outcome. Hence, there is not a definite variable with the highest predictive value for PE-related mortality in different populations.

Few studies with a limited number of patients have investigated the association between clot burden and left atrium size [12, 19]. A recent study by Aviram et al. proposed that LA and RA areas are associated with embolic extant, suggesting higher PAOI results in a larger RA and a smaller LA size [10]. However, our current study is the first to show that there is a correlation between almost all LA measurements and the PAOI in a number of PE patients. These findings confirm that assessing LA and RA dimensions could become an applicable tool for stratifying PE patients in daily clinical practice.

Studies had shown that although echocardiography should not be used as a routine modality for diagnosing PE, it can be useful for risk assessment in PE patients, especially those who may have poor prognosis due to RVD [20]. Lodato et al. investigated quantitative indices using echocardiography and proposed that RV/LV ratio has decent accuracy for diagnosis of PE [21]. Lim et al. compared the accuracy of echocardiography and CT in detecting of RVD in patients with acute PE [22]. Out of 14 patients with massive pulmonary embolism, echocardiography had detected RVD in 12 individuals, while CT had correctly identified 11 of 12 patients, resulting in a sensitivity of 91.6% and a specificity of 100% [22]. Moreover, He et al. evaluated qualitative assessment of qualitative assessment of RVD in patients with PE, on CT in comparison to echocardiography. CT had a sensitivity and specificity of 81% and 47%, respectively [23]. Since ventricular wall is significantly thicker than atrial wall, the effect of arterial obstruction on atrial size might be more noticeable. Our findings also suggest that RA area could be a sensitive parameter for the diagnosis of massive PE.

ECG-gated scanning technique was not used in our CT protocol. It is a lack for measurement of cardiac chambers. Also, echocardiography is better method for measurement of cardiac chambers. But in our study, correlation analysis between echocardiography and computed tomography measurements was not used. This point should be mentioned as a limitation of our study and recommended for future studies to be considered.

Furthermore, retrospective type of our study and small sample size are the other limitations of our study. Future investigations with large sample size can reveal new and detailed results.

In conclusion, we had investigated the association between pulmonary arterial obstruction index and atrial size in patients with acute pulmonary embolism. We found that atrial measurements are correlated with POAI, and they could be used as sensitive parameters in predicting heart failure in patients with PE. Further studies are needed to confirm this hypothesis.

References

[1] P. S. Marshall, K. S. Mathews, and M. D. Siegel, "Diagnosis and management of life-threatening pulmonary embolism," *Journal of Intensive Care Medicine*, vol. 26, no. 5, pp. 275–294, 2011.

[2] U. M. Nagamalesh, V. S. Prakash, K. C. K. Naidu, S. Sarthak, A. V. Hegde, and T. Abhinay, "Acute pulmonary thromboembolism: Epidemiology, predictors, and long-term outcome – A single center experience," *Indian Heart Journal*, vol. 69, no. 2, pp. 160–164, 2017.

[3] B. Ghaye, A. Ghuysen, V. Willems et al., "Severe pulmonary embolism:pulmonary artery clot load scores and cardiovascular parameters as predictors of mortality," *Radiology*, vol. 239, no. 3, pp. 884–891, 2006.

[4] U. J. Schoepf and P. Costello, "CT angiography for diagnosis of pulmonary embolism: state of the art," *Radiology*, vol. 230, no. 2, pp. 329–337, 2004.

[5] S. D. Qanadli, M. El Hajjam, A. Vieillard-Baron et al., "New CT index to quantify arterial obstruction in pulmonary embolism: comparison with angiographic index and echocardiography," *American Journal of Roentgenology*, vol. 176, no. 6, pp. 1415–1420, 2001.

[6] M. B. Çildag, M. Gok, and C. Z. Karaman, "Pulmonary artery obstruction index and right ventricular dysfunction signs in initial and follow up pulmonary computed tomography angiography in acute pulmonary embolism," *Journal of Clinical and Diagnostic Research*, vol. 11, no. 7, pp. TC21–TC25, 2017.

[7] K. E. Wood, "Major pulmonary embolism: review of a pathophysiologic approach to the golden hour of hemodynamically significant pulmonary embolism," *Chest*, vol. 121, no. 3, pp. 877–905, 2002.

[8] E. R. V. Buechel and L. L. Mertens, "Imaging the right heart: The use of integrated multimodality imaging," *European Heart Journal*, vol. 33, no. 8, pp. 949–960, 2012.

[9] K. Varol, C. Gumus, H. Yucel et al., "Correlation of right ventricular dysfunction on acute pulmonary embolism with pulmonary artery computed tomography obstruction index ratio (PACTOIR) and comparison with echocardiography," *Japanese Journal of Radiology*, vol. 33, no. 6, pp. 311–316, 2015.

[10] G. Aviram, A. Steinvil, S. Berliner et al., "The association between the embolic load and atrial size in acute pulmonary embolism," *Journal of Thrombosis and Haemostasis*, vol. 9, no. 2, pp. 293–299, 2011.

[11] R. W. van der Meer, P. M. T. Pattynama, M. J. L. van Strijen et al., "Right ventricular dysfunction and pulmonary obstruction index at helical CT: prediction of clinical outcome during 3-month follow-up in patients with acute pulmonary embolism," *Radiology*, vol. 235, no. 3, pp. 798–803, 2005.

[12] I. Ocak and C. Fuhrman, "CT angiography findings of the left atrium and right ventricle in patients with massive pulmonary embolism," *American Journal of Roentgenology*, vol. 191, no. 4, pp. 1072–1076, 2008.

[13] S. Grifoni, I. Olivotto, P. Cecchini et al., "Short-term clinical outcome of patients with acute pulmonary embolism, normal blood pressure, and echocardiographic right ventricular dysfunction," *Circulation*, vol. 101, no. 24, pp. 2817–2822, 2000.

[14] I. Mastora, M. Remy-Jardin, P. Masson et al., "Severity of acute pulmonary embolism: evaluation of a new spiral CT angiographic score in correlation with echocardiographic data," *European Radiology*, vol. 13, no. 1, pp. 29–35, 2003.

[15] A. S. Wu, J. A. Pezzullo, J. J. Cronan, D. D. Hou, and W. W. Mayo-Smith, "CT pulmonary angiography: quantification of pulmonary embolus as a predictor of patient outcome—initial experience," *Radiology*, vol. 230, no. 3, pp. 831–835, 2004.

[16] P. A. Araoz, M. B. Gotway, R. L. Trowbridge et al., "Helical CT pulmonary angiography predictors of in-hospital morbidity and mortality in patients with acute pulmonary embolism," *Journal of Thoracic Imaging*, vol. 18, no. 4, pp. 207–216, 2003.

[17] D. Collomb, P. J. Paramelle, O. Calaque et al., "Severity assessment of acute pulmonary embolism: evaluation using helical CT," *European Radiology*, vol. 13, no. 7, pp. 1508–1514, 2003.

[18] M. Pech, G. Wieners, P. Dul et al., "Computed tomography pulmonary embolism index for the assessment of survival in patients with pulmonary embolism," *European Radiology*, vol. 17, no. 8, pp. 1954–1959, 2007.

[19] Y. Hama, T. Yakushiji, Y. Iwasaki, T. Kaji, N. Isomura, and S. Kusano, "Small left atrium: An adjunctive sign of hemodynamically compromised massive pulmonary embolism," *Yonsei Medical Journal*, vol. 46, no. 5, pp. 733–736, 2005.

[20] S. Z. Goldhaber, "Echocardiography in the management of pulmonary embolism" *Annals of Internal Medicine*, vol. 136, no. 9, pp. 691–700, 2002.

[21] J. A. Lodato, R. P. Ward, and R. M. Lang, "Echocardiographic predictors of pulmonary embolism in patients referred for helical CT," *Journal of Echocardiography*, vol. 25, no. 6, pp. 584–590, 2008.

[22] K.-E. Lim, C.-Y. Chan, P.-H. Chu, Y.-Y. Hsu, and W.-C. Hsu, "Right ventricular dysfunction secondary to acute massive pulmonary embolism detected by helical computed tomography pulmonary angiography," *Clinical Imaging*, vol. 29, no. 1, pp. 16–21, 2005.

[23] H. He, M. W. Stein, B. Zalta, and L. B. Haramati, "Computed tomography evaluation of right heart dysfunction in patients with acute pulmonary embolism," *Journal of Computer Assisted Tomography*, vol. 30, no. 2, pp. 262–266, 2006.

Permissions

All chapters in this book were first published by Hindawi Publishing Corporation; hereby published with permission under the Creative Commons Attribution License or equivalent. Every chapter published in this book has been scrutinized by our experts. Their significance has been extensively debated. The topics covered herein carry significant findings which will fuel the growth of the discipline. They may even be implemented as practical applications or may be referred to as a beginning point for another development.

The contributors of this book come from diverse backgrounds, making this book a truly international effort. This book will bring forth new frontiers with its revolutionizing research information and detailed analysis of the nascent developments around the world.

We would like to thank all the contributing authors for lending their expertise to make the book truly unique. They have played a crucial role in the development of this book. Without their invaluable contributions this book wouldn't have been possible. They have made vital efforts to compile up to date information on the varied aspects of this subject to make this book a valuable addition to the collection of many professionals and students.

This book was conceptualized with the vision of imparting up-to-date information and advanced data in this field. To ensure the same, a matchless editorial board was set up. Every individual on the board went through rigorous rounds of assessment to prove their worth. After which they invested a large part of their time researching and compiling the most relevant data for our readers.

The editorial board has been involved in producing this book since its inception. They have spent rigorous hours researching and exploring the diverse topics which have resulted in the successful publishing of this book. They have passed on their knowledge of decades through this book. To expedite this challenging task, the publisher supported the team at every step. A small team of assistant editors was also appointed to further simplify the editing procedure and attain best results for the readers.

Apart from the editorial board, the designing team has also invested a significant amount of their time in understanding the subject and creating the most relevant covers. They scrutinized every image to scout for the most suitable representation of the subject and create an appropriate cover for the book.

The publishing team has been an ardent support to the editorial, designing and production team. Their endless efforts to recruit the best for this project, has resulted in the accomplishment of this book. They are a veteran in the field of academics and their pool of knowledge is as vast as their experience in printing. Their expertise and guidance has proved useful at every step. Their uncompromising quality standards have made this book an exceptional effort. Their encouragement from time to time has been an inspiration for everyone.

The publisher and the editorial board hope that this book will prove to be a valuable piece of knowledge for researchers, students, practitioners and scholars across the globe.

List of Contributors

Francesco Tramacere and Maurizio Portaluri
Radiation Oncology, Department of Radiotherapy, O. Policlinic "A. Perrino", Strada Statale 7 per Mesagne, Brindisi 72100, Italy

Artor Niccoli Asabella
Nuclear Medicine Unit, A. O. Policlinic "A. Perrino", Strada Statale 7 per Mesagne, Brindisi 72100, Italy

Corinna Altini and Cristina Ferrari
Nuclear Medicine Unit, Interdisciplinary Department of Medicine, University of Bari Aldo Moro, Piazza Giulio Cesare 11, Bari 70124, Italy

Lilia Bardoscia
Radiotherapy Unit, Clinical Cancer Centre, AUSL-IRCCS, Reggio Emilia, Italy

Angela Sardaro
Section of Radiology and Radiation Oncology, Interdisciplinary Department of Medicine, University of Bari Aldo Moro, Piazza Giulio Cesare 11, Bari 70124, Italy

Aisyah Mohd Rahimi, Intan Nurdin, Shahrina Ismail and Azira Khalil
Faculty of Science and Technology, Universiti Sains Islam Malaysia, 71800 Nilai, Negeri Sembilan, Malaysia

Athanasios Pavlou
St. Vincent's Medical Center, Bridgeport, CT, USA
Frank H. Netter MD School of Medicine, North Haven, CT, USA

Robert M. Kurtz and Jae W. Song
Hospital of the University of Pennsylvania, Philadelphia, PA, USA

Wanaporn Burivong, Thanatorn Sricharoen, Apichart Thachang, Sunsiree Soodchuen, Panitpong Maroongroge and Vichit Leelasithorn
Department of Radiology, Faculty of Medicine, Srinakharinwirot University, Bangkok, Thailand

Amin Saburi, Ramezan Jafari and Mostafa Ghanei
Chemical Injuries Research Center, Systems Biology & Poisonings Institute, Baqiyatallah University of Medical Sciences, Tehran, Iran

U. Joseph Schoepf
Department of Radiology and Radiological Science, Medical University of South Carolina, Charleston, SC, USA

Kyle A. Ulversoy
Augusta University/University of Georgia Medical Partnership, Athens, GA, USA

Fatemeh Eghbal
Birjand University of Medical Sciences, Birjand, Iran

Ramin Ghasemi Shayan, Maryam Oladghaffari, Fakhrosadat Sajjadian and Mona Fazel Ghaziyani
Radiology Department, Tabriz University of Medical Sciences, Tabriz 51368, Iran

Rashid Al Umairi
Department of Radiology, The Royal Hospital, Muscat, Oman

Maryam Al-khouri
Oman Medical Specialty Board, Muscat, Oman

Roy Munialo Machasio and Timothy Musila Mutala
University of Nairobi, Department of Diagnostic Imaging and Radiation Medicine, Kenya

Rose Nyabanda
Kenyatta National Hospital, Kenya

Boushab Mohamed Boushab
Department of Internal Medicine and Infectious Diseases, Kiffa Regional Hospital, Assaba, Mauritania

Noukhoum Kone
Department of Neurosurgery, Kiffa Regional Hospital, Assaba, Mauritania

Leonardo K. Basco
Aix-Marseille Univ, IRD, AP-HM, SSA, VITROME, Marseille, France
IHU-Méditerranée Infection, Marseille, France

Joshua Tambe
Division of Radiology, Department of Internal Medicine and Pediatrics, University of Buea, Buea, Cameroon
Department of Public Health, Centre for Research and Training in Graduate Studies in Life, Health and Environmental Sciences, The University of Yaoundé I, Yaoundé, Cameroon

Sylviane Dongmo
Division of Radiology, Department of Internal Medicine and Pediatrics, University of Buea, Buea, Cameroon

Yannick Onana
Department of Clinical Sciences, University of Ngaoundéré, Ngaoundéré, Cameroon

Georges Nguefack-Tsague
Biostatistics Unit, Department of Public Health, The University of Yaoundé I, Yaoundé, Cameroon

Pierre Ongolo-Zogo
Department of Public Health, Centre for Research and Training in Graduate Studies in Life, Health and Environmental Sciences, The University of Yaoundé I, Yaoundé, Cameroon
Department of Radiology and Radiation Oncology, The University of Yaoundé I, Yaoundé, Cameroon

Manuel Recio Rodríguez and Raquel Cano Alonso
Departamento de Diagnóstico por Imagen, Hospital Universitario Quironsalud Madrid, Madrid, Spain

Cristina Andreu-Vázquez and Israel J. Thuissard-Vasallo
Departamento de Medicina, Facultad de Ciencias Biomédicas, Universidad Europea de Madrid, Madrid, Spain

Carmina Bermejo López and Pilar Martínez Ten
Delta Ecografía, Madrid, Spain

Ines Tamarit Degenhardt
Departamento de Obstetricia y Ginecología, Hospital Universitario Quironsalud Madrid, Madrid, Spain

Yusuke Shimada, Ikuho Kojima and Masahiro Iikubo
Department of Dental Informatics and Radiology, Tohoku University Graduate School of Dentistry, 4-1 Seiryo-machi, Aoba-ku, Sendai 980-8575, Japan

Ali Kanj
Radiology Department, Hammoud Hospital University Medical Center, Saida, Lebanon

Ibrahim Ghosn
Fellow of Radiology, Radiology Department, Faculty of Medical Sciences, Lebanese University, Hadath, Lebanon

Assaad Mohanna and Georges Rouhana
Radiology Department, Faculty of Medical Sciences, Lebanese University, Hadath, Lebanon

Maryam Bahaloo, Mohammad Hossein Davari, Abolfazl Mollasadeghi, Seyyed Jalil Mirmohammadi and Amir Houshang Mehrparvar
Industrial Diseases Research Center, Shahid Sadoughi University of Medical Sciences, Yazd 89138-14389, Iran

Mohammad Sobhan
Department of Radiology, Shahid Sadoughi University of Medical Sciences, Yazd 89138-14389, Iran

Mohammad Taghi Jalalian
Department of Occupational Medicine, Shahid Sadoughi University of Medical Sciences, Yazd 89138-14389, Iran

Mohammad Javad Zare Sakhvidi
Department of Occupational Health, Shahid Sadoughi University of Medical Sciences, Yazd 89138-14389, Iran

Farimah Shamsi
Shahid Sadoughi University of Medical Sciences, Yazd 89138-14389, Iran

Sam Mirfendereski
Department of Radiology, Faculty of Medicine, Shahrekord University of Medical Sciences, Shahrekord 8815713471, Iran

Ajit Mahale, Shaloo Choudhary, Sonali Ullal, Merwyn Fernandes and Sonali Prabhu
Department of Radiodiagnosis, Kasturba Medical College Mangalore, MAHE Dakshina Kannada, Karnataka 575001, India

Elise Chua and Vincent Lam
Departments of Radiology, Northwick Park and Central Middlesex Hospitals, London North West University Healthcare NHS Trust, Watford Road, Harrow HA1 3UJ, UK

Annakan V. Navaratnam
Departments of ENT Surgery, Northwick Park and Central Middlesex Hospitals, London North West University Healthcare NHS Trust, Watford Road, Harrow HA1 3UJ, UK

Dominic St Leger
Departments of Radiology, Northwick Park and Central Middlesex Hospitals, London North West University Healthcare NHS Trust, Watford Road, Harrow HA1 3UJ, UK
Department of Radiology, Manchester Royal Infirmary, Oxford Road, Manchester M13 9WL, UK

Samit Unadkat
Royal National Throat, Nose and Ear Hospital, University College London Hospitals NHS Foundation Trust, 47–49 Huntley Street, London WC1E 6DG, UK

Alexander Weller
Departments of Radiology, Northwick Park and Central Middlesex Hospitals, London North West University Healthcare NHS Trust, Watford Road, Harrow HA1 3UJ, UK
Department of Radiology, St George's Hospital, St George's University Hospitals NHS Foundation Trust, Blackshaw Road, Tooting, London SW17 0QT, UK

Steven Raeymaeckers and Maurizio Tosi
Universitair Ziekenhuis Brussel, Laarbeeklaan 101, Jette 1090, Belgium

Johan De Mey
Universitair Ziekenhuis Brussel, Laarbeeklaan 101, Jette 1090, Belgium
Radiology, Vrije Universiteit Brussel, Laarbeeklaan 103, Jette 1090, Belgium

Guiswe Gnowe and Bonaventure Babinne Graobe
Higher Institute of Sciences, Health Technics and Management of Garoua, Garoua, Cameroon

Henri Paul Ekobena Fouda
University Technological of Institute, University of Ngaoundere, Ngaoundere, Cameroon

Mbo Amvene Jéremie
Faculty of Medicine and Biomedical Sciences of Garoua, Garoua, Cameroon

Takmou Pascal
General Hospital of Douala, Douala, Cameroon

Ninad Salastekar, Alexis Saunders, Kushal Patel and Katherine Willer
Department of Radiology, SUNY Upstate Medical University, 750 East Adam Street, Syracuse, NY 13210, USA

Lara Nassar, Amro Baassiri, Fatima Salah, Andrew Barakat, Elie Najem and Ghina Berjawi
Department of Diagnostic Radiology, American University of Beirut Medical Center, Lebanon

Fouad Boulos
Department of Pathology, American University of Beirut Medical Center, Lebanon

Anthony Baffour Appiah
Ghana Field Epidemiology and Laboratory Training Programme, University of Ghana, Accra, Ghana

Benjamin Dabo Sarkodie
Department of Radiology, University of Ghana, School of Medicine Sciences, Accra, Ghana

Dorothea Anim
Department of Radiology, Korle Bu Teaching Hospital, Accra, Ghana

Bashiru Babatunde Jimah and Philip Gorleku
Department of Medical Imaging, School of Medical Sciences, University of Cape Coast, Cape Coast, Ghana

Jose Manuel Sanz-Mengibar and José Hurtado-Aviles
Faculty of Medicine, University of Murcia, Murcia, Spain

Joaquín Roca-González
Technical University of Cartagena (UPCT), Technical School of Industrial Engineering, Cartagena, Spain
Director of the Industrial and Medical Electronics Section of the DINTEL Research Group, Cartagena, Spain

Konstantsin Sergeevich Kurochka
Head of Department of Information Technologies, Sukhoi State Technical University of Gomel, Gomel, Belarus

Fernando Santonja-Medina
Faculty of Medicine, University of Murcia, Murcia, Spain
V. de la Arrixaca University Hospital, Department of Traumatology, Murcia, Spain

Sana Shaikh
Radiology Department, Sindh Institute of Urology and Transplantation (SIUT), Karachi 74100, Pakistan

Afshan Rasheed
Oncology Department, Sindh Institute of Urology and Transplantation (SIUT), M. A. Jinnah Road, Karachi 74100, Pakistan

Hawon Lee
Montgomery Blair High School, Silver Spring, MD, USA
Division of Imaging, Diagnostics and Software Reliability, OSEL, CDRH, Food and Drug Administration, Silver Spring, MD, USA

Andreu Badal
Division of Imaging, Diagnostics and Software Reliability, OSEL, CDRH, Food and Drug Administration, Silver Spring, MD, USA

Elia Coimbra
Interventional Radiology Unit, Curry Cabral Hospital CHULC, Rua Beneficencia 8, Zip Code 1069-166, Lisbon, Portugal

Jose Hugo M. Luz, Filipe V. Gomes, Nuno V. Costa and Tiago Bilhim
Interventional Radiology Unit, Curry Cabral Hospital CHULC, Rua Beneficencia 8, Zip Code 1069-166, Lisbon, Portugal
Nova Medical School, Faculdade de Ciências Médicas, Universidade Nova de Lisboa, Lisbon, Portugal

Eric Kwasi Ofori and Seth Kwadjo Angmorterh
Department of Medical Imaging, School of Allied Health Sciences, University of Health and Allied Sciences (UHAS), Ho, Ghana

Andrew England
School of Allied Health Professions, Keele University, Staffordshire, Newcastle, UK

Sonia Aboagye
Department of Speech, Language & Hearing Sciences, School of Allied Health Sciences, University of Health and Allied Sciences (UHAS), Ho, Ghana

Peter Hogg
Directorate of Radiography, School of Healthcare Sciences, Allerton Building, University of Salford, Salford—Greater Manchester, UK

Taraneh Faghihi Langroudi, Maryam Sheikh and Morteza Sanei Taheri
Radiology Department, Modarres Hospital, Shahid Beheshti University of Medical Sciences, Tehran, Iran

Mohammadreza Naderian
Non-Communicable Diseases Research Center, Endocrinology and Metabolism Population Sciences Institute, Tehran University of Medical Sciences, Tehran, Iran
Cardiac Outcome Research and Education (CORE), Universal Scientific Education and Research Network (USERN), Tehran, Iran

Amir Ashraf-ganjouei
Students' Scientific Research Center (SSRC), Tehran University of Medical Sciences, Tehran, Iran

Isa Khaheshi
Cardiovascular Research Center, Shahid Beheshti University of Medical Sciences, Tehran, Iran

Index

A
Adult Patients, 29, 140, 51, 69, 139

Aneurysms, 60-66

Angiography, 17, 19, 21, 30, 44, 48-55, 57-58, 60, 64-66, 138, 224-229

B
Back Pain, 67

Bronchiectasis, 31-32, 39

C
Central Nervous System, 79-80, 85, 89

Cerebrovascular Disease, 60-61, 63-65

Chemotherapy, 23, 27-28, 68, 207

Chest Radiography, 23, 29, 80

Choline, 3-4

Clinical History, 34, 67, 216

Clinical Information, 44, 77, 225-226

Computed Tomography, 1, 11, 16, 21, 23, 29-30, 35, 39-42, 49-55, 57-58, 60, 67, 73, 77-78, 80, 102, 126, 128, 136-138, 154, 161, 174-175, 188, 191, 194, 200-205, 207, 212-213, 217, 224-226, 228-229

Coronary Artery, 19, 21, 51, 53-59

Coronavirus Disease, 1, 4, 18, 30, 39-41

D
Diagnostic Accuracy, 13-21, 51, 65, 79-83, 85, 88-89, 92, 97, 118-120, 122, 124-125

Diagnostic Evaluations, 42

Dose Comparison, 42, 191, 200, 204-205

Dose Reduction, 43-44, 200, 205

Dosimetry, 139-140, 145, 188-189, 192, 194, 205, 217

Dual-energy, 42-45, 47-52, 137

F
Febrile Neutropenia, 23-29

Fetal Ultrasound, 79-88

G
Gadolinium, 80, 89, 109, 113, 116, 119

Glioma, 109, 113, 116

H
Health Insurance, 73-78

Hematologic Malignancies, 23-25, 27

Hemorrhage, 47, 52, 60-61, 65

Histopathology, 98, 176-177

Hyperparathyroidism, 127, 136-138

Hypertension, 70, 144-145, 147, 224-227

Hypoplasia, 60, 66, 84-85, 89

I
Intracranial Pathology, 108

Ischaemic Stroke, 60, 64

K
Kinetic, 100, 149, 151, 212

L
Lesions, 24-25, 27-28, 31-33, 35-37, 52, 67-69, 82, 85-86, 104, 108-109, 113, 116-117, 122, 126-128, 134, 138, 147-149, 151-153, 184, 187

Leukemia, 25-27, 29

Logistic Regression, 7, 73-75, 137, 145, 177, 182

Lung Nodules, 30

Lung Severity, 32

Lymphadenopathy, 30-32, 36

Lymphoma, 25, 27, 120, 124

M
Magnetic Resonance Spectroscopy, 107

Magnetic Susceptibility, 101

Meningioma, 108-109, 111

Meta-analysis, 3-4, 17, 20, 77, 80, 83, 89, 125, 156, 159, 187, 223

Multiple Sclerosis, 19, 21, 108-109

Myeloma, 2-3, 25, 27

Myocardium, 52-55, 57

N
Nasal Cavity, 124, 126

Neutropenic Patients, 23-24, 28-29

O
Osteomyelitis, 71

P
Pandemic, 1-4, 122, 125

Parenchymal Lesions, 108-109, 113

Parotid Glands, 91-92, 97-98

Pathogenesis, 30, 36-39, 151

Pathology, 18, 20, 30, 38, 41, 60-61, 65, 67, 79-86, 89, 98, 108, 121, 126, 147-149, 151, 153, 205

Patient Selection, 13-14, 16, 20, 54, 122, 149

Pericardial Effusion, 31-32
Peritonitis, 88
Pleural Effusion, 31-32, 34-37
Pleural Thickening, 31, 36
Pneumonia, 29-41
Pneumothorax, 32-33
Postnatal Diagnosis, 79-85, 88
Prenatal Diagnosis, 79-82, 89-90
Prognosis, 1, 32, 34, 64-65, 71-72, 79-81, 83, 85-89, 124, 172, 213, 228
Pulmonary Embolism, 19, 21, 138, 224-225, 227-229
Pulmonary Infection, 23-24, 27-29

R

Radiographic Examinations, 143
Radiographic Interpretation, 28
Radiologic Diagnosis, 23-24
Radiology, 1, 5-11, 13-14, 16, 18-21, 23-24, 29-30, 32, 37, 39-43, 45, 51-53, 58, 65-66, 72-73, 77-80, 83, 89-91, 97-99, 102-104, 107, 116-117, 125-126, 136-140, 143-144, 147-149, 153-154, 156, 158-159, 166, 177, 187, 190, 204-206, 213-216, 223-225
Radiotherapy, 1-4, 11, 124, 204, 215-217, 219, 221-223
Risk Factors, 23, 31, 40, 55, 69, 144, 147, 162, 166, 222

S

Salivary Glands, 91-92, 94, 97, 189, 191, 200
Sclerosis, 19, 21, 82, 86, 108-109
Septal Thickening, 24, 31-32, 36-37
Sialography, 91-98
Sinuses, 119, 123, 125-126
Spatial Misregistration, 42

T

Tuberculomas, 108-109, 113
Tuberculosis, 67-72, 163